INSANITY, INSTITUTIONS AND SOCIETY, 1800–1914

Insanity, Institutions and Society presents and analyses the issues of recent and new social histories of insanity and the asylum.

The global retreat from institutional care for the mentally ill during the 1970s and 1980s has influenced the prevailing views of the asylum. These views are challenged by recent research which places less emphasis on the professional psychiatrists and the process of incarceration and devotes more attention to the complex social origins of insanity and the institutionalisation of those certified.

The English model is placed in a richer comparative context, in which the significance of ethnicity, race and gender as well as the impact of political and cultural factors are analysed. The book also develops these themes in studies set in Wales, Scotland, Ireland, India and South Africa, as well as the history of colonial medicine more generally.

Insanity, Institutions and Society is a valuable guide to current work in the social and cultural history of insanity, and provides a comprehensive summary of the debates on the growth of institutional care during the nineteenth and early twentieth centuries.

Joseph Melling is Senior Lecturer in the Department of Historical Studies and Director of the Centre for Medical History, and **Bill Forsythe** is Reader in the History of Crime and Punishment, both at the University of Exeter.

STUDIES IN THE SOCIAL HISTORY OF MEDICINE

Series Editors: Jonathan Barry and Bernard Harris

LIFE, DEATH AND THE ELDERLY
Edited by Margaret Pelling and Richard M. Smith

MEDICINE AND CHARITY BEFORE THE WELFARE STATE
Edited by Jonathan Barry and Colin Jones

IN THE NAME OF THE CHILD
Edited by Roger Cooter

REASSESSING FOUCAULT
Power, medicine and the body
Edited by Colin Jones and Roy Porter

MIGRANTS, MINORITIES AND HEALTH
Historical and contemporary studies
Edited by Lara Marks and Michael Worboys

FROM IDIOCY TO MENTAL DEFICIENCY
Edited by David Wright and Anne Digby

NUTRITION IN BRITAIN
Edited by David F. Smith

HEALTH CARE AND POOR RELIEF IN PROTESTANT EUROPE 1500–1700
Edited by Ole Peter Grell and Andrew Cunningham

MIDWIVES, SOCIETY AND CHILDBIRTH
Edited by Hilary Marland and Anne Marie Rafferty

THE LOCUS OF CARE
Edited by Peregrine Horden and Richard Smith

ILLNESS AND HEALING ALTERNATIVES IN WESTERN EUROPE
Edited by Marijke Gijswit-Hofstra, Hilary Marland and Hans de Waardt

INSANITY, INSTITUTIONS AND SOCIETY, 1800–1914

A social history of madness in comparative perspective

Edited by
Joseph Melling and Bill Forsythe

Routledge
Taylor & Francis Group
LONDON AND NEW YORK

First published 1999
by Routledge
2 Park Square, Milton Park, Abingdon, Oxfordshire OX14 4RN

Simultaneously published in the USA and Canada by Routledge
711 Third Avenue, New York, NY 10017

First issued in paperback 2014

Routledge is an imprint of the Taylor and Francis Group, an informa business

Typeset in Baskerville by Routledge

British Library Cataloguing in Publication Data
A catalogue record for this book is available from the British Library

Library of Congress Cataloguing in Publication Data
Insanity, institutions, and society, 1800–1914 / Joseph Melling and Bill Forsythe.
p. cm. – (Studies in the social history of medicine)
Includes bibliographical references and index.
1. Psychiatric hospital care–Great Britain–History–19th century 2. Social psychiatry–Great Britain–History–19th century 3. Mental health laws–Great Britain–History–19th century. I. Melling, Joseph. II. Forsythe, Bill. III. Series.
RC450.G7I57 1999
362.2'1'094109034–dc21 98–41827 CIP

ISBN 978-1-138-86824-3 (pbk)
ISBN 978-0-415-18441-0 (hbk)

CONTENTS

CONTRIBUTORS

Richard Adair is a Researcher at the Cambridge Group for the Study of Population and was Research Assistant on the Wellcome project on Institutions and Insanity at the University of Exeter, 1993–6. He wrote *Courtship, Illegitimacy, and Marriage in Early Modern England* (Manchester University Press, 1996).

Jonathan Andrews is a Wellcome Award Holder and Senior Lecturer in the History of Medicine at Oxford Brookes University. He edited (with Iain Smith) *A History of Gartnavel Royal Hospital* (1993) and has written (with Asa Briggs and others) *The History of Bethlem* (Routledge, 1997), and *The Scottish Lunacy Commissioners* (Wellcome, 1998).

Peter Bartlett is Lecturer in Law at the University of Nottingham. His book *The Poor Law of Lunacy* will be published by Cassell in 1999. He has co-edited (with David Wright) *Outside the Walls of the Asylum: The History of Care in the Community, 1750–2000* (Athlone, 1999).

Waltraud Ernst is a Wellcome Award Holder and Lecturer in History at the University of Southampton. Her current research involves a comparative history of psychiatry in British India and New Zealand. She wrote *Mad Tales from the Raj* (Routledge, 1991) and is co-editor (with Bernard Harris) of *Race, Science and Medicine* (Routledge, 1999).

Bill Forsythe is Reader in the History of Crime and Punishment at the University of Exeter and Dean of Academic Partnerships. He was co-director of the Wellcome Project on Institutions and Insanity. He has published widely in the field of history of penal institutions. His works include *The Reform of Prisoners 1830–1900* (Croom Helm, 1987).

David Hirst is Lecturer in Social Policy in the School of Sociology and Social Policy, University of Wales, Bangor. His research interests are in the history of health and social welfare.

Shula Marks is Professor of Southern African History at the School of Oriental and African Studies, London and has written and taught widely on South African history. Her most recent book is *Divided Sisterhood. Race, Class and Gender in the South African Nursing Profession.* She is currently working on *Mothers, Miners and Maniacs. A Social History of Medicine in South Africa.*

Hilary Marland is a Wellcome Award Holder Senior Lecturer in History at Warwick University and an editor of *Social History of Medicine.* She has published widely on the history of midwifery and is currently researching insanity of childbirth in the nineteenth century.

Joseph Melling is Senior Lecturer in Historical Studies and Director of the Centre for Medical History at the University of Exeter. He co-directed (with Bill Forsythe) a Wellcome project into Institutions and Insanity and his publications include studies on industrial health and welfare.

Pamela Michael was employed for three years on a Wellcome-funded project on the history of the North Wales Hospital, Denbigh, and is writing a book on the history of insanity in north Wales. She is a Welsh-medium lecturer in sociology and social policy at the University of Wales, Bangor.

Andrew Scull is Professor of Sociology at the University of California, San Diego. His recent books include *The Most Solitary of Afflictions: Madness and Society in Britain, 1700–1900* (Yale University Press), and (with Nicholas Hervey and Charlotte Mackenzie) *Masters of Bedlam* (Princeton University Press).

Leonard D. Smith is an Honorary Fellow of the Institute for Advanced Research at the University of Birmingham and is currently Principal Social Worker in a Community Mental Health Team in the West Midlands. He is author of *Cure, Comfort and Safe Custody: Public Lunatic Asylums in Early-Nineteenth-Century England* (forthcoming, 1999).

Akihito Suzuki is an Associate Professor in History at Keio University, Tokyo. He has written on the history of psychiatry in England and is completing a book on psychiatry and the family in nineteenth-century

London as well as researching the history of medicine in modern Japan.

Lorraine Walsh is a Teaching Fellow in American History at the University of Dundee. Her research interests include nineteenth-century urban and medical history with particular emphasis on medical charity. Her current research includes an analysis of class influences on admission to the Dundee Infirmary and the Lunatic Asylum.

Oonagh Walsh is Lecturer in History at the University of Aberdeen. She has published on the history of women in nineteenth- and twentieth-century Ireland and is currently researching the expansion of the asylum system in the west of Ireland.

David Wright is Wellcome Trust Lecturer in the History of Medicine at the University of Nottingham. His research interests include the history of psychiatric disorders, the social history of learning disability, and the history of the family. He has co-edited (with Anne Digby) *From Idiocy to Mental Deficiency* (Routledge, 1996) and (with Peter Bartlett) *Outside the Walls of the Asylum* (Athlone, 1999).

PREFACE

The idea for a collection of essays dedicated to a reappraisal of the social history of insanity originated in a seminar series held at the University of Exeter which was generously funded by the Wellcome Trust. These seminars were followed by a conference organised by the Centre for Medical History at Exeter and sponsored by the Society for the Social History of Medicine. We are grateful to David Allen and John Malin of the Wellcome Trust for their assistance and encouragement in organising the seminars, and to Tim Boon and his colleagues on the Executive of the Society for supporting what was a highly enjoyable and stimulating conference. Amongst those who helped in the organisation of the Exeter conference as well as contributing to the exchange of ideas were Michael Clark, Anne Digby, Mark Jackson, Roy Porter, Jonathan Sadowsky, Anne Shepherd, John Welshman and the numerous colleagues who acted as commentators in the different sessions. Many fine articles presented at that event would have filled a second volume on a different theme to the present collection. The contributions assembled here have clearly benefited from acquaintance with the wide range of research reported at the conference. In the surprisingly smooth transition from conference articles to publication we have gained from the excellent editorial support of Heather McCallum and Shankari Sanmuganathan at Routledge as well as the critical guidance of anonymous readers. We were fortunate in editing the essays of contributors who responded quickly and positively to requests and suggestions. The warmest thanks are due to Bernard Harris, as the SSHM Series Editor, for the invariably courteous, patient and meticulous manner in which he dealt with all our queries and concerns. We also gained much from his constructive criticisms in regard to the essays. Finally we wish to thank our respective partners Helen Rogers and Patricia Forsythe for their forbearance during the periods when we appeared beyond the reach of moral treatment.

Joseph Melling and Bill Forsythe
Exeter, January 1999

1

ACCOMMODATING MADNESS

New research in the social history of insanity and institutions

Joseph Melling

The social history of insanity is a recent growth area within medical history. Before the 1970s historians and social scientists showed relatively little interest in the history of psychiatry or the institutions where their patients were housed.[1] One explanation may lie in the limited prestige enjoyed by psychiatrists within a medical profession which had been greatly expanded by the growth of welfare states but which had devoted few resources to mental health provision.[2] As numerous scholars have noted, physicians who claimed a professional expertise in healing the insane were limited by the weakness of their scientific credentials and the evidence that large numbers of incurable patients were languishing in asylum care for decades.[3] Whilst psychiatric medicine struggled to establish its prestige within the wider medical profession after 1945, the renewed debates on the role of mental institutions in the regulation of deviance and the future of psychiatric care in the community raised profound reservations about the success of the facilities developed to care for the mentally ill.[4] These debates gave an urgency to the historical reappraisal of the asylum system which received a powerful stimulus from Michel Foucault's brilliant polemic against the Enlightenment, *Madness and Civilisation*.[5]

Most scholars would date the eruption of detailed investigations into the workings of asylums from the publication of Foucault's tirade against the pretensions of modern science and the appearance of the anti-psychiatry studies of the 1960s, which prefigured the revisionist accounts of Michael MacDonald, Roy Porter, Andrew Scull and many others.[6] As Scull comments in his contribution to the present volume, the Foucauldian vision of madness and society has always been subject to critical modification by such scholars whilst exerting a powerful influence on the revisionist interpretation of lunacy reform which swept the new social history of medicine in the 1970s–80s.[7] This new generation of revisionist historians was, therefore, at least as concerned to refine and correct the extravagant historical inaccuracies of Foucault's grand narrative of the history of madness as it was to integrate his profound insights into the processes of institutional growth and intellectual classification. The critical responses to Foucault have defined much of the literature in the social history of medicine since 1970. Within the rich and varied field of study devoted to the history of psychiatric practices and mental health institutions, scholars have presented at least three main criticisms of Foucault's work. One of the most fundamental difficulties in Foucault's account of the history of madness, which Scull, Porter and others have noted, is that it offers a model of modernisation without a compelling historical narrative.[8] Foucault often assumes a correspondence between intellectual engagement, institutional reform and a social environment which collapses the specific histories of different societies into a single chronology.[9]

Not only does Foucault's story leave us without a coherent, sustainable account of institutional reform in the process of modernisation, but his account also reduces the cast of contemporary actors to a few leading players whose intellectual pretensions are brilliantly exposed but whose importance in the historical drama of insanity reform is hardly challenged.[10] As Chartier has noted, Foucault's work offers an ambiguous reading of the relationship between power, resistance and agency, whilst cultural historians similarly focus on the production of texts and exclude the different ways in which specific audiences and communities appropriate these products for their own purposes.[11] More broadly, Foucault's brilliant essays obscure the fierce debates over asylum reform and the location of the asylum itself as a site of continuing social and political conflicts. His emphasis on the surgical division of space and the manufacture of the modern patient in the hands of the professional physician has given historians a distorted perspective from which to gaze at the institution, marginalising the agency of social classes, kinship networks and political movements in the shaping of the treatments offered for insanity at different periods in different societies.[12] For all his emphasis on the scope for opposition as well as the exercise of power, Foucault's work often implies that the rule of Reason determined the terms on which resistance could be mounted.[13]

A third aspect of Foucault's work which has presented difficulties for historians of institutions concerns the different forms in which he has posed the problem of power and rights within the modern state, including what contributors to the present volume have referred to as the history of 'asylumdom'. For Foucault often presents us with an institutional narrative that lacks a sense of institutional politics. Subsequent research on the historical relationship between the rise of the asylum and the elaboration of a penal system in modern societies has sought to provide at least some of this detail, though the analysis of the functions of the asylum in relation to the state's provisions for the poor has only recently been undertaken.[14] The contributors to the present collection continue to draw on Foucault in their studies, not least in studies of colonial medicine where the relationship between labour regulation, penal regulation and medical practices has been particularly apparent in the process of capitalist modernisation.[15] There is also a noticeable move away from Foucault's concern with the intellectual and physical mechanics of asylum life and towards a sharper contextualisation of the asylum's multiple functions within specific contemporary societies and communities.

It was within this setting of developing debate that Scull framed his initial contribution to the field with a deeply researched and provocative account of the growth of public asylums in England during the 'long nineteenth century'.[16] As his reflections in the present collection make clear, *Museums of Madness* was written in an attempt to provide a corrective to the imprecisions and distortions of Foucault's analysis whilst offering a substantive empirical grounding for many of his assertions. Scull completed detailed historical research on the growth of different institutions during the Victorian decades, whilst retaining a bold conceptual sweep of the English experience which offered an ambitious historical sociology of the making of insanity in modern society. The asylum was located in the landscape of industrialising Britain where the commercialisation of economic life and labour relations weakened many traditional ties and strained the resources of communities which could not cope with the growing numbers of social casualties. The upheaval which followed the commercial and consumer revolutions of the eighteenth century provided the new asylums with their key function in absorbing those individuals who could not function effectively within the new market environment. The purpose of the new asylums was to model social behaviour around the norms of rational bourgeois expectations. Damaged human capital was repaired and worthless labour was warehoused in the corridors of buildings which quickly became museums filled with lifeless artefacts of humanity.[17] The mad were managed by a new breed of superintendents who recognised that the stock of the private madhouses was falling under close scrutiny from humanitarian reformers such as Lord Ashley and that opportunities for professional advancement lay in the new public institutions which every county was compelled to introduce after the legislation of 1845. These mad-doctors laid claim to a large area of medical practice which was underpinned by the intellectual schema of moral treatment (pioneered by Tuke and others in the eighteenth century) and subsequently by the growing conviction that a significant residuum of the population was afflicted by hereditary insanity.

The importance of Scull's contribution lay in the construction of an imaginative historical sociology to explain the rising population of asylums and their place within modern commercial society, offering a critical account of the political economy of madness which many earlier historians had overlooked or rejected.[18] Recognising the limited analysis of class politics provided by Foucault, Scull posed the issue in part at least as one of class interests and working-class regulation by the new bourgeois intellectuals including the mad-doctors who were clearly anxious to join the elite groups of medical professionals in Victorian society.[19] In revising his analysis as *The Most Solitary of Afflictions*, Scull extended his arguments on the commercialisation of English society whilst reaching for a much bolder synthesis of scholarship to sustain a broad analysis of madness and modernity.[20] His thesis is laid out with characteristic clarity and verve in 1991.

> Over the course of the first half of the nineteenth century, in England, in Continental Europe and in North America, the typical response to the deranged underwent dramatic and radical changes.... Whereas in the eighteenth century only the most violent and destructive amongst those now labelled insane would have been segregated and confined apart from the rest of the community, with the achievement of what was widely portrayed as a major social reform, the asylum was endorsed as the sole officially approved response to the problem posed by mental illness. And, in the process, the boundaries of who was to be classified as mad, and thus was to be liable to incarceration, were themselves transformed.[21]

Here is the thrust of the revisionist interpretation of the history of psychiatry and of social reform which Scull has defended and refined in the face of often acerbic exchanges with professional psychiatrists and academic researchers.[22]

In the process of refinement Scull drew on original studies by Andrews, Digby, Finnane, Porter, Walton and many other scholars whose research enriched the analysis and revealed a host of historical actors who attended on the making of the lunatic in the eighteenth and nineteenth centuries.[23] The personalities of Scottish as well as English psychiatrists have been explored in the collective biographies of alienists who were assembled as *Masters of Bedlam*.[24] Subsequent empirical research has, as Scull acknowledges here, modified the interpretation offered in *Museums of Madness*. The foundations of the 'new' social history on which much of Scull's work rested have also been weakened by the seepage of post-modernist arguments into historical debates and the problematising of such core concepts as social class.[25] The contributions to the present volume reflect this wider transformation of the historian's practice, though Scull's own work remains the starting point for these current reappraisals of the social history of madness even if the methods adopted and conclusions reached may diverge.

Most of the essays gathered in this volume are devoted to some part of the long nineteenth century, i.e. 1780–1914, which Scull identifies *pace* Foucault as the critical period in the development of 'asylumdom'. Yet the authors often reach very different conclusions from those found in *The Most Solitary of Afflictions*. One important point of variance can be seen in the different perceptions of modernity which have developed in recent years. Historians are less confident about dating the emergence of a commercial society to the long eighteenth century, still less the long nineteenth century, and the consumer society which earlier historians found at the close of the 1700s has been relocated by scholars to earlier expansion 'irregular but incremental, of consumer cultures associated with commercial capitalism'.[26] If we view the growth of commercial society in a longer trajectory of economic and social change then the correspondence between lunacy reform and the expansion of capitalist markets becomes less compelling. Nor is it clear that the increased migration of labour, weakening community and kinship bonds and the spread of commodity relations during the first half of the nineteenth century, which provide the context for asylum growth in the work of Walton and Scull, had direct and consistent consequences for lunacy admissions in different regions of England and Wales.[27] The chapters on Wales, Scotland and Ireland as well as India and South Africa demonstrate the imperialist impetus behind the modernisation of institutions as well as the accommodation with the forces of tradition which marked the development of medical practice in different societies.

The crisp chronology of institutional innovation which is outlined in Scull and other work remains the subject of debate. L.D. Smith's chapter suggests that a mixed economy of provision had been a feature of the provision for the insane long before the passage of the legislation of 1808 and 1845, whilst the studies by Bartlett and others indicate the continuing importance of the Poor Law workhouse and various 'community' facilities for the care of pauper lunatics long after the seminal Acts of 1845. The paradox of the demise of commercial madhouses and the growth of state provision in the midst of intense commercialisation becomes less pronounced as more researchers reveal the variety of options which were used to house the insane in Victorian Britain.[28] The chapter on Devon indicates that the Lunacy Commissioners' grip on the administration of pauper lunacy was tightened steadily in the period, though it was only in the 1880s that local boroughs were finally pressed into building the asylums envisaged in the original lunacy legislation. This work casts some light on the neglected area of borough asylums and the impact of central–local state relations in changing the environment of lunacy regulation at the end of the nineteenth century.

The interest shown by new researchers in a longer historical perspective on Poor Law provision and the mixed economy of pauper provision owes much to the scholarship not only of MacDonald and Porter but also methods utilised by demographic and family historians such as Richard Smith to chart the evolution of community welfare since the late medieval and early modern periods.[29] The theoretical orientation of such writers is often very different from Scull and *marxisant* interpretations, since Richard Smith is concerned to chart the micro-politics of Poor Law provision for the elderly in terms of the search for rational solutions to community problems as society undergoes economic and social change.[30] This emphasis on the historical adjustment between the supply of public services and the changing demands of local communities is also a strong theme in much of the new research on nineteenth-century lunacy care, including David Wright's study of the role of kinship and family ties in the release as well as admission of inmates at the Buckinghamshire Asylum. Such accounts echo and refine Walton's stress on family preferences in determining the dispatch and retrieval of lunatics in Victorian Lancashire and illustrate the capacity of working-class and lower-middle-class kinship groups to utilise these institutions at different points in the family life cycle. They also present the growth of asylum care as the outcome of transactions between a range of social agents in the community and authority rather than the imposition of a medical hegemony during this period.[31]

Not only are lunacy historians increasingly aware of the complex demographic and kinship relations which formed the context of Poor

Law provision for insanity in the nineteenth and twentieth centuries, but they are more inclined to view the mixed economy of care as the product of a set of contractual and bargaining relationships where commercial calculations were only one feature of a continuing process of institutional negotiation. Even more fundamental than the refinement of our analysis of the workings of the Poor Law may be the evidence gleaned from Devon sources that the county asylum catered for a much broader social constituency than the very poorest groups identified by Scull as the mass of the asylum population. For Scull's thesis rests on the assumption that the forces of commercialisation and the intensification of labour drove hard-pressed families to deposit their awkward and unproductive relatives in the new county asylums. Affluent and middling groups had very different experiences and the divide between private and state institutions reflected, it is argued, a basic class division within English society during the nineteenth century. The essays in this volume provide a range of views on the question of the social and class construction of the insane during the long nineteenth century. Peter Bartlett locates the experience of the pauper lunatic within the workings of the Victorian Poor Law and largely shares a Foucauldian perspective on the function of the asylum as a regulatory agency. Jonathan Andrews illustrates the significance of class dynamics in the segmentation of the institutional market place in Scotland, as the 'royal' institutions were reserved for the more respectable and affluent. The chapter on Exminster suggests a more uneven picture where substantial farmers, entrepreneurs, commercial trades people and even professionals found their way to the Devon County Asylum with the tacit consent of Poor Law Guardians and medical physicians.[32] The significance of the county asylum may not have been so much its capacity to reinforce the hierarchy of class society as the service offered to different social groups who could utilise its provision without acquiring the stigma of idleness and improvidence associated with workhouse residence. Here may be found one of the more important implications of the decision to establish the county (and to a lesser degree borough) asylums as legally autonomous from the Poor Law authorities whilst creating an administrative framework in which a close relationship between the Unions and the asylum was essential to its effective operation. (The Unions were parishes which grouped together for the administration of the Poor Law of 1834.) Such a reading of asylum administration is clearly at variance with the class/commercialisation model found in earlier work, though it would still register the importance of economic transformation and class relationships in defining the functions of such institutions.[33]

Scholars are now more likely to question the necessary relationship between economic and institutional change whilst economic historians are increasingly prone to emphasise the remote origins of commercialisation and consumer societies and the uneven impact of such patterns of change across continents and regions. It is even more common for cultural historians (drawing on Foucault and other post-modernist theorists) to argue that the construction of class and gender boundaries and even the hegemony of capitalism itself were contingent rather than fixed, dependent on the capacity of different groups to mobilise around a particular rhetoric of rights and interests.[34] Different pathways to the modernisation of social institutions may be traced in relation to distinct political and cultural reference points as much as to the material expansion of the capitalist economy.[35] Some of these emphases can be found in the chapters of Lorraine Walsh and Jonathan Andrews, where the peculiarities of Scottish provision are illustrated in relation to the robust vitality of voluntary and charitable provision for lunatics. The Presbyterian church continued to occupy a key role in the dispensation of Poor Law relief, whilst the newly created charitable 'royal' asylums were monuments to the mobilisation of urban coalitions as well as civic virtue and a professional ethos.[36] The exchanges between Andrews and Scull indicate the scope for debate around this point of national divergence, though Andrews also demonstrates the significance of class identities in the strategic market move of the older royal asylums to cater for the better-heeled patient. Each of the Celtic studies suggests the importance of gender as well as class identities in the treatment offered in the later nineteenth century and Hilary Marland gives us a detailed analysis of how the incidence of puerperal insanity was recognised and handled by medical practitioners in the Victorian decades.

Whilst it is fair to say that many of the contributions to this volume would encourage a sceptical response to the ambitious model of institutional transformation in modern Europe and North America offered by writers such as Scull, there is considerable support for the view found in much recent scholarship that the modernisation of medical facilities formed part of a philosophical and political project directed by the powerful.[37] The interesting question posed by Foucault is how were the powerful constituted and what techniques comprised the exercise of power. Again the Celtic case studies suggest that psychiatrists were often less important as moral entrepreneurs in this venture than were clergymen, landowners, Poor Law Guardians, and the business and professional groups who formed an urban gentry at some of the most important sites of institution building. A key determinant in the shaping of lunacy provision appears to have been the strength of voluntary associations in civil society and the degree of autonomy from central direction which volunteer citizens exercised in the control of such state agencies as the Poor Law. Whilst the highland Scots suffered the trauma of land clearances in the modernisation of the agrarian economy, the lowland heritors and kirk sessions negotiated the terms on which pauper provision should be given to those who could find no voluntary support.

The foundation of lunatic asylums in the peripheral nations of the United Kingdom therefore formed part of a cultural engagement between the metropolitan forces of civilisation and the non-anglicised subjects of the Crown. Pamela Michael and David Hirst show that the institution of a North Wales Asylum was seen by some of its early advocates as part of a civilising process where the ethnic Welsh should be cleansed of their insanity by the removal of their native tongue. The essay reveals that this view was far less significant amongst the leading protagonists than their concern to provide the humanitarian counsel of psychiatry. Oonagh Walsh argues that the administrative structure of the Irish asylums starkly reflected the greater power of the colonial British state *vis-à-vis* its subject populations and the political weakness of the Roman church in which a large majority of the population worshipped. Rather different patterns were to be found in the distinctive colonial environments of India and the Cape surveyed by Waltraud Ernst and Shula Marks respectively. In these societies the imperial state was not inclined to recognise or register a problem amongst native subjects as worthy of an institutional response, whilst insanity amongst the settler elites was lower than that recorded in England and Wales. Such absences indicate that one of the pre-requisites for asylum building was some calculation that insanity was a problem worthy of an investment to diagnose its extent and the dedication of specialist facilities for its cure or containment. For most colonial subjects this was an experience of the twentieth rather than the nineteenth century.[38] Ernst emphasises the symbolic importance of the new asylums in India as monuments to imperial benevolence and scientific superiority. They could also function to remind the colonial elite of the standards expected and provide a means for the rapid repatriation of those whose conduct threatened scandal.

The distinctive experiences of care even within southern Africa during the later nineteenth and early twentieth centuries illustrate the point that even in colonial societies the politics of lunacy were made by human beings rather than pre-ordained by economic or state structures. If the modernisation of institutions for the insane took many forms in different societies, the institutional politics involved in caring for the pauper lunatic engaged a wide variety of ideas and interests. We have seen that in Scotland the landed and middle classes were anxious to devise voluntary rather than statist solutions to many social problems and did not always welcome the higher taxes involved in public projects. In southern England the leading landowners often championed the cause of the public county asylum against the opposition of liberals in both urban and rural areas who wanted the asylum brought under the close control of the Poor Law.[39]

Here lies a second main point of difference between most of the new research reported here and much earlier scholarship, which situated the new lunatic asylums in a historical landscape of class struggle where they functioned to secure the values of possessive individualism. Whilst the leading author of *Masters of Bedlam* displays an unrivalled knowledge of the personal and political biographies of the leading psychiatrists of the nineteenth century, he has usually seen the defensive sensibilities of the mad-doctors in terms of their strategic role as advocates of a liberal social order and promoters of a Whiggish vision of scientific progress.[40] Recent historians of the welfare state tend to express greater scepticism about the bid for professional power via state medicine by physicians, noting the persistence of private medical interests opposed to state control and also the hesitant response of these 'reluctant imperialists' to society's demand for medical men as social arbiters.[41] It is also apparent that psychiatrists have long viewed the presence of the most seriously and chronically ill amongst their patients as impediments to the effective cure and management of the insane within medical establishments.[42] This is not to underestimate the quality of the research which Scull and other scholars have undertaken on the institutional practices and the political context in which European psychiatry developed during the mid-century decades.[43] The issue is whether we can usefully read the foundation of the Victorian asylum and the practical work of early psychiatry as the product of a peculiarly bourgeois view of the world which underwrote bourgeois hegemony by filling the corridors of these new institutions with the unproductive labouring poor and imposing medical authority on the broader mass of working people who never entered the asylum but feared that they might.

The chapters which follow provide a mass of evidence that public asylums in different countries remained saturated with an ethos of labour, sobriety and individual responsibility long after the promise of moral treatment had faded from view. Yet the contributors also reveal a large cast of actors and a variety of practices influencing the dispatch and treatment of the insane from the years surveyed by Smith to

Suzuki's Bethlem and on to the Valkenberg Asylum examined by Marks. Andrews and Wright suggest how the micro-politics of family provision were enmeshed in a changing environment of innovation and reform which shifted as new provisions were made by the state throughout the long nineteenth century. Evidence from Devon and other areas indicates that the golden age of asylum building was in fact a period when the control of these institutions was still contested and many county asylums were carved out of the pastoral landscape as monuments to the virtues of aristocratic leadership rather than as pillars of bourgeois morality. In certain respects the architecture and governance of the public lunatic asylum pointed towards a rural idyll that historical sociologists have termed the 'Beau Ideal' of the English historical landscape and which formed part of a conservative reaction to commercialisation rather than a celebration of the free labour market.[44]

The value of the concept of moral entrepreneurship used by Scull and others is that it enables us to extend our vision of the purpose of the asylum into the arena of popular politics during the years when class leadership itself was being contested by millenarians, Owenites and Chartist radicals, each competing in the political and cultural market place to stamp their own programmes for the 'reformation of character' and improvement of manners on the body politic. Whilst most of the chapters on the United Kingdom register the significance of both the Old Poor Law and the New Poor Law in the history of English lunacy administration, this relationship was often held in place by tensions and conflicts rather than a shared sense of purpose. Such frictions were vividly apparent in the political struggles of the 1830s and 1840s, which defined the terms on which the state provided services such as lunacy treatment for its citizens during the second half of the nineteenth century. The remarkable contrast to be made in the social reforms of the 1840s is between the intense controversy aroused by the introduction of the New Poor Law and the relative quiescence which met the introduction of the radical Lunacy Acts of 1845. Much of Lord Ashley's success lay in his ability to exploit the Tory–radical alliance which had been forged out of the northern campaigns against the Poor Law and hardened by the Factory Movement and Ten Hours struggle of the Chartist years.[45]

The hostility of the Conservative press towards the 'Malthusian' science of the New Poor Law is evident in such newspapers as *The Bolton Chronicle*, one of a battery of provincial journals to attack the Poor Law for the iron logic of 'classification' which overlooked the fact that some of the supposed misdemeanours of the poor were committed by those of weak intellect whose place was 'more properly in a lunatic asylum'.[46] Urban Tories who were elected to local Poor Law boards were anxious to appear to be close friends of economy and hesitated openly to support the erection of county asylums, whilst also seeking to present themselves as the most faithful poor man's guardian. Similar ambiguities are apparent in the more sophisticated analysis of such radical newspapers as the Chartist *Northern Star* during the passage of the 1845 Lunacy legislation. Such papers certainly attacked the New Poor Law as well as the commercialisation of agriculture which had 'caused the landlords and farmers to act more like the inmates of a lunatic asylum than as men of ordinary sanity'.[47] The attack continued on the jobbery associated with the new institutions, with the radical journalists complaining that,

> there are all the County-rates, and the building of prisons, and houses of correction, and tread-wheels, and lock-ups, and court houses, and the erection and maintenance of County bridges; there are all the expenses of prosecuting misdemeanants, and of keeping them while in prison; there are...all the County Lunatic Asylums, erecting, maintaining, and sustaining, with all *their* tribes of paid officials...[48]

Yet the Tories and radicals appear to have found common ground not only in the factory movement and attacks on the Poor Law but also in promoting the model lunatic asylum. At a time when the English and also Scottish Poor Law legislation produced a storm of protest amongst Tories and working-class radicals, Ashley's Lunacy proposals of 1845 appear to have passed without serious controversy. It would appear that the asylum issue had been effectively de-politicised by the end of 1845 and did not form a significant part of the discourse of class conflict and political engagement even in these years of Chartist agitation.[49]

The contrast between the popular reception of the Poor Law and that of the Lunacy legislation again indicates how difficult it is to read the dynamics of bourgeois hegemony into the institutional politics of insanity. It also raises questions about the degree to which asylums were an integral part of a system of penal regulation of the poor in industrialising Britain. Chartists who pressed for universal male enfranchisement as the expression of rational citizenship may have found it difficult to oppose the introduction of reforms which claimed to emancipate as well as humanise the mad, though the rise of the specialist asylum can equally plausibly be seen as a triumph for the politics of aristocratic humanitarianism promoted by Ashley and the Tory traditionalists. The consequence of this accommodation between radical politics and moralised economics was a golden age of asylum building sustained by the promise of moral treatment for the individuals who entered such places.

The extent to which medical practice was informed by both class and gendered conceptions of the body has been a powerful theme in feminist accounts of the Victorian period and one of the most vivid images from contemporary literature remains that of the mad *woman* who occupied an ambivalent class position.[50] The studies by Suzuki and Marland illustrate both the growing power of the medical professional as forensic detective and the different pathologies of childbirth being offered during the Victorian decades. In common with the analysis of Valkenberg by Marks, these chapters address the complex problem of how historians might deconstruct the diagnoses and therapeutic strategies pursued in the long nineteenth century. The lexicon of insanity, madness and lunacy which contemporaries deployed can be translated into modern psychiatric language, though the contributions to this volume share with most social historians a reluctance to engage in broad generalisations on the biological origins of disease. As Nancy Theriot has suggested, we can best understand the rise and fall of such diagnoses as puerperal insanity as the outcome of an interplay between growing medical knowledge, altered relations between medical professionals and patients, and a change in gender relations in wider society.[51]

One conclusion to draw from such work is that the discourses of treatment as well as the political practices which gave birth to the asylum remained a contested space between different actors and there were divergent conceptions of the responsibilities for the lunatic pauper. These contests extended into different areas of lay authority long after 1845. The 'mixed economy' of care for the insane remained the responsibility of a variety of institutions and individuals, as is shown by the continued residence of hundreds of lunatics, imbeciles and others in the massive Bolton Workhouse at the end of the nineteenth century.[52] The chapters by Andrews, Bartlett and Forsythe *et al.*, reveal the continuing struggles over the political control of the insane and the Exminster case in particular suggests that central government regulation tightened in the second half of the century as the Lunacy Commissioners pursued a Chadwickian agenda of more specialist provision for different groups of pauper lunatics, including 'deficient' children who were the subject of both voluntary and state initiatives before 1914.[53]

This detailed work on the actors engaged in the making of the institutionalised lunatic raises the question of historical agency and identity, which forms the third main point of difference between much earlier research and the fresh crop of studies which are represented in this volume. As Scull notes in his reflections on these new studies, there is an inclination for recent scholarship to award agency to even the most vulnerable and marginalised groups in an attempt to retrieve the voice of the poor. It is equally important to register the influence of those who did not participate in the formal discourse of scientific diagnosis but whose commonsense experience formed part of a logic of institutionalisation which is described in these chapters.[54] Institutions provided some of the most obvious and important rules and conventions for social behaviour, though they could not (and cannot) prescribe all of the practices and stratagems which families and other groups exploited in playing the rules of the game to their own ends.[55]

The machinery of the Poor Law does indeed reveal some of the massive inequalities in power and resources which determined access to medical services in this period. To follow Roberts and detect in the workings of the Victorian lunatic asylum the benign origins of a modern health service would be to lapse into a kind of late Whiggism which obscures the discontinuities in institutional care.[56] Many authors would also emphasise the concentration of legal power in the hands of a county and borough magistracy who certified the insane, often controlling the local Poor Law Unions as well as the lunatic asylums and prisons before the local government reforms of the 1880s.[57] The pauper lunatic was doubly disqualified from exercising the rights of citizenship, even where not excluded by gender and age. Suzuki's analysis of Bethlem psychiatric treatment suggests that the medical professionals steadily extended their hold over the interpretation of the lunatic's voice, and lay opinion, at least in the form of a commonsense narrative of the causes of the individual's madness, was slowly pushed to the margins of diagnosis. In contrast to the more sympathetic treatment of family influence offered by Wright amongst others, Suzuki views the growing autonomy of the medical men as a step towards more enlightened treatment. Even if other authors discover that the approach of the bedside psychiatrist at Bethlem was more urgent than that recorded in provincial asylums where lay authority persisted in various forms far longer, it would seem that the rise of the medical professional and the salaried bureaucrat had eclipsed both the charismatic moral healer and the traditional authority of the magistracy by the outbreak of war in 1914.

The continuing controversy over the use and abuse of professional power by the mad-doctors of the long nineteenth century also cautions us against hasty generalisation in regard to the progress of psychiatry and this point is underlined by many contributors to this volume.[58] In contrast to early Foucauldian studies, scholars now emphasise the limitations imposed on modernising intellectuals by the force of tradition, the dispersion of institutional authority, and the capacity for resistance which Foucault himself located within the exercise of power. Lorraine Walsh's work suggests that medical professionals formed a weak element in the coalition of professionals and propertied groups considering asylum provision in Dundee as compared to their formidable influence in Edinburgh and Glasgow. Andrews emphasises the limited successes of Scottish psychiatrists whilst Marks shows the impact of Scottish training in universalist libertarian notions of moral therapy on individual superintendents in the Cape at the end of the century. As noted above, Suzuki portrays the growing influence of the psychiatrist at the bedside of the patient, gently elbowing aside the relatives and friends whose lay testimonies had previously provided the authoritative history of the illness. Whereas Wright's chapter illustrates the vital importance of family influence to the lunatic's escape from the asylum, Suzuki and Marland both suggest that the medical professional was an increasing presence as the century progressed. In general, the essays alert us to the marginal role which psychiatrists often enjoyed in relation to the initial classification of the insane as well as the importance of philosophical and institutional differences within the profession. Towards the end of the period we can see psychiatrists as well as physicians asserting their corporate professional autonomy in dealings with the lay authorities. The lunatic inmate gradually became the mental hospital patient under the care of the physician. This did not necessarily denote a benign step towards modernity, since the medical practitioners of different societies were also attuned to the emergence of social and political ideologies concerning effective citizenship, human efficiency, class degeneration and racial purity.

These themes are evident in contributions which show the contribution of psychiatry and the asylum to the making of the normative nation and notions of responsible citizenship in different countries. Oonagh Walsh as well as Michael and Hirst indicate the degree to which patriarchal notions of appropriate behaviour were coupled with assumptions about the use of language, race, ethnicity, gender and religion. Crude if often casual Darwinian notions of Irish racial characteristics stare out from the Ballinasloe case notes quoted by Walsh as do stereotypes of gender. Whilst families sought to intervene with some success in the passage of their members to and from the workhouse or asylum, medical practitioners contributed their own views on heredity and domestic arrangements to the formation of notions of the normal family, reshaped by state legislation before 1914, as well as the obligations of male breadwinners and female domestic carers. The translation of psychiatric practices in societies where race and the classification of the 'native' peoples formed the guiding principles of political rule is explored in Ernst's chapter on colonial India and Marks's study of Valkenberg Asylum in the Cape. Megan Vaughan noted how European psychiatrists characterised the environment of the African native as both primeval and exotic, alongside the existence of genuine debate amongst psychologists and psychiatrists on the importance of racial differences in human consciousness.[59] Nancy Leys Stepan has provided an illuminating discussion of the relationship between ideas of race, gender and citizenship in the promotion of scientific method since the European Enlightenment in an exploration of the ways in which these conceptions informed medical practices.[60] Important research by Harriet Deacon and Sally Swartz on psychiatric practices in southern Africa has registered the growth of racialist and gendered classifications within the medical profession during the late nineteenth and early twentieth centuries.[61] Swartz has also made an imaginative attempt to retrieve the imagery of madness expressed by patients in Cape asylums by close analysis of patient records to examine how racial classifications and prejudices were assimilated into the 'delusional systems' mapped out in the case notes.[62] However, the low figures for the admission of non-Europeans to insane asylums in both African and Indian colonies during the nineteenth century suggest that the diagnosis of insanity worthy of institutional treatment was mainly confined to the colonising Europeans and a limited number of non-whites who presented some recognisable threat by violence or other means to the stable order.[63]

The research of Marks acknowledges the gradual racialisation found by Deacon and Swartz whilst stressing the residual importance of a liberal universalist outlook which had pervaded the Scottish asylums from which some of the leading figures in Cape psychiatric treatment were recruited. The separate spheres occupied by the coloniser and colonised are even more graphically evident in Ernst's wide-ranging survey of the treatment of the employees of the East India Company and later settlers who were brought back to England for treatment, usually in private asylums far removed from the county pauper asylum and the colonial environment where their illness was recognised. As both Ernst and Marks note, there were very few provisions made for non-Europeans in these colonies and various ideas were raised that 'natives' were less susceptible to mental disorder than the inhabitants of more civilised countries.[64] These chapters identify different themes in the moral mission of psychiatry developed in such colonies and again extend our analysis of institutional treatment into the rhetorics of race, gender, nation and class which Stepan has elucidated in her recent discussion of medicine and citizenship.[65] For the language of race and nation pervaded not only colonial discourses but also contemporary discussions on the 'sunken race' of poor Irish peasants, outcast slum dwellers of the urban slum districts and degenerate women who debilitated the military forces by infection. Their visitations by physicians and philanthropists were often dramatised as explorations into darkest England, a comparison often made with medical expeditions in remote and exotic regions of the world.[66] The moral authority for such benign medical policing of the poor and the legal intrusion into private spaces and civil liberties was disputed in the controversy over the Contagious Diseases legislation as feminist historians have shown.[67]

The spectacle of foreign bodies raised in discussions of medical care for the mass of the population in the United Kingdom and its colonies alerts us to the importance of Scull's argument that the micro-histories of particular institutions and community networks need to be informed by a theoretical and comparative perspective rather than descending into ever-decreasing circles of 'exceptional' cases.[68] Whilst the new research on the history of insanity calls into question the model of modernisation and class politics outlined in some earlier work, there is a common emphasis on the importance of the material environment and social relationships as a context for understanding the institutional politics of lunacy provision. The experience of different countries within and beyond the UK suggests the significance of institutions not only as registers of the balance of power within societies but also as groups of actors who were capable of resisting as well as initiating change. Attempts by eighteenth-century modernisers to reform Sweden's medieval asylums to service the needs of a changing labour market were stubbornly resisted by local communities who controlled these institutions, whilst efforts to fund rival private facilities for more affluent groups also faltered in the nineteenth century.[69] The outcome of these struggles set the scene for the pattern of specialist lunacy provision made by the Swedish state at facilities such as the Danvikens Asylum (near Stockholm), which continued in possession of its own resources and in considerable autonomy from a state poor law system and private benefactors.[70]

Such conflicts between traditionalists and modernisers in civil society marked out the ground on which state facilities were built during the nineteenth century. They were not simply imposed by the logic of capitalist expansion *or* by the unfolding structures of state administration which some scholars have stressed.[71] Even after the passage of key state reforms such as the lunacy legislation of the 1840s and 1850s in the United Kingdom, the institutional provision for the insane remained a contested terrain on which different groups sought to promote their ideas and interests. As states sought to exert greater central control over the classification and treatment of lunatics by the elaboration of administrative regulations and statistical information, local agents and professional bodies asserted their own capacity to identify and manage the insane.

Conclusions

After three decades in which almost every developed country has abandoned the mass institutionalisation of the mentally ill, it seems an appropriate point to reflect on the origins of these systems in Europe and America during the long nineteenth century. The renewed debates on the historical development and functions of the psychiatric services can be traced to the radical critique of medical theory and clinical practices of the 1960s as well as Foucault's assault on the pretensions of modernity. Scholars quickly registered the importance of these new paradigms for the history of insanity but found Foucault's account of modernisation, institutional politics, the exercise of power and historical agency deeply problematic. It was partly in response to such omissions that historians such as Scull developed a well-researched historical sociology of madness, focusing on the central importance of the asylum and the scope which these institutions offered for the exploitation of an expanded trade in lunacy by a rising group of powerful mad-doctors who assumed control of a growing population of inmates. This interpretation provided a social and political landscape for the building of these new structures in the great transformation to commercialised class society where the mobility and efficiency required of the labour force left the awkward and unproductive without resources. Many earlier narratives of lunacy reform have therefore been organised around two key points: that lunatic asylums were institutions which met the needs of the economy and society as perceived by the powerful, and that they formed part of an ideological project of civilisation through medical intervention.

One of the most important implications of this revisionist debate was a renewed interest in the historical construction of insanity and the relationship between the environment in which a person was identified as mad and the scientific evidence of their organic and somatic disorders. Foucault stressed the growing incarceration of the insane as a specific category of disorderly person which the rational scientific order could not tolerate, whilst Scull has emphasised the degree to which the building of the new asylums during the long nineteenth century served to reduce family and community tolerance of awkward and unproductive behaviour. Behaviour which might not qualify a person for institutionalisation in the eighteenth or the twentieth centuries was the basis for certification in the decades which the present volume encompasses. The contributors are generally more cautious than earlier revisionist scholars in asserting a clear and consistent theme in the classification of the insane and more concerned to demonstrate the different elements which contributed to the process of institutionalisation. There is little attempt to recalibrate contemporary discussions according to more recent psychiatric classification.[72] Most authors replicate the contemporary usage of terms such as insanity, madness and lunacy without attempting an authoritative discussion of the nosologies of psychiatry which earlier authors have provided. The essays seek rather to locate these terms within the context of the legal and practical transactions which secured the passage of the lunatic from community to asylum and back again.

The arguments laid out in the scholarship of the past two decades have therefore set many of the terms of the debates on the history of the care of the insane and remain the starting point for most chapters in this volume. The authors share many important positions in seeking to reappraise institutional provision for the insane in different societies during the long nineteenth century. Drawing on Foucault's insights into the intellectual construction of the insane and the primary importance of new institutional regimes, most of these essays offer a more empirically detailed and historically complex analysis of the function of the asylum within a network of power which encompassed the traditional as well as the modern and the lay witness alongside the professional expert. The contributors therefore share a concern to combine an understanding of the specific content and context of the politics of insanity with an understanding of the workings of the institutions created in these years. This requires a subtle institutional perspective that takes cultural references and political formations seriously, alongside the structure of states, economies, family household structures and other demographic factors. Foucault not only interrogated but also deployed the dramatic images of chain-breaking and chain-making in an attempt to demonstrate the links between the asylum and the penal system, thereby fixing steps in the rise of modernity and the place of institutions within the scientific age. In dramatising his anti-narrative of institutional oppression he concentrated attention on the technologies of asylum building and seriously obscured his own critical insights into the elaborate circuits in which power is exercised. Such a master narrative disrupts the continuities in institutional provision which these essays have emphasised and understates the function of such institutions as sites for competing rhetorics of humane accommodation. Modernity is always a contested space, and not merely amongst rationalising intellectuals. As Roy Porter has noted, the power of an institution such as Bethlem Asylum should be understood (like the Bastille) more in its capacity to generate a mythology of madness and images of desperation than in its physical techniques of incarceration during the eighteenth and nineteenth centuries.[73]

The position of the asylum within a complex of state institutions and a market place for the treatment of the insane returns us to Foucault's arguments on the penal regulation of the labouring poor and the role of the Poor Law identified in Bartlett's pioneering work on insanity provision. There were close links by law and administrative practice between the lunatic asylum and the Union workhouse as various chapters note. Yet we should be careful of reading into the politics and practice of the lunacy administration under the Poor Law a narrow conception of pauperism or of institutional growth. The Poor Law was absent in India and South Africa, with their highly distinctive settler populations and very large non-European populations as compared to colonised areas such as Canada and Australasia.[74] Almshouses may have functioned in the United States in a similar way to the Poor Laws in Europe, though an analysis of the social function of different institutions must include the role of non-state associations in civil society and the political context of state action. It is possible to view the county asylum as a monument to the continuities of aristocratic and land-holding power (at least until the reform of local government) as much as a landmark in the spread of bourgeois commercialisation. One of the strongest themes to emerge from this collection is the configuration of lunacy administration within the social politics of the long nineteenth century, as tensions between central regulation and local autonomy enabled different groups to claim responsibility for pauper lunatics and to limit the power of the asylum.

Nor can the asylum be seen as simply the product of class management. The essays emphasise the multiple functions of the asylum in the nineteenth century rather than privileging the custodial warehousing of the mad. The relationship between the growth of 'asylumdom' and the spread of capitalist market relations in different societies was defined by a range of environmental conditions. Important differences emerge not only between England, Scotland and Ireland but also between England

and Wales, and even within different regions of England, according to the balance of social and political forces which mobilised around the Lunacy legislation. We can see distinctive economic and demographic forces shaping different regions within states even as governments sought to impose similar models of the modern institution on their populations. The resilience of voluntary provision was a key factor in the mixed economy of provision as was the power of national and colonial states. As numerous scholars have argued, the asylum failed the protagonists of moral treatment and could claim limited success as a curative institution in the period. In the light of the overcrowding found in numerous county and borough establishments, the recalcitrance of Poor Law Guardians and the growing scepticism of leading psychiatrists themselves becomes comprehensible.

The contributions therefore indicate something of the complexity and permeability of the institutional politics of insanity, involving different groups with varying resources. Even an institution as forbidding as the Poor Law workhouse could be approached and utilised if not manipulated by local communities and families seeking solutions to the problems of managing those who were identified as mad. The emphasis in current research on the detailed reconstruction of the community, familial and cultural contexts of lunacy provision has enabled us not only to explore the micro-politics of care but also the limits of medical control within what remained a highly mixed market of commercial, state and voluntary provision.[75] We find a large cast of actors involved in the construction of lunacy during the nineteenth century and clear scope for accommodation, evasion and resistance within the system of pauper lunacy. Rather than the arrival of the asylum marking the dawn of an era of close control and intense regulation, the process of committal and discharge can be characterised as one of asymmetrical bargaining in which different actors had unequal power resources and capacities but could exert *some* degree of choice if not control over their environment.[76] The condition of insanity was legally defined in ways which constrained the pauper lunatic as the inverse of the positive citizen. This implied complete exclusion from rational choice and participation in civil society, although it should be noted that the legal protection of those identified as lunatics, idiots, imbeciles and mentally defective was strengthened at the end of the nineteenth century. These changes contributed to the transition in clinical status of the individual from asylum inmate to mental patient.

The reappraisal of the institutional treatment of the insane provided in these essays has also opened up fresh avenues of debate and inevitably left many issues of interpretation unresolved. Scholars are seeking to reconstruct the experience of the asylum from the perspective of the patient by tracing the network of relations which made up the micro-histories of insanity using detailed analysis of case notes and record linkages with a range of other sources.[77] Contributors such as Smith, Suzuki and Wright appear to follow Gerald Grob in viewing the asylum essentially as a therapeutic establishment which responded to community problems and needs by providing an alternative to earlier and less adequate services.[78] Bartlett and Andrews offer a more austere view of the asylum and its relationship to the Poor Law whilst other chapters on Scotland, Ireland, India and South Africa appear to share at least some of Scull's concern with the contribution of the asylum to a class-based imperialist order where the defence of existing power relations was implicit within the institutional project. These variations in the analysis of the asylum point again to the need for a careful historical contextualisation of institutions and their functions within distinct societies. Different perspectives are also evident in the depiction of the medical profession and the position of the psychiatrist. Chapters by Suzuki and Marland are two of the contributions which suggest how we might carefully excavate the different layers of meaning within the archaeology of expertise that make up the system of legal certification and clinical case notes, whilst exposing the power relations between the medical interrogator and his subject. The influence of the psychiatrist is questioned, usually implicitly, in many of the other chapters. Marks explores the ways in which notions of citizenship informed psychiatric practice in the peculiar conditions of Valkenberg.

A number of the essays attempt a close reading of the textual sources provided by the asylums themselves, including Oonagh Walsh's chapter on Ireland. Any attempt to reconstruct the experience of the certified lunatic and the relationship between patient and physician requires great skill, as Suzuki's account reveals. Marland traces the history of a particular diagnosis and distinguishes the usage found in text books from the recorded incidents in asylum registers. Rather than decoding the specific usage of a term such as 'lunacy' in great detail, most of the contributors necessarily deploy the contemporary descriptions with as much detachment as possible in summarising developments across time and space. In attempting to chart what we might term the interior landscapes of these institutions and the processes which led to an individual's admission, most contributors have sought to read the formal texts against some discernible material environment in which to locate the meaning of the information and to place the actions which apparently secured an outcome of admission and discharge. Cultural historians and historical sociologists have alerted us to the conventions and devices which the authors of our primary sources used in their production and the point has been made above that historians of psychiatry as well as historical psychiatrists often reached for the dramatic or literary image to embolden their analyses. As Porter has demonstrated, the poetics of Bedlam entailed a particular politics of lunacy which formed part of the visual economy of the eighteenth and nineteenth centuries. The capacity of scholars to reconstruct narratives from such historical materials must be restricted not only by the vocabularies used in primary documents but, as Carolyn Steedman has noted, by our own familiarity with a particular kind of psychoanalytical and confessional narrative that may be very different from the imagery which poor people use to understand their state.[79] The circumstances in which insanity was identified, or disguised, are likely to remain obscure and difficult to construe and cases are often reported at the time in terms of the incomprehensibly uncivilised conditions in which individuals had been held.[80]

The contributors to this volume have generally responded to these daunting challenges by engaging with a variety of original texts to investigate the meanings of insanity and by seeking to ground these statements (and their authors) in the specific material cultures of their households, communities and societies. The building of the lunatic's identity depended on a number of formative influences but the legal identification and accommodation of the insane required an institutional process that has been the subject of these chapters. Our main theme has been that to understand this process we need to uncover the institutional politics of madness and the historical conditions under which asylums came to be defined as necessary to the welfare of the body politic itself.

Acknowledgements

An earlier version of this chapter was presented at the University of Exeter and the Economic History Institute, University of Uppsala. I am grateful to seminar participants including Mats Morrell, Goran Ryden, Lena Sommerstad and my colleague Jane Whittle for their comments. Particular thanks are due to Bernard Harris as Series Editor for his meticulous and incisive reading of earlier drafts, and to my co-editor Bill Forsythe and Helen Rogers for their criticism, advice and encouragement.

NOTES

1 R. Porter, 'History of psychiatry in Britain' *History of Psychiatry*, 2, 1991, pp. 271–9, especially 270–4. The familiar exceptions such as MacAlpine and Hunter, K. Jones and others are noted by Porter. Recent additions include H. Freeman and G.E. Berrios, eds, *150 Years of British Psychiatry: Volume II. The Aftermath*, London, Athlone, 1996.

2 C. Webster, *History of the National Health Service: Volume 2*, London, HMSO, 1997.

3 A. Scull, 'Psychiatry and social control in the nineteenth and twentieth centuries' *History of Psychiatry*, 2, 1991, p. 164; see L.J. Ray, 'Models of madness in Victorian asylum practice' *European Journal of Sociology*, 22, 1981, pp. 221–64, cited p. 157, n. 40.

4 J. Welshman, 'Community care: the policy background in England and Wales, 1948–74'. Paper presented to the SSHM Conference on Insanity, Institutions and Society, April 1997, University of Exeter [hereafter SSHM Exeter]. I am grateful for permission to cite this paper. B. Luckin, 'Towards a social history of institutionalisation' *Social History*, 8, 1, 1983, pp. 91–3 and *passim*, provides a critical note on institutions, medicine and community.

5 M. Foucault, *Madness and Civilisation: A History of Insanity in the Age of Reason*, New York, Random, 1985 edn; see P. Levi, *If This is a Man*, London, Abacus, 1987, p. 15, for a view of the role of 'unspoken dogma' rather than reason in the origins of the total institution of Auschwitz-Birkenau.

6 A.T. Scull, *Museums of Madness: The Social Organisation of Insanity in Nineteenth Century England*, London, Allen Lane, 1979; M. MacDonald, *Mystical Bedlam: Madness, Anxiety, and Healing in Seventeenth-Century England*, Cambridge, Cambridge University Press, 1981, particularly pp. 72–111; R. Porter, *Mind Forg'd Manacles: A History of Madness in England from the Restoration to the Regency*, London, Athlone, 1987; W. Bynum, R. Porter and M. Shepherd, eds, *The Anatomy of Madness: Essays in the History of Psychiatry*, particularly volume 2, London, Tavistock, 1985. Shula Marks notes that Africa is one region which has only recently gained its historians of insanity. D. Wright, 'Getting out of the asylum: understanding the confinement of the insane in the nineteenth century' *Social History of Medicine*, 10, 1, 1997, pp. 137–55, offers a recent survey of the field.

7 P. Major-Poetzl, *Michel Foucault's Archaeology of Western Culture. Toward a New Science of History*, Brighton, Harvester, 1983, pp. 105–48; M. Poster, *Foucault, Marxism and History*, Cambridge, Polity, 1984, pp. 95–120.

8 Scull, 'Psychiatry and social control', pp. 150, 153–4, 'the massive internment of the mad is essentially a nineteenth-century phenomenon'.

9 A. Suzuki, 'Lunacy in seventeenth and eighteenth-century England: analysis of Quarter Session records' *History of Psychiatry*, 2, 1991, pp. 437–57 and 3, 1992, pp. 29–44, provides a commentary on Foucault's methodology applied to the institutions of the old Poor Law and the legal system.

10 R. Chartier, 'Writing the practices' *French Historical Studies*, 21, 2, 1998, pp. 258–9, acknowledges the ambivalence in Foucault's discussion of the relationship between knowledge, power and resistance.

11 Ibid., pp. 259–61 and *passim*.

12 A. Digby, 'The changing profile of a nineteenth-century asylum: the York Retreat' *Psychological Medicine*, 14, 1984, pp. 739–48, provides an important

early analysis of social and geographical profiles; G.N. Grob, 'The social history of medicine and disease in America' *Journal of Social History*, 10, 1977, pp. 391–409. Grob's work includes an important emphasis on the role of American almshouses in the development of asylum facilities. The broader literature is too large to summarise though the *History of Psychiatry* provides an excellent range of studies.

13 G. Wickham, 'Power and power analysis: beyond Foucault?' in M. Gane, ed., *Towards a Critique of Foucault*, London, Routledge, 1986, for discussion in relation to biopolitics, the location of power and resistance, particularly pp. 163–7.

14 J. Saunders, 'Institutionalised offenders: a study of the Victorian institution and its inmates with special reference to late nineteenth-century Warwickshire', University of Warwick, Ph.D., 1983; D. Garland, *Punishment and Welfare: A History of Penal Strategies*, Aldershot, Gower, 1985, for a discussion of the penal–welfare complex; M. Thomson, 'Sterilisation, segregation and community care: ideology and solutions to the problems of mental deficiency in inter-war Britain' *History of Psychiatry*, 3, 1992, 473–98; P. Bartlett, 'The Poor Law of Lunacy: the admission of pauper lunatics in mid-nineteenth century England with special reference to Leicestershire and Rutland', University College, London, Ph.D., 1993; F. Driver, *Power and Pauperism: The Workhouse System, 1834–1884*, Cambridge, Cambridge University Press, 1993.

15 A. Butchart, 'The Industrial Panopticon: mining and the medical construction of migrant African labour in South Africa, 1900–1950' *Social Science Medicine*, 42, 2, 1996, pp. 185–97, particularly 194–5, provides a valuable application of the Foucauldian model to labour regulation in an economy which is the setting for the work of Shula Marks in this volume and elsewhere.

16 The literature cited in the chapters which follow indicates the fundamental contributions to the social history of insanity made by many scholars, not least those who have modified or rejected *marxisant* approaches. Particular attention is paid to Scull's work here both because of his undoubted influence within the field and because his major surveys have summarised a range of research findings in this area.

17 A. Scull, *Social Order/Mental Disorder*, Berkeley, 1989, p. 94 'defective human mechanisms were to be repaired so that they could once more compete in the marketplace', quoted in G.N. Grob, 'Marxian analysis and mental illness' *History of Psychiatry*, 1, 1990, p. 225.

18 The degree to which the nineteenth century saw a remarkable growth in the numbers of insane has been the subject of some debate, indicated in chapters below.

19 The discussion of gender in Scull's account remains rather muted. E. Showalter, *The Female Malady: Women, Madness, and English Culture, 1830–1980*, New York, Pantheon, 1985, offers an influential interpretation.

20 A. Scull, *The Most Solitary of Afflictions: Madness and Society in Britain, 1700–1900*, New Haven, Yale University Press, 1993.

21 Scull, 'Psychiatry and social control', p. 149. Scull identifies G.N. Grob as a 'scholarly ally' of the psychiatric profession, p. 153, ns 17–20.

22 A. Scull, 'Psychiatrists and historical "facts". Part two: rewriting the history of asylumdom' *History of Psychiatry*, 6, 1995, pp. 387–94, for exchanges with Mersky and Carr.

23 Some of the work of Andrews and Porter has been published as J. Andrews, A. Briggs, R. Porter, P. Tucker, and K. Waddington, *The History of Bethlem*, London, Routledge, 1997. A. Digby, *Madness, Morality and Medicine: A Study of the York Retreat, 1796–1914*, Cambridge, Cambridge University Press, 1985; J. Walton, 'Lunacy and the industrial revolution' *Journal of Social History*, 13, 1979; M. Finnane, *Insanity and the Insane in Post-Famine Ireland*, London, Croom Helm, 1981, for examples of the massive literature which now exists.

24 A. Scull, C. MacKenzie and N. Hervey, *Masters of Bedlam: The Transformation of the Mad-doctoring Trade*, Princeton, Princeton University Press, Chapter 4.

25 P. Joyce, 'The return of history: postmodernism and the politics of academic history in Britain' *Past and Present*, 158, 1998, pp. 225–9 and *passim.*

26 P. Glennie, 'Consumption within historical studies' in D. Millar, ed., *Acknowledging Consumption*, London, Routledge, 1995, p. 165.

27 R. Adair, J. Melling and B. Forsythe, 'Migration, family structure and pauper lunacy in Victorian England: admissions to the Devon County Pauper Lunatic Asylum, 1845–1900' *Continuity and Change*, 12, 3, 1997, pp. 373–401.

28 L.D. Smith, 'Close confinement in a mighty prison: Thomas Bakewell and his campaign against public asylums, 1810–1830' *History of Psychiatry*, 5, 1994, pp. 191–214.

29 R. Smith, 'Charity, self-interest and welfare: reflections from demographic and family history' in M. Daunton, ed., *Charity, Self-interest and Welfare in the English Past*, London, University College Press, 1996, pp. 23–4, 27–8; R. Smith and P. Horden 'Introduction' to *The Locus of Care*, London, Routledge, 1998.

30 Cf. E.H. Hunt, 'Paupers and pensioners' *Ageing and Society*, 9, 1990, pp. 407–30; S. King, 'Reconstructing lives: the poor, the Poor Law and welfare in Calverley, 1650–1820' *Social History*, 22, 3, 1997, pp. 318–38, especially p. 320, for the small numbers who came into contact with the Poor Law in Calverley: 'Relief obtained by those who did need communal support was at best meagre.' King stresses the importance of alternatives to 'harsh communal welfare', particularly kinship ties.

31 D.H. Alderman, 'Integrating space into a reactive theory of the asylum: evidence from post-Civil War Georgia' *Health and Place*, 3, 2, 1997, pp. 111–22, provides a community-reaction analysis in contrast to 'social control' perspectives such as those deriving from Foucault.

32 See also J. Melling, R. Adair and R. Turner, 'Occupations and insanity', Centre for Medical History, University of Exeter, 1996.

33 P. Mandler, 'The making of the new Poor Law *redivivus*', *Past and Present*, 117, 1987, and Driver, *Power and Pauperism*, 1993, chapters 2–3, for valuable discussion of such continuities. R. Adair, B. Forsythe and J. Melling, 'A danger to the public? Disposing of the pauper lunatic in Victorian and Edwardian England: the Exminster Asylum, 1845–1914' *Medical History*, 42, 1, 1998, pp. 1–25.

34 L. Hunt, 'Introduction: history, culture, and text' in *Cultural History*, particularly pp. 7–11 for an assessment of Foucauldian analysis; P. Joyce, *Visions of the People: Industrial England and the Question of Class*, Cambridge, Cambridge University Press, 1990.

35 W.H. Sewell, 'Language and practice in cultural history: backing away from the edge of the cliff' *French Historical Studies*, 21, 2, 1998, pp. 250–1 and *passim*, attempts to combine semiotic and mechanistic explanations of historical transformations.

36 'The English bastile' *Social Science Review*, 3, 1865, noted that the English county lunatic asylum resembled 'a large mansion' whilst the Union workhouse or 'bastile' had the appearance of 'a factory or huge store-house'. Quoted in Driver, *Power and Pauperism*, p. 1.

37 S. Marks and N. Andersson, 'Typhus and social control: South Africa, 1917–1950' in R. Macleod and M. Lewis, eds, *Disease, Medicine and Empire*, Routledge, 1988, pp. 257–83, for example.

38 J. Sadowsky, 'Colonial psychiatry' comment at SSHM Conference, Exeter, 1997, and *Imperial Bedlam: Institutions of Madness and Colonialism in Southwest Nigeria*, Berkeley, University of California Press, 1998.

39 B. Forsythe, J. Melling and R. Adair, 'The New Poor Law and the county pauper lunatic asylum' *Social History of Medicine*, 9, 1996, pp. 335–55.

40 G.N. Grob, 'Marxian analysis and mental illness' *History of Psychiatry*, 1, 1990, especially pp. 225–8 for similar criticisms.

41 A. de Swaan, 'The reluctant imperialism of the medical profession' *Social Science Medicine*, 28, 11, 1989, pp. 1,165–70. De Swaan draws heavily on Elias's notion of the civilising process and the kind of rational choice models which Richard Smith also discusses. See note 29 above.

42 W.H. Fisher and B.F. Phillips, 'Modelling the growth of long-stay populations in public mental hospitals' *Social Science Medicine*, 30, 12, 1990, pp. 1,341–2 and *passim*.

43 I. Dowbiggin, 'Alfred Maury and the politics of the Unconscious in nineteenth-century France' *History of Psychiatry*, 1, 1990, pp. 255–87, especially pp. 258–9 for Maury's influence on Freud.

44 For rural idyll and the Beau Ideal see L. Davidoff, J. L'Esperance and H. Newby, 'Landscape with figures: home and community in English society' in J. Mitchell and A. Oakley, eds, *The Rights and Wrongs of Women*, Harmondsworth, Penguin, 1976, particularly pp. 163–7.

45 *Bolton Chronicle* [*BC*] 18 October 1845 for description of Ashley as a 'persevering and disinterested' advocate of factory legislation.

46 *BC*, 16 August 1845. See also *BC*, 26 July 1845.

47 *Northern Star* [*NS*] 25 January 1845, p. 4, cl. 3.

48 *NS*, 15 February 1845, p. 4, cl. 4.

49 *NS*, 17 April 1845, p. 8, cl. 4. For the comment of a coroner on the death of a male lunatic, William Holden, in the care of Alexander Patrick Stuart at Peckham House Asylum, that 'Criminals are better off than lunatics, but a new bill is about to be introduced that will remedy the evil.' Peckham is one of the asylums discussed in the chapter by Len Smith below. For opposition of Duncombe to the Bill and reference to the petition of the Surgeon of Pentonville against the Bill see *NS*, 19 July 1845, p. 8, cl. 4.

50 J. Melling and B. Forsythe, 'Madness, marriage and mortality: gender and admission to the pauper lunatic asylum in Victorian and Edwardian England', forthcoming, provides a discussion of the scholarship of Showalter, *The Female Malady*.

51 N.M. Theriot, 'Diagnosing unnatural motherhood: nineteenth-century physicians and "puerperal insanity" ' in H. Cravens, *et al.*, eds, *Technical Knowledge in American Culture: Science, Technology and Medicine Since the Early*

1800s, Tuscaloosa, University of Alabama Press, 1996, pp. 78–9 and *passim*.

52 I.A.J. Percival, 'Lunacy within the workhouse: an investigation into lunatic paupers institutionalised within the workhouse with reference to the Fishpool Institution, Bolton 1861–1900', BA Honours Dissertation, University of Exeter, 1995, p. 3.

53 J. Melling, R. Adair and B. Forsythe, ' "A proper lunatic for two years": pauper lunatic children in Victorian and Edwardian England' *Journal of Social History*, 30, 4, 1997, pp. 371–405.

54 Sewell, 'Language and practice', pp. 243–7 and *passim*, considers de Certeau's and Chartier's claims for the significance of non-verbal practices including the logic of common sense experience.

55 Chartier, 'Writing the practices', pp. 262–3, for a distinction (from de Certeau and Bordieu) between the logics of formal discourses and of practices.

56 D. Roberts, *The Victorian Origins of the British Welfare State*, New Haven, Yale University Press, 1960; also D. Fraser, *Evolution of the British Welfare State: A History of Social Policy Since the Industrial Revolution*, London, Macmillan, 1984. Much 'revisionist' scholarship on popular politics also emphasises a long trajectory of radicalism and shared political culture rather than conflict and discontinuity. For example, E.F. Biagini and A.J. Reid, eds, *Currents of Radicalism: Popular Radicalism, Organised Labour, and Party Politics in Britain, 1850–1914*, Cambridge, Cambridge University Press, 1991. The politics of lunacy reform is only one of many areas where a radical–conservative alliance proved more significant than radical–liberal links.

57 J. Saunders, 'Quarantining the weak minded: psychiatric definitions of degeneracy and the late Victorian asylum' in W.F. Bynum, R. Porter and M. Shepherd, eds, *Anatomy of Madness: Volume Three*, London, Tavistock, 1988, pp. 273–96; Bartlett, The Poor Law of Lunacy, 1993; N. Finzsch and R. Jutte, eds, *Institutions of Confinement: Hospitals, Asylums and Prisons in Western Europe and North America 1500–1950*, Cambridge, Cambridge University Press, 1996; J. Melling, B. Forsythe and R. Adair, 'Families, communities and the legal regulation of lunacy in Victorian England' in P. Bartlett and D. Wright, eds, *Outside the Walls: Community Care in Britain and Ireland*, London, Athlone, 1999, forthcoming.

58 Scull, 'Psychiatrists and historical "facts" ', pp. 387–94, for a flavour of the exchanges.

59 M. Vaughan, 'Idioms of madness: Zomba Lunatic Asylum, Nyasaland, in the colonial period' *Journal of Southern African Studies*, 9, 2, 1983, pp. 218–38, particularly pp. 226–7.

60 N.L. Stepan, 'Race, science and medicine: citizenship and the natural'. Paper presented at SSHM Conference on Race, Science and Medicine, Southampton, 1996. I am grateful for permission to cite this paper.

61 H.J. Deacon, 'Madness, race and moral treatment: Robben Island Lunatic Asylum, Cape Colony: 1846–1890' *History of Psychiatry*, 7, 1996, especially pp. 288–9; S. Swartz, 'The black insane in the Cape, 1891–1920' *Journal of Southern African Studies*, 21, 3, 1995, pp. 399–415.

62 Swartz, 'The black insane', pp. 404–6.

63 Ibid., p. 408, where Swartz notes that the ratios of 1:678 white insane in the Cape in 1909 compared to 1:1,994 non-white insane to non-white population 'reflect the extent to which insanity amongst the black popula-

tion was either hidden from, or ignored by colonial authorities'. Comparable figures for England and Wales in 1901 was 1:288.

64 The ambiguities of psychiatrists towards civilisation long pre-dates Freud. See A. Scull, ed., *The Asylum As Utopia: W.A.F. Browne and the Mid-Nineteenth Century Consolidation of Psychiatry*, London, Routledge, 1990.

65 Stepan, 'Race, science and medicine'.

66 C. Hall, *White, Male and Middle-Class: Explorations in Feminism and History*, Cambridge, Polity, 1992, for essay on the Governor Eyre controversy.

67 J. Walkowitz, 'The making of an outcast group: prostitutes and working women in nineteenth-century Plymouth and Southampton' in M. Vicinus, ed., *A Widening Sphere: Changing Roles of Victorian Women*, London, Methuen, 1980, pp. 72–93 for discussion of the Contagious Diseases Acts; H. Rogers, *Authority and Authorship: Radical Women and Popular Politics in Nineteenth-Century England* (forthcoming, 2000). I am grateful for permission to cite this manuscript.

68 A. Scull, 'Psychiatry and its historians' *History of Psychiatry*, 2, 1991, pp. 242–3 for a criticism of Rothman and Grob for stressing the exceptionalism of the American experience.

69 M. Morell, *Studier I den svenska livsmedelskonsumtionens historia. Hospitalhjonens livsmedelskonsumtionens, 1621–1872*, Uppsala, Studies in Economic History, Uppsala University, 1989.

70 E. Eggeby, *Vandringsman, har ser du en avmalning av varlden. Vardade, vard och ekonomi pa Danvikens darhus 1750–1861*, Stockholm, 1996, pp. 258–60 and *passim*; R. Qvarsell, 'History of psychiatry in Sweden' *History of Psychiatry*, 2, 1991, pp. 315–20.

71 Skocpol provides an alternative state-centred model of welfare development in direct contrast to that of socially derived analyses of social policy; which is applied in J.R. Sutton, 'The political economy of madness: the expansion of the asylum in Progressive America' *American Sociological Review*, 56, 1991, pp. 665–78. For a critique of the Skocpol and the rational-choice models see J. Melling, 'Industrial capitalism and the welfare of the state: the role of employers in the comparative development of welfare states' *Sociology*, 25, 1991, pp. 219–39.

72 R.L. Numbers and J.S. Numbers, 'Millerism and madness: a study of "religious insanity" in nineteenth-century America' *Bulletin of the Menninger Clinic*, 49, 4, 1985, pp. 289–320, particularly Table 4, p. 303, which is one of numerous important attempts to combine quantitative and qualitative historical evidence with modern psychiatric diagnostic classifications.

73 R. Porter, 'History of Bethlem/Histories of Bethlem', SSHM Conference Exeter, April 1997. I am grateful for permission to cite this paper.

74 See S. Garton, *Medicine and Madness: A Social History of Madness in New South Wales, 1880–1940*, Kensington, Australia, N.S.W. University Press, 1988.

75 D. Jodelet, *Madness and Social Representations: Living With the Mad in One French Community*, Berkeley, University of California Press, 1991, a close analysis of Ainay-le-Chateau, for example.

76 An analogy might be drawn with the bargaining models familiar to labour economists in which the parties have unequal information and resources but where everyone's rationality is necessarily bounded by what can be known about the rules and each other. It is not suggested that the certified person has free choice but there are instances of individuals expressing

preferences concerning their admission and release to physicians as well as relatives advocating their entry or exit from the asylum.

77 Various contributors cite the excellent standards set by N. Tomes and M.E. Fissell, see particularly, N. Tomes, *A Generous Confidence: Thomas Story Kirkbride and the Art of Asylum-Keeping, 1840–1883*, New York, Cambridge University Press, 1983; and M.E. Fissell, 'The disappearance of the patient's narrative and the invention of hospital medicine', in R. French and A. Wear, eds, *British Medicine in an Age of Reform*, London, Routledge, 1991, pp. 92–109.

78 G.N. Grob, *Mental Institutions in America: Social Policy to 1875*, New York, Free Press, 1973, provided a pioneering analysis which can be directly contrasted with the more Foucauldian view of D.J. Rothman, *The Discovery of the Asylum*, Boston, Little, Brown, 1971.

79 C. Steedman, *Landscape for a Good Woman: A Story of Two Lives*, London, Virago, 1986, pp. 74–6, including discussion of Freudian methods in psycho-analytical history. This problem is imaginatively explored in the work of MacDonald, Tomes, Fissell and others cited above.

80 De Certeau calls attention to the existence of 'non- or pre-verbal domains in which there are only practices without any accompanying discourse'. Quoted in Sewell, 'Language and practice', p. 244. One set of practices relevant to a study of insanity might be, for example, incest conventions within a family, kinship or community grouping. It was extremely rare for such behaviour to figure in the admission documents, if the Devon Asylum is representative of other asylums. For rather different application of the concept of domains of formal discourse involving the interplay between a moralised and a scientific construction of the female body, see M. Poovey, *Making a Social Body: British Cultural Formation, 1830–64*, Oxford, Oxford University Press, 1996; and J. Melling 'The body in question?' *Journal of Victorian Culture*, forthcoming, 1999.

Part I

THE ENGLISH EXPERIENCE OF THE COUNTY LUNATIC ASYLUM

2

THE COUNTY ASYLUM IN THE MIXED ECONOMY OF CARE, 1808–1845

Leonard D. Smith

The decades after 1845 in England have attracted much attention from historians of psychiatry and of the asylum. The legislation of that year made public asylum provision mandatory, and within a few years county asylums had attained a dominant position in the management and care of mentally disordered people. Rather less attention has been given to the period between 1808 and 1845, which was a unique one in the history of institutional provision for the insane. Wynn's Act of 1808 enabled, but did not require, county justices to establish and operate a lunatic asylum. Ever since Kathleen Jones' pioneering work on the history of lunacy legislation, the Act's real practical consequences have tended to be underestimated.[1] Between 1808 and 1845, as many as fifteen counties had provided asylums, some on their own and some in conjunction with voluntary subscribers. Eight county asylums were in place by 1825, with a further seven completed by 1845.[2] This group of early county asylums operated in largely uncharted territory. The lack of universal provision meant that they had to take their place alongside private madhouses and public subscription asylums. This was very much a transitional period, when county asylums were forced to participate in what today would be called a 'mixed economy of care', involving the public, private and voluntary sectors. At this juncture the county asylums were, though significant, not the major players in the system.

The early county asylums could not operate in isolation. Their managers had not only to take account of the other types of provision, but had to adapt to and compete with them. More than at any other time before the National Health reforms of the 1980s, the publicly funded facilities were required to function in a climate where commercial considerations were intimately intertwined with aspects of the provision of health care for those in need. This chapter will consider how county asylums adapted to this mixed economy, and how it impacted on their management and operational policies.

The incipient system

A mixed economy in the care of lunatics had effectively been in existence since the later seventeenth century, with the emergence of private madhouses offering an institutional alternative to Bethlem Hospital. During the eighteenth century, there was significant development in both private and public provision. More private madhouses were opened around the country to meet the growing demand for confinement of unmanageable relatives of the well-to-do. It was largely because of concern about abuses taking place in some madhouses, as well as their lack of provision for the poorer classes, that the movement to establish public subscription asylums began. London's St Luke's in 1751 was followed by asylums in Newcastle in 1764, Manchester in 1766, York in 1777, and then others in regional centres like Liverpool, Leicester and Exeter. These 'lunatic hospitals' were set up on similar lines to the subscription infirmaries being developed in major towns. Their projectors emphasised their philanthropic intent, in comparison to the commercial motives of madhouse proprietors. The trustees of Manchester Infirmary in 1763, for example, sought to offer a place where the 'terribly afflicted' relations of people of 'middling Fortunes' could be preserved 'from the Impositions of those who keep private Mad-Houses'. An element of active competition with the private sector was clearly envisaged.[3]

The lunatic hospitals were intended primarily to cater for people whose relatives could not afford private care – members of the artisan, trading and lower professional classes. In the later eighteenth century the patterns of demand for institutional care of the insane were changing perceptibly. Parish officers, faced with paupers alleged to be insane, whose families were unable to look after them and who were unmanageable in the poor house, increasingly sought their removal from the community. Some found their way into the public asylums, but limited capacity resulted in the consignment of growing numbers to private madhouses. The demand of parish authorities for placement of pauper lunatics brought a significant new element into the market for care. Some madhouse proprietors met the opportunities offered by contracting with them to accept paupers at charges well below those received from private patients, with comparable differences in the nature of care and accommodation provided.[4]

The rising perception of a problem of pauper lunacy, with its associated threats of public nuisance and violence to others, brought a willingness to contemplate a degree of state intervention and social engineering which only the containment of criminals had hitherto aroused. The movement to establish county asylums developed out of the perceived success of the eighteenth-century public subscription asylums. Reformers considered that their example demonstrated a clear alternative to the private madhouse, increasingly being viewed as undesirable and exploitative. The legislation that emerged in 1808 was based on the conclusions of a select committee in 1807, which had been greatly influenced by the work of Sir George Onesiphorus Paul, the Gloucestershire prison reformer. Paul had studied the operation of the subscription asylums, particularly that at York, and advocated the dissemination of their model.[5]

Under Wynn's Act of 1808, or the County Asylums Act, funding from the county rates was to be made available to stimulate the building of one of two alternative types of asylum. The first option was an institution intended solely for county paupers. The second was a joint facility of the county and a charitable body, to cater for paupers, charity patients and private patients. The latter model, which Sir George Paul had advocated, effectively provided the means to subsidise the efforts of voluntary subscribers who had previously been unable to raise the necessary sums to proceed with the building. In the first wave of asylums under the Act, four were of this type – those for the counties of Nottingham, Cornwall, Stafford and Gloucester. Another four were purely for pauper patients – in the counties of Bedford, Norfolk, Lancashire and the West Riding of Yorkshire.[6]

The promoters of the new county asylums had first to persuade uncertain county justices and then a sceptical public that the considerable expenditure was worthwhile. The philanthropic component was heavily emphasised, as by the trustees of the proposed Staffordshire Asylum in 1812:

> In a county where to alleviate the affliction of the unfortunate, a general inclination has ever prevailed, it is not doubted but that the same benevolent disposition will be manifested, when of all calamities that which it is now proposed to relieve, is the worst that man can suffer.[7]

Subscribers and ratepayers would not only be flattered as to the extent of their prospective generosity, but also encouraged to provide an elegant asylum as tangible evidence of civic munificence and a progressive spirit. As another of the Stafford Asylum's supporters suggested in 1818, they would 'leave it to posterity an enviable monument of the humanity and liberality of the present enlightened age'. These new institutions would be something altogether superior to the differently motivated private alternatives, challenging them on philosophical as well as on economic grounds.[8]

In the market place

The new county asylums openly entered into competition with the steadily expanding private sector, on price as well as on principle. Not surprisingly some of the private proprietors, whose custom could become vulnerable, hit back. One of the more enlightened practitioners was Thomas Bakewell whose asylum at Stone in Staffordshire had been established in 1808. Once his business was operating successfully, he was prepared to offer the facilities to a limited number of pauper patients at a favourable rate. The projected erection of a county asylum at nearby Stafford, accepting also private and charitable patients, severely threatened his market. Bakewell did not merely take measures to defend his business, but mounted a strident campaign against the whole premise of a large public asylum and its inevitable therapeutic failure. The county justices, embarrassed but impressed with the evident knowledge and experience of a local man, on more than one occasion invited him to become the asylum's superintendent. Bakewell rejected their blandishments and went on to widen his campaign, developing it into a protracted and damaging critique of the principles and practices of all public asylums.[9]

The early group of county asylums certainly did not initially have things all their own way. The optimistic expectations of their promoters as to the likely demand for their services were not immediately met. Many local parish officers were singularly reluctant to commit the expenditure necessary to maintain their pauper lunatics in the institution, preferring the cheaper options of retaining them within the parish, supported on outdoor relief or, if more troublesome, placed in the workhouse. This was seen to impede the asylum's therapeutic effectiveness, for the doctrine had already been established that cure related to the early detection of insanity and speedy despatch to the asylum. The withholding of suitable candidates also seriously threatened the asylum's financial base. Remonstrations through the press and circulars to parish officials had only limited effect. The asylums' advocates were able to use their influence in parliament to secure legislation in 1815 and 1819, which gave justices powers to call for committal of eligible patients and to impose fines on recalcitrant parish overseers. The position of the county asylum was, in consequence, at least somewhat strengthened.[10]

Asylum managers sought diversification to raise their income. The amended legislation empowered all county asylums to accept private patients, as well as paupers from outside the county or from independent boroughs which did not contribute to the county rates. Although the expressed justification for widening the clientele was to make the superior system of asylum care more widely available, commercial considerations were paramount. Legislative sanction was given for paupers from external counties or boroughs, without the benefit of their own asylum, to be charged at higher rates. Subject to comparable pressures to relocate their disruptive pauper lunatics, but not having shared in the necessary capital outlay for an asylum, parishes in these counties would find themselves having to pay the differentials. Charges for private patients were yet higher, though still competitive with the private sector. The asylum's additional income from these sources could subsidise the upkeep of county paupers, thus reducing the charges to its hard-pressed parishes. Those county asylums partly funded through charitable subscription, like Nottingham, Stafford and Gloucester, had an additional motive for maximising income from private patients. It could subsidise provision for the charitable patients, those above the rank of pauper but unable to afford private care, the relief of whose plight was the chief object of the voluntary subscribers. Over the next few years most of the county asylums entered energetically into the trade in lunacy, actively seeking to attract both private and out-county pauper patients.[11]

The preparedness of county asylums to receive private patients differed. The joint asylums had been designed to cater for their anticipated requirements. The private patients would be accommodated in the imposing central part of the building, while the paupers were consigned to the wings and charitable patients occupied the areas in-between. Special rooms and apartments might be made available for private patients, with extra facilities available for those able to pay more. At Stafford and Gloucester asylums, private patients could have additional rooms, wine with their meals and a personal servant, if they paid supplementary rates. Charges might range from fifteen shillings up to three guineas per week. In the early asylums funded entirely from the county rates, it was more difficult to provide accommodation attractive to the families of private patients, and their charges were consequently lower. Distinct provision was, however, made at those asylums like Chester, Suffolk and Dorset, which were opened in the later 1820s or early 1830s.[12]

The degree of success in attracting private patients was variable. The Stafford Asylum, despite Thomas Bakewell's strictures, managed quite well; by the mid-1820s there were normally around twenty-five private patients in the house at any one time. Nottingham also received a significant amount of private custom. The Gloucester Asylum, architecturally the grandest of all the early asylums, had more difficulties. For several years, its Visitors lamented their failure to recruit private patients and consequent inability to admit charity patients at subsidised rates. They attributed this to a prevalent 'erroneous idea'...'that the unfortunate inmates of Lunatic Asylums not only cease, when incurable, to be objects of kindness and solicitude, but are even treated with inhumanity'. This suspicion of public asylum provision among the better classes restricted referrals for admission. Private care was still seen by many as inherently more desirable, despite the well-publicised evils of private madhouses. Eventually, by 1830, the prejudices were lessening and private patients came to Gloucester in larger numbers, enabling the charitable fund to operate properly for poorer private patients.[13]

A contract culture

The attraction of pauper patients from outside the county or from boroughs within the county proved not to be difficult. Not only did this provide additional income, but also some economies of scale from filling empty beds without comparable increases in expenses. There were advantages also for the committing parishes, who actively sought placement of their unmanageable lunatics in the asylum of a neighbouring county. Although they had to pay higher rates than county parishes, these were still usually competitive with those of private asylums that accepted paupers. In addition, a county asylum offered a reasonable likelihood of a standard of care superior to that of a private establishment.

Managers of county asylums entered into the commercial spirit by offering favourable or discounted rates to particular parishes or counties by negotiation. For example, the Stafford Asylum agreed special arrangements with the parish officers of Birmingham in December 1818. While county paupers were being received at 10s. per week, arrangements were made to accept a large group of Birmingham paupers at 12s. per week. Birmingham had previously had a block contract with the private asylum at Droitwich, but transferred their patients to Stafford for largely commercial motives. In July 1821, Stafford agreed to receive paupers from Worcestershire at 11s. per week (Staffordshire parishes were now paying 9s.); others were received from Leicestershire, Derbyshire and Shropshire. At the beginning of 1822, the rates for Staffordshire and Birmingham paupers were reduced to 7s.6d., with those from Birmingham to be accorded preference over all other external admissions. By the mid-1820s, the asylum's population had reached near capacity. Nevertheless, the lure of additional income was hard to resist. In 1828, a further thirty-seven Birmingham paupers were transferred from Droitwich Asylum, at 12s. per week, compared to the 8s. being received for Staffordshire paupers.[14]

Other county asylums came to similar arrangements with their neighbours. The Cheshire Asylum attracted patients from North Wales. The Cornwall Asylum at Bodmin reached agreements with Devon parishes, notably Plymouth and Devonport, with rates on a sliding scale according to the numbers received. The Norfolk and Suffolk Asylums accepted 'boarders' from the various autonomous boroughs within their counties, at suitably enhanced rates. Nottingham Asylum received a significant number of patients from Derbyshire. The spread of commercialism was infectious and public asylums even found themselves in competition with one another. The Nottingham Asylum's director, Thomas Morris, wrote to his friend George Jepson at the York Retreat in 1820 to lament the consequences:

> Our house is not full neither can we expect it should be, there being many Institutions now established around us for the same laudable though melancholy purpose as our own.

Nottingham's custom had been adversely affected by the opening of the Lincoln subscription asylum, which was also accepting private, charitable and pauper patients from the wider East Midlands region.[15]

Parliamentary returns in 1836 show the general continuation of differential charging arrangements. Nowhere was this more evident than at the Chester Asylum, where the charges of 4s.8d. for county paupers were among the lowest of any county asylum, while paupers from other counties were accepted at 12s. The difference was almost as great at the Stafford Asylum, with county parishes charged at 6s. and external parishes at 12s. However, the asylum was coming under pressure to admit increasing numbers from within Staffordshire, and the Visitors were being forced to allow the numbers of lucrative out-county pauper patients to gradually decline (from forty-one in 1831 to twenty-seven in 1835). Elsewhere, as at the asylums for Kent, Lancashire and Suffolk, the disparities were smaller. They too were having to begin restricting the admissions of people from outside the county.[16]

Market forces influenced asylum management in other ways. Indeed, the 'contract culture' made itself apparent in several aspects of the institution's operation. The original construction and equipment of the buildings were normally carried out following competitive tender. Subsequently, the purchase of provisions and equipment was conducted on a similar basis, with annually renewable contracts, advertised through the county press. The system was taken to unusual lengths at the Cornwall Asylum, opened in 1820. The justices decided to contract out the whole of the asylum's management. Its governor, Dr Richard Kingdon, was to receive the patients' maintenance payments on a sliding scale, according to numbers of paupers admitted (from 14s. per week down to 9s.). Of the 112 places, ten were to be for subscription patients at no more than 14s., but up to thirty could be for private patients, for whom Kingdon could set his own charges by negotiation. He was responsible for employing and paying staff, feeding the patients, and for maintaining the building and equipment. The arrangement must have proved problematic, however, for when he left in 1824 he was replaced by a salaried governor.[17]

'Strict economy'

The pursuit of 'economy' in financial management became a preoccupation of the justices. In several instances, the consideration belatedly followed extravagant initial expenditure on a grand and prestigious building. The Suffolk justices, however, were conscious of their responsibilities to the ratepayers from the beginning, having kept their outlay to the minimum by converting a disused former house of industry (workhouse) at Melton, near Woodbridge. In completing the work they exercised 'the strictest economy compatible with the quality and durability of the requisite materials'. Once the asylum was operational, they promised that 'every endeavour' would be exerted 'on the most economical scale'. Similar operational principles were commonly adopted, partly with a view to keeping down the charges in order to encourage parishes to send eligible people. At the Dorset Asylum, opened in 1832, they were written into the rules and regulations, which insisted on 'the most particular regard to a strict, but judicious system of economy'.[18]

The drive for economy showed itself in attempts to limit key areas of costs – salaries and wages, and provisions. In some counties, a Poor Law-orientated ideology, which emphasised the pauper status of patients and the commensurate standard of care they should receive, had gained an ascendancy. In the mid-1830s, Norfolk and Suffolk asylums openly vied with one another as to who could feed their patients the cheapest. The Norfolk Asylum had particularly low charges, based on poorly paid and ill-qualified management, a minimal level of staff receiving low wages and a sparse dietary provision. Envious of their neighbour's success in holding down costs, the Suffolk justices in 1835 sought to emulate them and attempted to instigate a drastic programme of reduced food allowances and lower staff numbers and wages. Their zeal for economy was, however, checked by alarm from within their own ranks at the possible consequences, and by well-publicised warnings from John Kirkman, the superintendent, of adverse effects on the asylum's cure rates.[19]

Other asylums took measures to reduce their charges as low as possible. William Ellis at Wakefield, and later at Hanwell, prided himself on the steady reductions he brought about in the weekly charges, which were as low as 6s. by when he left Wakefield in 1830. Partly he managed this by a 'strict economy', particularly in the diet. More significantly, it was achieved by the elaborate arrangements for the employment of patients which he developed. Although the intention of his system of work was primarily therapeutic and curative, it became increasingly significant as an element in reducing costs. Financial benefits came from the partial saving of wages of domestic, cooking and laundry staff, and from home-produced food, clothing, bedding and so on.[20]

There were, of course, consequences to a rigid adherence to a policy of minimising running costs. Justices, like those in Kent, were fully aware of the likely conflict between their pursuit of a 'well regulated economy' and the need to ensure that the asylum was 'well conducted' and 'its suffering inmates properly treated'. Not only were there the risks to health that John Kirkman of the Suffolk Asylum had highlighted, when he argued pointedly that 'Of all economy an ill regulated dietetic economy is the very worst.' There were also clear effects on practices of care and treatment. In several instances, economies on staffing levels could be clearly linked to the extent of the use of mechanical restraint. George Poynder, the superintendent of the Kent Asylum, in 1840 blamed 'a system of economy so rigid' as to be 'any thing rather than wholesome' for his institution's embarrassing exposure over its excessive employment of restraint.[21]

Purchasers and providers

The entry of the new county asylums into the 'mixed economy' had offered an important new option both to the parish authorities and to families. Surviving admission and case records illustrate that many county asylum patients, private and pauper, had previously been committed to private madhouses or to public subscription asylums. Some were transferred directly when the new county asylum opened. Of the initial group of admissions to Stafford Asylum in 1818, thirteen came from Thomas Bakewell's house at Spring Vale and several others from madhouses in Lichfield and Bilston. A similar phenomenon was apparent at the Gloucester Asylum, after its opening in 1823, with patients transferred from the private asylums at Droitwich, Hook Norton and Brislington House (near Bristol). After the Kent Asylum opened outside Maidstone in 1833, twenty-nine patients were transferred from Rix's Asylum at West Malling, and a further twenty-seven from the large metropolitan madhouses at Hoxton, Peckham and Bethnal Green, in addition to four from St Luke's and three from Bethlem.[22]

There were many people admitted to the county asylum for the first time after relapse of their disorder, following previous episodes of treatment in other institutions. George Harrison (aged 39), a carpenter admitted to Wakefield in July 1821, had previously been confined in the York Asylum and in a private asylum at Spinkwell, his initial onset of insanity attributed to 'loss of property & a very bad tempered wife'. Susanna Lyne (aged 61), the wife of a 'decayed farmer', admitted to Gloucester in December 1825 after several days and nights of wandering around the country, had previously spent periods at St Luke's and at Joseph Mason Cox's madhouse near Bristol. A first-class private patient, Reverend J. Montgomery Mercer of Leicestershire, admitted to Nottingham Asylum in March 1825, due to 'deep melancholy and religious despair', had previously been at the Leicester subscription asylum and at the private madhouse of a Dr Hill. The advent of the county asylum afforded a new alternative facility for care and treatment.[23]

With a greater choice available to purchasers of care, commercial considerations could take their place alongside attempts to match needs to services. Part of the success of some county asylums in attracting private custom was due to the standard of accommodation offered at a competitive price. Purchasers of care for pauper patients, the parish authorities and, later, boards of Guardians, had been coming under increasing legislative pressure (in the Acts of 1811, 1815, 1818 and

1828) to send lunatics to asylums, rather than attempt to maintain them on outdoor relief or within the workhouse. The Poor Law Amendment Act brought further pressure with section 45, which required that all lunatics who were dangerous had to be sent to an asylum. Although some Guardians tried to circumvent this by extending or blurring the boundaries of dangerousness, the demand for asylum places grew markedly. Naturally, they would seek the most economical placement.[24]

The decision of the parish, or the family of a private patient, to seek committal to the county asylum would be based on a combination of economic, social and therapeutic considerations. Where there was not a county asylum which Guardians were required to use, they had a choice between a private asylum, another county's asylum, or in some instances a public subscription asylum like Lincoln. Before the 1830s, they could make their decision on price, as well as on standards of care. After that time, however, with all the county asylums subject to overcrowding, their managers increasingly restricted themselves to acceptance of paupers from within their own county. For local purchasers it then became more a question of locating a place wherever available, as cheaply as possible. If this meant moving people from one asylum to another, or sending them considerable distances from home, this was accepted with few qualms. A new generation of large private asylums emerged to meet the demand, catering almost exclusively for pauper patients – like Duddeston Hall in Birmingham and Hunningham Hall near Leamington Spa. The apogee of the commercialisation of care was the massive Haydock Lodge in Lancashire, with capacity for over 400 patients.[25]

The mixed economy of mental health care, which had flourished for over thirty years after the legislation of 1808, was struck a severe blow, at least for the time being, by the Lunacy Acts of 1845. The reformers clearly intended both to attack the evils of commercialism and to promote the alternative of enlightened statutory provision. The Metropolitan Commissioners in Lunacy had also looked askance at the operation of public asylums with their mixture of social classes, arguing that the paupers suffered from the contiguity of people who were receiving a higher standard of accommodation, better food and so on. The new legislation required that each county provide an asylum for its pauper lunatics. Although some counties made limited provision for non-pauper patients in their asylum, the presence of private patients in county asylums declined steadily. Several of the original joint asylums were reconstituted during the 1850s, and the private and charitable patients were removed to new asylums, leaving the paupers behind in the original old, and increasingly unsuitable, buildings. County asylums ceased to be significant direct participants in the market for non-statutory care.[26]

Conclusions

The period between 1808 and 1845 saw the incremental development of the county lunatic asylum system. The principle of the county asylum had been established, but its acceptance was far from universal. A 'mixed economy' situation emerged for several reasons. The problem of where to place socially undesirable pauper lunatics had become general, but the options were limited. Even where there was a county asylum, parish parsimony restricted the early uptake of the facility. At the same time, the well-publicised short-comings of private madhouses contributed to a growing demand for placement of private patients in properly regulated public facilities. The interaction of these diverse patterns of demand in a context of limited and patchy provision of public asylum places encouraged their managers to adopt a commercially orientated approach.

There might be some interesting parallels with the present situation in mental health care. County asylums were one element in a range of options. There was clear competition between the publicly funded, the voluntary and the private sectors. In order to compete effectively, county asylums had not only to show price sensitivity, but also sought to demonstrate a superiority of philosophy, of standards of practice and of outcomes. They evidently succeeded at least sufficiently to provide the lunacy reformers with the rationale for the creation of the universal county asylum system.

Acknowledgements

I wish to acknowledge the generous assistance of the Wellcome Trust in funding the research for this essay.

NOTES

Abbreviations: BPP – British Parliamentary Papers, CRO – County Record Office

1 K. Jones, *Lunacy, Law and Conscience; 1744–1845*, London, 1955, pp. 73–6; Leonard D. Smith, *'Cure, Comfort and Safe Custody'; Public Lunatic Asylums in Early Nineteenth Century England*, London, 1999, forthcoming, will deal with this period in some detail.

2 *Report of the Metropolitan Commissioners in Lunacy to the Lord Chancellor*, London, 1844, pp. 8–20.

3 J. Woodward, *To Do the Sick No Harm: A Study of the British Voluntary Hospital System to 1875*, London, 1974; R. Porter, *Mind Forg'd Manacles: A History of Madness in England from the Restoration to the Regency*, London, 1987, chapter 3; W.L. Parry-Jones, *The Trade in Lunacy; A Study of Private Madhouses in England in the Eighteenth and Nineteenth Centuries*, London, 1972; A. Digby, *From York Lunatic Asylum to Bootham Park Hospital*, University of York, Borthwick Papers, No. 69, 1986, pp. 1–6; Manchester Royal Infirmary Archives, 'An account of the proceedings of the trustees of the Public Infirmary, in Manchester, in regard to the admission of lunaticks into that hospital', *c.*1763.

4 Parry-Jones, *The Trade in Lunacy*, pp. 13–14, 50–1.

5 BPP 1807, Vol. 1 *Select Committee on the State of Criminal and Pauper Lunatics*, Gloucester Reference Library J7.22; *An Abstract of Proceedings Relative to the Institution of a General Lunatic Asylum in or Near the City of Gloucester*, Gloucester, 1794; G.O. Paul, *A Scheme of an Institution and a Description of a Plan for a General Lunatic Asylum for the Western Counties*, Gloucester, 1796.

6 48 Geo. III, Cap. 6, *An Act for the Better Care and Maintenance of Lunatics, Being Paupers or Criminals in England*; *Report of Metropolitan Commissioners in Lunacy*, 1844, p. 9.

7 *Staffordshire Advertiser*, 21 March 1812.

8 *Staffordshire Advertiser*, 18 July 1818.

9 L.D. Smith, 'To cure those afflicted with the disease of insanity: Thomas Bakewell and Spring Vale Asylum', *History of Psychiatry*, 4, 1993, pp. 107–27 and 'Close confinement in a mighty prison; Thomas Bakewell and his campaign against public asylums, 1810–1830', *History of Psychiatry*, 5, 1994, pp. 191–214; T. Bakewell, *A Letter to the Chairman of the Select Committee of the House of Commons Appointed to Enquire into the State of Madhouses*, Stafford, 1815.

10 *Gloucester Journal*, 9 February 1824; *Wakefield and Halifax Journal*, 23 October 1818; *The West Briton*, 20 September 1822; *Wolverhampton Chronicle*, 7 October 1818; Cornwall CRO, DDX 97/1, 14 November 1820; Suffolk CRO, Acc 2697, 27 April 1829; 55 Geo. III, Cap. XLVI; 59 Geo. III, Cap. CXXVII.

11 55 Geo. III, Cap. XLVI, Sections VII, XII; *Metropolitan Commissioners*, 1844, p. 31; Bedfordshire CRO, LB/1/8, 3 June 1815, 14 October 1828; Suffolk CRO, B106/10/4.4 (1), Report of Suffolk Lunatic Asylum (1839), p. 8; Norfolk CRO, SAH 2, 23 December 1815, SAH 3, 29 July, 28 October 1816; Gloucestershire CRO, HO22/8/1, Gloucester Asylum, Annual Reports, 1824–1830; J.T. Becher, *Resolutions Concerning the Intended General Lunatic Asylum Near Nottingham*, Newark, 1810; *An Address to the Public Concerning the General Lunatic Asylum Near Nottingham*, Nottingham, 1811, x; *The Articles of Union for the General Lunatic Asylum Near Nottingham*, Nottingham, 1825, pp. 6–11.

12 L.D. Smith, ' "Levelled to the same common standard"? Social class in the lunatic asylum, 1780–1860', in O. Ashton, R. Fyson and S. Roberts, eds., *The Duty of Discontent: Essays for Dorothy Thompson*, London, 1995, pp. 142–66; J. Hemingway, *History of the City of Chester*, Chester, 1831, Vol. II, p. 228; Staffordshire CRO, D550/1, 13 July 1820, D550/4, 6 July 1829; Gloucs CRO, HO22/1/1, 8 July 1833; Suffolk CRO, Acc 2697, 1 April 1834; Beds CRO, LB/1/8, 3 June 1815.

13 Staffs CRO, D550/62, 3 April 1824, 1 October 1825; Nottingham Ref. Library, qL3648, Nottingham Asylum, 4th Annual Report (1814); *Notting-*

ham Journal, 21 October 1826, 10 November 1827; Gloucs CRO, HO22/8/1, Annual Reports 1825–30 (quote 1826).

14 Staffs CRO, D51, 2 November 1818, 11 July 1821, 16 January 1822, 16 July 1828, D550/62, D550/63.

15 Chester City Record Office, HW 190; Cornwall CRO, DDX 97/1, 26 May 1828, 9 May 1831; *The West Briton*, 6 April 1838 – this referred to the loss of the 'profitable patients' from Devonshire, who paid almost twice as much as county paupers; Suffolk CRO, Acc 2697, 1 April, 24 June 1834, 8 April 1839, 19 June 1840; Norfolk CRO, SAH 2, 4 August 1815, SAH 3, 25 July 1821, SAH 5, 29 February, 25 March 1836; Notts CRO, SO/HO/1/9/1; University of York, Borthwick Institute, C/1, 30 April 1820, Thomas Morris to George Jepson.

16 BPP 1836, Vol. XLI, County Lunatic Asylums, Returns, pp. 5, 9, 11, 22, 29; Staffs CRO, D550/1, 3 July 1833, D550/5, 31 August, 27 October 1837.

17 Staffs CRO, D550/1–5; Gloucs CRO, HO22/1/1, HO22/3/1–2; Notts CRO, SO/HO/1/1, SO/HO/1/3/2–3; Suffolk CRO, Acc2697; Cornwall CRO, DDX 97/1, 16 November 1818, 23 February, 11 October 1819, 1 February 1820, 9 February, 12 July 1824; C.T. Andrews, *The Dark Awakening: A History of St Lawrence's Hospital, Bodmin*, Bodmin, 1978, pp. 32–5, 47.

18 Suffolk CRO, Acc 2697, 14 July 1828; Dorset CRO, *Rules and Regulations for the Management of the Pauper Lunatic Asylum for the County of Dorset*, Dorchester, 1833, p. 9.

19 Norfolk CRO, SAH 1, 28 April 1814, SAH 5, 27 March 1835, 25 April 1836; Suffolk CRO, Acc 2697, 30 December 1834, 31 March, 23 June, 13 October 1835, B106.10/4.4, Annual Reports 1839, pp. 7–9, 1840, pp. 3–6.

20 West Riding CRO Wakefield, C85/107, Annual Reports of West Riding County Lunatic Asylum, 1819–1830; Greater London Record Office, H11/HLL/A7/1, *Reports of the Resident Physician of the County Lunatic Asylum at Hanwell*, London, 1842.

21 Centre for Kentish Studies, Q/GCL/1, 16 April 1839, U1515/OQ/L1, 6 November 1848, George Poynder to John Adams; Suffolk CRO, B106/10/4.4, Suffolk Asylum, Annual Reports 1839, p. 9, 1840, pp. 3, 6.

22 Staffs CRO, D5, Apothecaries' Day Book, 29 September–21 December 1818; Gloucs CRO, HO22/70/1, Gloucester Asylum, Case Books, nos 5, 8–11, 16–18, 21, 27, 28, 36; Centre for Kentish Studies, MH/Md/2/Ap1, Kent Asylum, Admissions Book, 1833–4.

23 Notts CRO, SO/HO/1/9/1, no.598; Gloucs CRO, HO22/70/1, no. 179; West Riding CRO, C85/936.

24 51 Geo. III, Cap. LXXIX; 55 Geo. III, Cap. XLVI; 59 Geo. III, Cap. CXXVII; 5 Geo. IV, Cap. LXXI; 9 Geo. IV, Cap. XL; Parry-Jones, *Trade in Lunacy*, pp. 62, 86, 104, 277–80; K. Jones, *A History of the Mental Health Services*, London, 1972, p. 125; L.D. Smith, 'The pauper lunatic problem in the West Midlands, 1815–1850', *Midland History*, 21, 1996, pp. 101–18.

25 Parry-Jones, *Trade in Lunacy*.

26 Metropolitan Commissioners, 1844, pp. 30–1; Smith, 'Social class in the lunatic asylum', pp. 147–8; 9th Report of the Commissioners in Lunacy, 1855, App. B, p. 67; Birmingham Reference Library, *Reports of the Committee of Visitors of the Lunatic Asylum for the Borough of Birmingham*, 2nd Report, February 1853, pp. 6–7, 6th report, January 1857, pp. 28–9; Warwickshire CRO, CR 1664/30, Warwickshire County Lunatic Asylum, Annual Report

1859, p. 6; *Charitable Institution for the Insane of the Middle Classes: Proceedings of a Public Meeting*, Stafford, 1851 (Copy held in William Salt Library, Stafford); D. Hunter, *A History of the Coppice, Nottingham*, Nottingham, Author, 1918, pp. 22–7.

3

THE ASYLUM AND THE POOR LAW

The productive alliance

Peter Bartlett

At least until recently, twentieth-century scholars have tended to view the care of the insane in nineteenth-century England in the context of the history of psychiatry. In these accounts, the Enlightenment reached the insane at some time in the eighteenth century, and the bestial images of lunacy which accompanied the whips and chains of earlier establishments gave way to new forms of treatment which acknowledged the humanity of the lunatic.[1] This transition was concurrent with the rise of the medical profession. Metaphors of demonic possession gave way to diagnoses of illness as doctors consolidated their sole authority in the field of lunacy. Concurrent in turn with this professionalisation had been the rise of a trade in madness in eighteenth-century England, as medical men turned their authority to business advantage by opening profit-motivated private madhouses for the care of the insane. The care provided in these private facilities was increasingly challenged by humanitarian reformers as cruel in nature and inadequate in scale. Asylums established as philanthropic endeavours on the model of voluntary hospitals were unable to provide care on a sufficient scale. As governments were convinced of the need for more and better regulated care, new county asylums were built, staffed by medical specialists. It was, at least initially, a triumph of reform. The triumphalism was short-lived, however. Historians tend to view the asylum in the later nineteenth century as a failure, full of incurable cases and unable to fulfil the humanitarian promise of the reformers. The promised cures never materialised. At best, ideals of individualised cure had given way to impersonal care in the huge institutions of the end of the century; at worst, the asylum had become merely a 'convenient place to dump the troublesome'.[2] Things had somehow gone horribly wrong.

This factual structure is remarkably consistent between traditional and revisionist accounts. Those versions differ not on the basic factual structure, but rather on the interpretation to be put on those facts. Apologists emphasise the horrors of the eighteenth-century madhouse and the humanitarian objectives of the reformers. For them, the eventual failure lay outside the realm of the essentially benevolent medical specialists and reformers. Shortage of funding is often pivotal in these accounts: parsimonious local authorities did not send cases to the asylum until they were past hope of cure, and insufficient expansion of the system was funded to allow prompt treatment of all those in need. Occasionally, the stifling effect of legal regulation is noted.[3] Revisionists are more likely to stress the unfortunate results of these benevolent motivations,[4] the professional interests of the psychiatrists,[5] or the social control implications of the process.[6] Either way, the narrative takes the form of a classic tragedy, with the asylum in the role of hero: a rise to prominence, full of promise, a tragic flaw, and the inevitable failure. The debate is on the nature of the flaw.

My concern in this chapter is not about the factual basis of these accounts, although that has been challenged elsewhere.[7] Instead, this chapter challenges the centrality both of the specialist medical profession and the uncomplicated version of humanitarianism which are at the core of the accounts in question. Recent scholars, including several represented elsewhere in this volume, have moved away from a unitary view of the asylum as the locus of medical professional development and specialisation, and have begun to examine more closely the administrative structures both within the asylum, and surrounding the asylum in the broader community.[8] Such an approach creates a very different picture of the place of medical knowledge and the medical profession in the asylum structure. Consistent with these broader approaches, this chapter argues that the administrative and legal structures surrounding the nineteenth-century asylum movement identified the county asylum as a Poor Law institution, in which the role of specialist medical professionals has been overplayed. I will then examine the place of the asylum in the Poor Law imagery of the nineteenth century. Here, it will be argued that the imagery of the asylum was inconsistent, reflecting various strands of Victorian social policy and Poor Law debate. Finally, I question how the 'success' or 'failure' of the asylum is to be gauged, given the inconsistency in understanding of its purpose.

The county asylum as a Poor Law institution

Connections between the county asylum and the Poor Law are suggested by a simple survey of the individuals confined. Reliable statistics start being kept in the mid-1840s. County asylums became mandatory in 1845, and the number of paupers confined rose from 3,611 in 1844 to 9,412 in 1852. The numbers of paupers in county asylums increased fivefold between 1852 and 1890, that is, to 51,910. In 1890, paupers represented 98 per cent of those in the county asylum system.[9]

This connection is consistent with the statutory framework. The first statute allowing asylums to be constructed on the county rates was passed in 1808. Its title, 'An Act for the Better Care and Maintenance of Lunatics, Being Paupers or Criminals in England',[10] specifically identifies it as directed to the poor, and the long titles of county asylum acts continue to refer explicitly to paupers at least until 1863.[11] The 1808 statute made no provision for the admission of privately paying patients to county asylums at all, and while such provision was made in 1815,[12] such admissions were conditional on there being excess space in the asylum, and on terms which suggested that the primary purpose of the provision was to ease the economic burden on the institution. In practice, patients who were formally designated as 'private' never formed more than a relatively small proportion of those in county asylums. Instead, the focus remained on patients who were legally categorised as 'paupers'. The two Yorkshire asylums printed the following clause on their admission documents, in italics:

> *The asylum is for paupers only, and the justices are earnestly requested not to permit overseers or relieving officers to send any lunatics who are not actually chargeable as paupers.*[13]

While the 1808 Act is reasonably seen as the starting point of the county asylum system, it was not the first mention of the insane poor. The eighteenth-century Poor Law provided for corporal punishment of poor persons refusing to work. A Poor Law statute of 1714 provided that paupers who were 'furiously mad' were to be exempt from such corporal punishment, and were instead to be confined.[14] This legislation did not establish a place of confinement, however. The 1808 Asylum Act provided specifically that those confined under the eighteenth-century legislation were to be confined in a county asylum, if one were constructed,[15] and the 1808 legislation can therefore be seen as growing directly out of the Old Poor Law. The so-called 'Old', or pre-1834 Poor Law had generated a variety of institutions since its introduction in the sixteenth century, including workhouses, almshouses and houses of correction. The asylum was a part of this trend.

Like other institutions under the Old Poor Law, at the top of the administrative pyramid were the local Justices of the Peace, who both ran the facilities and made the decisions regarding admissions and discharges. Until 1834, it was the local overseers of the poor who were in charge of organising the applications for admission to the asylum, a role given to the Poor Law relieving officers when the New Poor Law was introduced. Surveillance of the pauper insane by the Poor Law gradually increased. Commencing in 1845, when county asylums became mandatory, Poor Law medical officers were required to visit and report quarterly on those pauper lunatics not in an asylum,[16] and commencing in 1853, a fee of two shillings and sixpence per visit was to be payable to the medical officer to ensure compliance with this section.[17] These medical officers were given the authority in 1853 to sign the medical certificate required to admit the pauper to the asylum, and their involvement in this way quickly became the norm.

By comparison, the asylum superintendent, the medical professional in lunacy, had no role in asylum admissions. He was specifically precluded from signing admission certificates, and effectively admitted those patients for whom the Justices signed orders. Release from the asylum was also under the control of the Justices of the Peace, in the legal form of the Visitors of the Asylum. While my research into the situation at the Leicestershire and Rutland County Asylum up to 1870 would suggest that the asylum staff had influence here, there are also instances when people were released over the objections of the asylum staff, generally at the instigation of the local Poor Law authorities.

The county asylum was therefore an institution legally based in the Poor Law, with Justices of the Peace in charge, and reliant on Poor Law officials to control and process admissions. It was directed at and actually contained paupers to the virtual exclusion of others. It was in essence a Poor Law institution. This connection remains fast throughout the nineteenth century; indeed, if anything, it was fortified, for the Old Poor Law was staffed with parish volunteers. It was only with the introduction of professional Poor Law relieving officers and medical officers after 1834 that the intensive administrative provisions of the Asylum Acts became remotely realisable, and the asylum system could flourish.

Chronologies and contexts

The interrelation between asylums and the remainder of the Poor Law is complex. The 1808 County Asylums Act had laid out the basic rules for construction of asylums and for admission of lunatics. While these rules were developed, they were not fundamentally altered for the remainder of the century. County asylums did not become mandatory, however, until 1845. Only twelve county asylums were built prior to 1834, and they were relatively small in size. The big expansion of the system happened after 1834, and particularly after the 1845 Act. Between the establishment of the legislative structure and the growth in scale was the introduction of the New Poor Law in 1834. Thus the structure of the asylum law is under the Old Poor Law, but its expansion and application part of the new.

The success of the county asylum under the New Poor Law initially appears surprising. The 'Oliver Twist' image of the 1834 Act does not at first blush appear to create a fertile ground for the expansion of the benevolent county asylum network. This seeming anomaly is not merely a twentieth-century illusion. Some nineteenth-century advocates were proud to distinguish the asylum from the punitive workhouse. Yet the thriving of the asylum under the Poor Law was far from coincidental. The asylum was attractive to advocates and opponents of the New Poor Law, Whigs and Tories alike, and could readily be justified according to the evangelical, paternalist and utilitarian ideologies which informed the debates around the New Poor Law. Inconsistencies in the pictures of the asylum drawn by its advocates resulted, but the inconsistencies created a space where the asylum could flourish.

The remainder of this chapter will examine the attractiveness of the asylum in these contexts, and consider the ways in which the images of the asylum and its place in the Poor Law structure were reflected in the descriptions contained in the admission documents and case books of patients. There were of course pragmatic reasons for agreement between asylum and Poor Law partisans. The fundamental administrative reason has already been noted: the asylum advocates needed a large and effective local administration to put into effect their desired system of admissions. The Poor Law bureaucracy provided this, and there was no one else. The system of admissions after 1834 was also a delicate balance of interests: Justices of the Peace continued actually to authorise admissions, thus keeping the traditional local elites content. The carriage of the applications by comparison rested with the New Poor Law bureaucracy, providing them with consolidated power in the Poor Law arena. At Westminster, the Poor Law Commissioners and the

Lunacy Commissioners were established at a time when centralised administration remained controversial. Open disagreements would be risky and, in any event, co-operation was needed to ensure the best use of what little persuasive power each board had at the local level.

Rather than focusing on these purely pragmatic considerations in greater detail, however, this chapter will discuss the ideological, or at least discursive, points of intersection between the asylum and the Poor Law. In this context, it is convenient to identify three different strands of argument. The first two strands would both place the asylum as operating in tandem with the workhouse and other Poor Law institutions to achieve a common set of socially defined goals and as an outgrowth of the same Victorian social policy. The third portrays the asylum as a refuge within the Poor Law for those opposed to the New Poor Law rhetoric.

The analysis which follows adopts the version of social policy presented in David Garland's book, *Punishment and Welfare*.[18] In this analysis, official Victorian social policy was centred on the working class. The strategy was one of dividing this class. At the lower end were the poor, the lumpenproletariat, the criminal classes, the social residuum. These were contrasted with the 'large middle sectors of the working classes, who were generally in employment and fairly respectable',[19] but were still not socially or economically secure. Regarding this middle working class, Garland states:

> Composed mainly of semi-skilled workers, low-grade clerical staff and tradesmen in seasonal or casual trades, these sectors formed a kind of 'perishing class' subject to the effects of trade cycles, seasonal unemployment and economic depression, and continually in danger of 'demoralisation' and social 'failure'. By comparison, the residuum was seen to form a permanent danger, a constant source of contamination always ready to 'foul the record of the unemployed' and to 'degrade whatever they touch'.[20]

The aim of the 1834 Poor Law theorists was to root out and dismantle a culture of poverty, perceived in terms of immorality, intemperance and promiscuity, and replace it with a culture of self-help, respectability, sobriety and hard work. A stick and carrot approach was employed. The stick was directed to the lowest social class. The Victorian penal institutions, which in this context include not only prisons but also workhouses, were to enforce morality upon what later came to be identified as the residuum. The carrot was offered to the middle sector of the working class in the form of county schools and private agencies of moralisation.

The asylum is conspicuously absent from Garland's discussion. If the asylum is to be understood as a part of the New Poor Law, the question is whether it was to be directed to the residuum, and thus similar in nature to the workhouse ideal, or to the middle working class, making it more comparable to a county school. As indicated above, there is support for both these characterisations.

The asylum and the 'residuum'

The very title of the asylum acts themselves suggests an intent to associate the asylum with the social residuum: recall that the titles refer to 'lunatics, being paupers or criminals' in England and Wales. Criminal lunatics were admitted to county asylums in Leicester and elsewhere, particularly prior to the completion of Broadmoor, and at least in Leicester there is no indication of any segregation to ensure that they would not 'infect' the other inmates of the asylum. This would suggest that the other inmates of the asylum might also be considered as of the residual class. However, by the 1860s, pauper lunatics, including the criminal lunatics remaining in the asylum, were segregated off from inmates admitted by a charity associated with the asylum, reinforcing the image of the pauper lunatic as a creature distinct from the respectable poor.[21]

Attempts to construe the term 'pauper' narrowly suggest a juxtaposition between the target clients of the asylum and the more respectable poor. According to the Poor Law orthodoxy, pauper status implied that the individual should have no means of support: an ability to repay the costs of confinement would preclude pauper status, and thus preclude admission to the asylum.[22] Consistent with a different strand of Poor Law argument, discussed in the next section of this chapter, the Lunacy Commissioners took a different view, but it was not until 1875 that they got a legal opinion favourable to their viewpoint.[23] The previous orthodoxy seems to reflect the Poor Law concern about restricting availability of poor relief, and the importance of self-sufficiency.

Such a restricted view is also reflected at the local level. The lack of facilities for those just above the pauper class was a source of concern to the lunacy authorities, who understood that the law applied only to the lowest class of paupers. The existence of a number of charities to cater for this near-residuum class can be seen as reinforcing the role of the asylum as caring for the lowest of the low. Such a charity was justified in the case of the Leicestershire and Rutland County Asylum in the following terms:

> The public can scarcely be aware of the extent of the benefit to the indigent Insane this charity confers; THE LAW PROVIDES ONLY FOR *ACTUAL PAUPERS*: but the numerous class of the population who are poor, and many of them the poorest, whose families have struggled not to be upon the parish, would in cases of insanity be totally without assistance, if the Institution [i.e. the Charity] did not open its doors to afford it to them.[24]

The asylum was encouraged to separate these charitable near-paupers from the actual pauper class, again suggesting that the 'true' paupers are to be understood as being in Garland's underclass.

This vision is further consistent with some of the descriptions of the paupers confined in the asylum. The culture the Poor Law attempted to stamp out was based in immorality, intemperance and promiscuity. These were connected with insanity by both the admitting officials and by the Lunacy Commissioners. Thus Lord Shaftesbury testified in 1858 to a parliamentary committee that 'one half, and perhaps more, of the cases of insanity that prevail among the poorer classes arise from their habit of intoxication'.[25] The Commissioners were similarly concerned about idiot women and bastardy, and the risks of having two lunatic men sleeping in the same bed (or indeed, of having precisely two men sleeping alone in the same room). These were people that needed morality imposed upon them.

At the local level, there was similarly no shortage of the moralising tone directed at the individual pauper that one associates with the hardest line of the Poor Law. The case book entry for John Healey, admitted to the Leicester Asylum in 1851, provides a particularly clear, but none the less illustrative, example:

> The Patient's temper is very vindictive, and his disposition bad, his conduct has been very irrational, and his propensities dangerous to others....The habits of this Patient, for years past have been very irregular, he has had no home, or settled abiding place, but has been a wanderer and a vagabond, he had a similar attack four years ago [for which he was apparently not confined] his life has been one of intemperance, idleness, and vice, his conduct to his mother has been most unnatural, and cruel...he is very restless, taciturn, and cun-

> ning, and his countenance bears the stamp of undisguised villainy.[26]

Upon his readmission, the point was even clearer:

> This Patient's appearance, on his readmission, was more unfavourable, and forbidding than on the previous occasion, if possible. He was more disreputable in appearance, more diabolical in aspect, and certainly in worse health. There was not so much mental excitement, but in its place was a large amount of animal cunning, low trickery, and all the paltry, and petty devices of an abandoned character, his habits had become those of a confirmed drunkard, idle, dissolute, and intemperate, his conduct most irrational, his propensities violent and, toward his Mother, dangerous and most unnatural.[27]

Descriptions of this type do not suggest respectable poverty, but rather the 'principles of 1834' at their most moralising.

The Leicester admissions from 1845 to 1870 show a considerable representation of inmates admitted directly from workhouses. Between 1861 and 1865, about 27 per cent of pauper admissions came to the asylum through this route. Removal to the asylum in this context seems to have been triggered when the workhouse inmate became troublesome. The asylum in this context was an escape valve for the workhouse. The asylum's place relative to the workhouse thus became ambiguous. It can sometimes be seen as the final stage in the pauper's slide to moral depravity. The case book says of Marianne MacHale, admitted to Leicester Asylum in 1846:

> [She was] placed in a respectable situation as soon as she left the Asylum on the 5th of August 1845 where she might have gained a decent livelihood had she conducted herself with propriety. She soon, however, left it; frequented her old haunts of vice and profligacy, took to drinking and soon beggared herself. She was subsequently sent to the Union where she addicted herself to theft and became the terror of all the inmates, and in consequence of her excessive violence she was soon removed to this establishment.[28]

While advocates from within the asylum system itself might be unwilling to portray the asylum as one rung below the workhouse in its selection of clientele, they were content to argue that the insane caused disruption in workhouses, and ought therefore to be removed to the asylum. While avoiding some of the moralising language, they still placed the asylum as a necessary adjunct of the workhouse, a requirement if a well-ordered workhouse was to be maintained. This argument thus adopts the categorical structure of the workhouse ethic: it is an argument from within the 1834 framework, not opposed to it.

The asylum and the respectable worker

Under this strand of images, the asylum was directed to assist the middle working class, and is thus more similar to county schools and infirmaries, and in juxtaposition to the punitive workhouse. Certainly, this view can be perceived among the Lunacy Commissioners. Consider for example the following statement in their 1854 annual report:

> [I]n our Pauper Lunatic Asylums, many inmates are to be met with who have formerly held a respectable station in society, and who, in point of education and manners, are greatly superior to the inmates of a workhouse.[29]

Much of the structure of the asylum does seem calculated to appeal to the respectable poor. Thus the trades at which the inmates worked were those of the middle lower class: domestic work and cleaning for the women, farming, shoemaking and carpentry for the men. The entertainments provided were likely also to appeal to members of such a class. Often, there were weekly dances. In Leicester there was a brass band composed mainly of staff, but with some patient involvement as well, and the Leicester Dramatic Society played at the asylum on various occasions. Outings were made periodically, to places such as the Leicester Forest and agricultural fairs, and bowls and quoits were played on the lawn.

Much of the argument here invokes the inverse positions to the first strand. Thus while the orthodoxy of the Poor Law may have required paupers to be destitute for purposes of asylum admission, it seems clear that most Unions did not insist on such a high standard. Lunatics 'found wandering at large or not under proper care and control' might be admitted under the asylum act even if not paupers. Some documents regarding the Leicestershire Asylum show at least compliance of Poor Law authorities, if not outright connivance, in expanding the definition of 'not under proper care and control' to allow recovery of part of the maintenance funds from families who were poor but not destitute.[30]

This is notwithstanding the periodic claims by the asylum, noted above, that Poor Law admissions were restricted to the destitute.

Just as the image of the asylum as a house of detention fits in with the argument that the residuum was the target population, so the asylum as a house of cure fits in with the vision of the asylum as aimed at the more respectable. The loss of employment or the 'reverse of circumstances' was understood by the Leicester Asylum as a cause of madness, and one of the roles of the asylum in this context seems to have been to set people back on their feet, through a regimen of good food, work and appropriate recreation. In Leicestershire, the asylum authorities would occasionally even find people jobs prior to leaving the asylum, or hire them when the former patient had a slump in work. The asylum can here be seen as a parallel to the county school, attempting to fit people for life in the world, or of other charitable organisations of the nineteenth century tiding the respectable poor over in their hour of need.

Typical of these cases are persons admitted in frail physical health. For example, it was not uncommon in Leicester that women considered insane consequent upon childbirth would be admitted to the asylum for a few months. Often, these women already had large families, and it seems a not unreasonable speculation that they were exhausted, and they needed time away from their domestic duties in order to recover some energy. These women were generally discharged within a few weeks or months, 'recovered'.

For cases such as these, there is a marked absence of the judgmental tone in the case book. Sometimes they are perceived as the victims of circumstance. This attitude is in stark contrast to the attitudes in the case book noted above, regarding the residuum. Social engineering is not absent from this model, however, for the nature of the cure reflected the priorities of the Poor Law itself: it was to make the individual fit into his or her place in society. The placement of the individual in suitable employment at the end of their stay in the asylum was but the final stage of this. The main treatment offered by the asylums was 'moral management', of which work was to be a cornerstone. This need not be viewed in a malevolent light: employment would be essential to the individual's successful return into society, after all. It none the less suggests a particular agenda in the structuring of the asylum, bringing the pauper to understand the Victorian precept, 'a place for everything, and everything in its place'. This itself could be understood as therapeutic. A particularly clear example of this can be seen in the testimony of Sir George Robinson, to the Parliamentary Select Committee on Lunatics in 1858. He was a magistrate on the board of the Northampton Asylum, an asylum which atypically accepted both private and pauper admissions. In that asylum, poor men carted sand and did farm work, poor women did needlework and worked in the laundry, and the rich played cricket:

> 3400. [Sir G. Grey] Has any inconvenience arisen from the mixture of the two classes of patient in the asylum? [Robinson] I think decidedly not. I should say that great convenience has arisen. It may be prejudice or fancy, but I believe it agrees with the opinions of very many eminent men, that the more you can assimilate the state of society inside an asylum to that which Providence has placed a person outside, the more likely are patients to be comfortable and happy. I believe in my own heart and conscience that it has a very good effect, as the two classes of patients witness, to a certain extent, the lives of each other. The class patients walk about and see the paupers at their employments, and they are interested in it. Then, on the other hand, the pauper patients are glad to be noticed by the class patients.
>
> 3401. [Grey] What degree of intercourse takes place between them? [Robinson] They are mixed up very much. We have a lady of the highest rank in that asylum; she has been there for many years, and one of her fancies is that she never would mix with any but the pauper women, and we could not get her to go to her own rooms, but she is now rather improved, and she mixes rather with her own class.[31]

What we see here is a peculiar blend of Toryism and utilitarianism. The Toryism is obvious. The utilitarianism works in a different fashion from the workhouse test principles. The genius of the workhouse test was that it would function with minimal administrative interference: paupers' free choice would ensure that only those in real need would apply for relief. The mechanisms of the asylum were different: at least in theory, there would be intensive surveillance of the population, with justices, police, Poor Law medical officers and other Poor Law staff on continual and vigilant watch for insane persons to be improved in the asylum. This is reminiscent of Bentham's proposals for privatised Poor Law, where the poor could if necessary be forced into the pauper panopticon, for their own good, of course. The proactive intervention in equipping the insane person for later life similarly has to it the ring of Benthamite love of planning and systems, and, for the new social engineers of the nineteenth century, this aspect would have its appeal.

The asylum as the challenge to 1834

The third strand can be characterised in various ways. While the sections above have sketched the similarities between the Poor Law theory and the role of the asylum, the difficulty remains that there are some glaring inconsistencies between the asylum discourse and any form of the Poor Law theory as outlined. The third strand can instead be seen as establishing the asylum as an anti-Poor Law institution, an institution which, although part of the Poor Law, challenged the essential theory of the Poor Law.

The New Poor Law was founded on the principle of less eligibility. As a protection of the free market in employment, life in the workhouse was to be less desirable for any able-bodied person than any existence outside it. The public image which the asylum system created for itself was fundamentally different. Consider the following description of the Leicester Asylum, from a document it circulated to the local justices in charge of the admissions:

> Placed on an eminence, and commanding one of the most beautiful views in the County of Leicester, extending over the valley of the Soar, and bounded by the hills of Charnwood Forest, there is everything in its position to soothe and cheer the patient; the grounds belonging to the Asylum comprise in the whole twenty acres, part of which is laid out in walks and pleasure grounds, and the remainder, save such part as is occupied by the building and the yards for the exercise of the Patients, is cultivated as much as may be by the inmates themselves; labour in the open air being found of all employments the most conducive to health of the great majority of the insane; not, however, that the comforts of those who are necessarily debarred from this exercise, are neglected, no effort is left untried to cheer the melancholy, and soothe the excited, the great object being to make this Asylum a HOUSE OF CURE, and not a HOUSE OF DETENTION.[32]

This sounds more like a holiday camp than an institution under the New Poor Law. Admittedly the rule of less eligibility was intended by the Poor Law Commissioners to apply to able-bodied people (and more particularly males) only, and would thus not apply to the asylum. It is also to be remembered that descriptions may or may not correspond to the reality encountered by the individual patient. None the less, the contrast between the above description and the doctrine of the Poor

Law is still striking. The following response from the Poor Law Guardians in Leicester to the Building Committee for a new asylum in 1866 is thus unsurprising:

> This Board however cannot conceal its regret, that in the Town Council there appears to be a desire for external ornament in the proposed building, which in the opinion of this board would be somewhat out of character in a Pauper Lunatic Asylum.
>
> The chief object of such Institutions is the recovery of the Patients, and this Board would therefore, with all respect submit, that while every convenience and appliance that will further this object should be provided; it should ever be borne in mind that the inmates of such an Institution will for the most part, if not exclusively, be Paupers, and that to provide a building for their reception, with much external decoration, would be both impolitic and unwise.[33]

Far from attempting to discourage the poor from receiving relief, the positive images were, if anything, intended to have the reverse effect, so that in Leicestershire, the superintendent reported with pride in 1862 that 'There is now but little reluctance felt by the poor in availing themselves of the advantages of your asylum.'[34]

Similarly, when assessing the causes of insanity, the asylum might pick out social factors rather than pin blame on the individual. Thus poverty itself was generally seen as a physical cause of insanity, not a moral one, with blame not necessarily attaching to the individual for their own poverty. Similarly, poor employment conditions were recognised as sometimes leading to madness. Thus it was said of Elizabeth Spawton,

> This patient has worked, for many years, as a factory hand in a crowded and vitiated atmosphere, where, no doubt, she contracted her disposition to pulmonary disease, and the predisposing one of her Insanity.[35]

There is a distinctly Old Poor Law, charitable flavour here. Consider the following comment of Francis Burdett MP, in his advocacy of the 1828 statute: 'Being paupers as well as lunatics, they had a double claim on general humanity.'[36] The vision of paupers as having a claim on general humanity is far too generous for the New Poor Law, and if the traditional view of the New Poor Law is correct, this would have been a highly improbable statement ten years later. Yet this is perhaps unsurprising, as the foundation of the county asylum movement predated the New Poor Law. As noted above, the original enabling legislation was passed in 1808, with a largely similar statute being passed in 1828, the latter being six years in advance of the New Poor Law. In this interpretation, the apparent contradictions between asylum law and New Poor Law are a result of momentum created before the New Poor Law came into being.

It is unsurprising that this strand of imagery remains, for the New Poor Law itself was controversial for years. *Oliver Twist*, which commenced publication in serial form in 1837, is but one example. *The Times* campaigned against the new system for a decade. The Andover scandal broke in 1845, with its reports of workhouse inmates sucking the rotting marrow of the chicken bones they were set to break for fertiliser. This forced the resignation of the Poor Law Commissioners. The older, gentler attitude to the poor did not die in 1834. That attitude can be seen in this third strand of images.

The older and gentler strand must be approached with some cynicism in the context of the county asylum, however, for it was not simply charitably motivated. As noted above, the county asylum administrative structure was not fundamentally altered by the introduction of the New Poor Law in 1834: Justices of the Peace remained in charge. The asylum system was here at variance with much of the rest of Poor Law, where the Justices were replaced by Boards of Guardians. While Justices did sit *ex officio* on these boards in rural areas, the boards were otherwise elected, and an implied challenge to the magistrates' authority. The Victorian asylum, with its attractive imagery and ornate architecture, can here be seen as a visible and political symbol of and monument to that authority, remaining in the Poor Law.

This strand of imagery also serves as a reminder, however, that the older vision of Poor Law never entirely died out, even in the New Poor Law itself. The rationale for the inclusion of good works in the Poor Law altered in the early nineteenth century to include utilitarianism and market-based economics, but it never disappeared. It was, after all, the Poor Law authorities who were charged with the enforcement and implementation of the Vaccination Act and the Nuisances Act. Considerable energy was spent over the century in attempting to improve general Poor Law medicine and, later, the housing of the poor. In addition, the Poor Law authorities seem to have made honest attempts at improving apprenticing of pauper youths, and improving workhouse schools. While there may be reason to doubt their success on these issues, there is no obvious reason to doubt their motives. Avoiding pauperism was never lost as an objective of the Poor Law. The more mainstream Poor Law voices might thus favour the asylum as the provision of benevolence on utilitarian grounds, since a cured pauper, permanently out of the Poor Law system, resulted in a saving to the parish. While these voices would be likely to shrink from the excesses of language noted above, they might none the less perceive the asylum in this other line of constructive solutions offered to the poor.

Conclusion

There is no point in pretending these strands can somehow be rendered consistent: they cannot. The images are too conflicting, and the theories too divergent. There was no single, consistent vision of what the county asylum was to be, or who it was to serve, in the nineteenth century. And yet the placement of the asylum in a Poor Law context does provide a framework, if not a solution, to understanding the institution.

To begin with, it is clear that the historical narrative focused on the boom and bust of humanitarian reform must be viewed critically. That is not to say that there was no humanitarian impulse in the creation of the asylum system. The third stream of imagery above is most overt in its humanitarianism, but the other two streams are not without humanitarian resonances. One of the objectives of the New Poor Law, after all, was to terminate pauperism. The belief of the framers of the 1834 legislation was that it would force paupers to choose a life of employment and morality. The residuum would, within a generation or so, wither on the vine. The approach toward the residuum may have been one of 'tough love', but a view to the greater, long-term good is not necessarily to be portrayed simply as callous. Similarly, the view of the asylum as directed to the respectable poor is consistent with a humanitarian set of values.

Instead, it is to acknowledge that the humanitarianism of the asylum was neither pure nor simple. Humanitarianism was framed by beliefs in market economics, theology or utilitarianism. The arguments were intimately connected with professional and personal interest, whether the interest of the Poor Law staff in furthering their professional prospects, or the belief of the justices in maintaining their power in the Poor Law structure. And as we have seen, notwithstanding the inconsistencies between the images, the three strands of discourse identified above occur at both central and local levels, frequently in the same actors. In the nineteenth century, as much as the twentieth, it would appear that individuals lived with their own contradictions.

These were not, of course, debates that circulated merely regarding asylums. That point has already been made regarding the third strand: that was, in part, one aspect of an anti-Poor Law animus which remained a part of the Poor Law debate for years. It is equally true regarding the first two lines of imagery, for, notwithstanding the optimism of the framers of the 1834 amendments, the New Poor Law never functioned as had been anticipated. Workhouses were intended to penalise the able-bodied poor; yet the bulk of able-bodied poor were always relieved outside the workhouse, and the majority of those in the workhouse were aged or infirm. The result was, from the beginning, ambiguity in the application of the theory to practical situations. As one might anticipate, the same sorts of imagery noted above circulated equally about the remainder of the pauper population.

Where in this lies 'success' or 'failure'? It should be clear by now that to judge the asylum on an uncritical test of humanitarianism is inappropriate. The benevolence of the asylum advocates was set in a complex context of personal and professional interests and theoretical perspectives. Assessment of the asylum without accounting for those contexts is anachronistic, yet the contradictions in the contexts make it difficult to see how an evaluative standard might arise.

Yet despite the anomalies, the asylum system grew, and grew monumentally, both in terms of the number of paupers it contained, and in terms of resource allocation. The varying perspectives tended to result in justifications of the asylum, not condemnations. Whether based in private interests of professionals and justices, Poor Law theory, utilitarianism, humanitarianism, market economics, Tory paternalism or evangelicalism, the intersection point in Poor Law argumentation was that the county asylum was a required part of the system. The variety of discourses may make it difficult to provide an appraisal of the 'success' of the asylum in any normative sense, but the intersection of the Poor Law discourses would suggest that growth of the asylum in the nineteenth century is unsurprising.

Acknowledgements

Previous versions of this chapter were read to the conference of the Society for the Social History of Medicine (University of Exeter, 1997), a colloquium on 'Insanity and Institutions' (University of Exeter, 1996), and the 'Work in Progress' seminar at the Wellcome Institute (London, 1992). I am grateful to all participants for comments, and particularly to David Wright for his specific comments at the 1997 event. Funding for much of the research in this paper was provided by the Wellcome Trust.

NOTES

1 The precise periodisation is debated. The traditional account views the most significant progression occurring at the end of the eighteenth century and beginning of the nineteenth, with the founding of the York Retreat in 1796, the passage of the first County Asylums Act in 1808, and the scandal over the care of James Norris in 1815 being taken as convenient markers. More recently, eighteenth-century historians of medicine have challenged the orthodoxy, objecting to the uncritical use of what they see as a nineteenth-century caricature of the eighteenth-century treatment of the insane: see, for example, R. Porter, *Mind-Forg'd Manacles*, Harmondsworth, Penguin, 1990, pp. 276 ff. and *passim*. For the discussion which follows, the precise periodisation is not important.

2 A. Scull, *The Most Solitary of Afflictions*, New Haven and London, Yale University Press, 1993, p. 245.

3 See, for example, Kathleen Jones, *Asylums and After*, London, Athlone, 1993, chapters 6 and 7, regarding law as undercutting the reforms made in the mid-nineteenth century.

4 For example, David Rothman, *The Discovery of the Asylum*, Boston, Little Brown, 1971 and *Conscience and Convenience*, Boston and Toronto, Little Brown, 1980.

5 Andrew Scull has argued this position most forcefully in the context of nineteenth-century England; see for example *Museums of Madness*, Harmondsworth, Penguin, 1982; 'Humanitarianism or control? Some observations on the historiography of Anglo-American psychiatry', in S. Cohen and A. Scull, eds, *Social Control and the State*, Oxford, Blackwell, 1985, p. 118; 'Mad-doctors and magistrates: English psychiatry's struggle for professional autonomy in the nineteenth century', *Arch. Europ. Sociol.*, 17, 1976, p. 279; *Social Order/Mental Disorder*, London, Routledge, 1989; *The Most Solitary of Afflictions*, New Haven and London, Yale University Press, 1993. For continuation of these themes into the twentieth century, A. Scull, *Decarceration*, 2nd edn, Englewood Cliffs, Prentice Hall, 1984.

6 See the works by Scull, above. Michel Foucault can also be seen in this vein: *Madness and Civilisation*, trans. Richard Howard, New York, Random House, 1965, especially chapter 9.

7 The recent literature on cure rates in asylums is summarised in D. Wright, 'Getting out of the asylum: understanding the confinement of the insane in the nineteenth century', *Social History of Medicine*, 10, 1, 1997, p. 137, at p. 143. Regarding funding and delays in sending patients, see P. Bartlett, 'The Poor Law of Lunacy: confinement of the insane poor in mid-nineteenth-century England with special emphasis on Leicestershire and Rutland', diss., University of London, 1993, at pp. 37–42, 201–2, app. II, tables 5 and 6.

8 See for example A. Suzuki, 'The politics and ideology of non-restraint: the case of the Hanwell Asylum', *Medical History*, 39, 1, 1995, p. 1; D. Wright,

'Getting out of the asylum: understanding confinement of the insane in the nineteenth century', *Social History of Medicine,* 10, 1, 1997, p. 137; D. Wright, ' "Childlike in his innocence": lay attitudes to "idiots" and "imbeciles" in Victorian England', in D. Wright and A. Digby, eds, *From Idiocy to Mental Deficiency*, London, Routledge, 1996, p. 118; D. Wright, 'A beam for mental darkness: a history of the National Asylum for Idiots, Earlswood, 1847–1886', diss., University of Oxford, 1993; W. Forsythe, J. Melling and R. Adair, 'The New Poor Law and the county pauper lunatic asylum – the Devon experience 1834–1884', *Social History of Medicine,* 9, 3, 1996, p. 335; P. Bartlett, 'The Poor Law of Lunacy: the administration of pauper lunatics in mid-nineteenth-century England with special emphasis on Leicestershire and Rutland', diss., University of London, 1993.

9 Source of statistics: annual reports of Poor Law Commissioners and Poor Law Board, printed annually in Parliamentary Papers.

10 48 George III (1808), c. 96.

11 26/27 Vict. (1863), c. 110; cf. the view offered in the essay in this volume by Forsythe *et al.*

12 55 George III (1815), c. 46, s. 12.

13 See for example documents admitting John Willows to the Leicestershire County Asylum transferred from the West Yorkshire Asylum on 22 June 1869, LRO DE 3533/230. Italics in original.

14 12 Anne (1714), c. 23. The provisions of this act were essentially re-enacted in 1744: v. 17 George II (1744), c. 5, esp. s. 20.

15 48 George III (1808), c. 96, s. 19.

16 8/9 Vict. (1845), c. 126, s. 55.

17 16/17 Vict. (1853), c. 97, s. 66.

18 D. Garland, *Punishment and Welfare*, Aldershot, Gower, 1985.

19 Ibid., p. 39.

20 Ibid., p. 39. Footnote omitted.

21 Regarding such charities in other institutions, see L. Smith, ' "Levelled to the same common standard"? Social class in the lunatic asylum, 1780–1860', in O. Ashton *et al.*, eds, *The Duty of Discontent*, London, Mansell, 1995, pp. 146–9. Smith cites segregation of charitable from 'pauper' classes by the second decade of the nineteenth century: pp. 152–6.

22 PRO MH/51/755.

23 See PRO MH 51/772. Compare with PRO MH 51/755 (1863).

24 1864 Annual Report of Leicester and Rutland County Lunatic Asylum, LRO DE 3533/13. Emphases in original.

25 Report of the Select Committee on Lunatics; Together with the Proceedings of the Committee, Minutes of Evidence, Appendix, and Index', PP 1859 1st Session (204) III 75, p.7.

26 LRO DE 3533/186; adm. 16 June 1851.

27 LRO DE 3533/186; adm. 15 April 1852.

28 Adm. 2 May 1846. Case book LRO DE 3533/184.

29 PP 1854–5 (240) XVII 533, p. 35.

30 For the same situation regarding Surrey, see PRO MH 51/755.

31 'Report of the Select Committee on Lunatics; Together with the Proceedings of the Committee, Minutes of Evidence, Appendix, and Index', PP 1859 1st Session (204) III 75, p. 278.

32 Leicestershire and Rutland Lunatic Asylum, 'Rules for the General Management of the Institution, with Prefatory Remarks by the Committee of Visitors', Leicester, n.p., 1849, p. 19.

33 Minute book, Leicester Board of Guardians, 3 April 1866, LRO G–12–8a/12.

34 Leicestershire and Rutland County Asylum, Report of Medical Superintendent (J. Buck) for 1862, LRO DE 3533/84.

35 Admitted to Leicestershire and Rutland County Lunatic Asylum, 14 March 1851. Case book, LRO DE 3533/186.

36 *Hansard* (2nd ser) vol. 17, p. 1265 (13 June 1827, HC). Burdett in fact opposed the New Poor Law, see *Hansard* (3rd ser), vol. 23, cols 822–24.

4

POLITICS OF LUNACY

Central state regulation and the Devon Pauper Lunatic Asylum, 1845–1914

Bill Forsythe, Joseph Melling and Richard Adair

Introduction

Historians of medicine and social policy have long been interested in the workings of the walled institutions in which so much of the social policy was acted out. One response to Foucault's seminal writings on 'total' institutions was an impressive range of studies which demonstrated the complexity and porosity of bodies created in the nineteenth century, showing that such organisations were far from the dominant, self-enclosed and isolated establishments found in many of the seminal revisionist texts published in the 1970s.[1] An earlier literature had interrogated the model of administrative growth and centralisation given in MacDonagh's study of the revolution in government.[2] From these two strands of writing there has emerged a growing recognition of the importance of central–local relations to the exercise of power within society. On one hand there was an almost frenetic construction of new inspectorates, boards and commissions in the mid-nineteenth century whilst in contrast at local level there was a strong sense of their novelty and a fear that they would undermine deeply respected local autonomies and customs. Whilst radical scholars have emphasised the growing dominance of local communities by the forces of regulation emanating from the centre,[3] others have emphasised the degree to which the permissive and enabling legislation of the Victorian period allowed the survival of local autonomy within the British state.[4] Not only were localised interests often responsible for the initiatives which resulted in statutory provision, they decided many of the forms in which legislation was implemented.[5] Indeed it is important to remember that the actual powers of intervention held by many of these new central boards were strictly limited and depended on the ability of their officials to win over local interest groups who were often highly distrustful.

State provision of the treatment of lunatics in the nineteenth and early twentieth centuries forms an important reference point in this debate on the locus of power within institutions and society. Andrew Scull viewed the growth of lunacy legislation and central control of asylums as an essential complement to the spread of commercialisation and the erosion of the local regulation of deviance.[6] Roy Porter likewise saw the Poor Law of 1834 and the Lunacy Act of 1845 as important steps in the central regulation of measures for the lunatic.[7] Such an interpretation can be contrasted with Hervey's study of the Lunacy Commission (the central regulatory authority created in 1845), which recognises the real progress made by the Commission in setting standards and checking abuses but also portrayed the Commissioners as avoiding confrontation and compromising or even retreating in the face of contentious issues.[8] Peter Bartlett's research revealed the local Justices and Poor Law officials as the key actors in the administration of pauper lunatics whilst the Lunacy Commission fulfilled an essentially conciliatory function within the system.[9] Bartlett suggests that the Commissioners were weak in dealing with intransigent local interests and parsimonious authorities which refused to build asylums.[10] The anaemic response of the Commission was contrasted in Bartlett's account with the robust activities of the central Poor Law authorities[11] and Mellett in an earlier essay was emphatic that the Lunacy Commission had little room for effective manoeuvre or intervention.[12]

Our essay is designed as a contribution to the discussions on the distribution of power and the growth of government in Victorian and Edwardian Britain, as well as an assessment of the relations between an important medical institution and its regulatory authorities in this period. The prevailing view of the Lunacy Commission as a passive and conciliatory body is not sustained in research on the Devon County Pauper Lunatic Asylum and by the end of the Victorian era (if the Devon experience was representative) the county institutions were subjected to a remarkable degree of central regulation. The Lunacy Commission interacted effectively and subtly with local interest groups to secure its desired policy outcomes and, within the context in which it existed, it was authoritative and successful. The Commissioners exercised a significant and increasing influence on the administration of pauper lunacy in Devon, though the terms on which the central state could regulate county asylums were substantially altered by both the Local Government Act of 1888[13] and the Lunacy Act of 1890.[14] By contrast the Poor Law Board, which regulated the administration of the Poor Law, appears to have been ineffective in dealing with pauper lunacy, failing to support the Lunacy Commission and weak in the face of local Poor Law officials and interest groups. Only at the end of the nineteenth century did the Local Government Board (successor to the Poor Law Board), join the Lunacy Commission in directly monitoring the conduct of business at the pauper asylums as a result of their responsibility for the new county councils, including their financial affairs. At the level where pauper lunatics were most obviously deployed and directed, i.e. the workhouse and the Union, the Local Government Board continued to be little more decisive in directing local affairs and ensuring adequate certification procedures than its predecessor.

Whilst the personnel who governed the Devon Asylum continued to be substantially drawn from an elite who provided the magistrates, aldermen and councillors before and after the 1888 legislation, their room for manoeuvre and autonomy were clearly circumscribed by the terms of reference and regulatory authorities under which they now served. Far from medical men and magistrates deriving great professional power and autonomy from the growing numbers of lunatics institutionalised within the county asylums, we find those most responsible for the conduct of the Devon Asylum subjected to enormous external pressures in consequence of the unrelenting expansion seen in the Victorian years.

Successful beginnings

Throughout the years 1845 to 1888, when the Local Government Act brought the administration of the Asylum under the direct control of the Devon County Council, Exminster was governed by a Committee of Visiting Justices directly appointed by the County Quarter Sessions and accountable to them. This committee of initially fifteen magistrates met monthly at the asylum in order to approve applications for discharge, ensure effective administration of the asylum and advise the Quarter Sessions on its correspondence with the Home Secretary and the Lunacy Commission. It was the alliance between Tory and Whig county aristocracy on one side and central authorities on the other which had earlier enabled the Earls of Devon to overcome backwoods resistance to the founding of the Asylum near Powderham Castle at Exminster in 1845.[15] There are echoes here of the alliance between aristocratic paternalists and electors that Bartlett found elsewhere, though the use made of the Poor Law was clearly complex.[16] In Devon the St Thomas Union was not only the seat of the Earls of Devon but the power base from which they controlled the Asylum itself. The institution at Exminster was the only pauper lunatic asylum within the county until the opening of the Exeter Borough Asylum in 1886 and the Plymouth Borough counterpart at Moorhaven in 1892.

In the years 1845–85 the new Lunacy Commission was greatly influenced by its formidable first chairman, Lord Shaftesbury, who guided his fellow Commissioners through the period of legislative implementation and the regular inspection of institutions recognised and licensed to house the insane.[17] Shaftesbury was driven by an ethical and religious conviction that private madhouses should be eradicated and replaced by comprehensive public provision.[18] At the apex of the system of lunacy provision overseen by the new Commission stood the new county pauper asylums which were intended by the Commissioners to fulfil the vision of sanitary, humane and protective sanctuary foreseen by the reformers of 1845.[19] Clearly the Lunacy Commission was much more than just Lord Shaftesbury and developed a systematic bureaucracy administered by figures such as Robert Lutwidge its indefatigable secretary between 1845 and 1856. Lord Shaftesbury's general views chimed with most of the views of the dominant school of lunacy reformers in mid-century. In particular, his faith in public provision and detestation of private enterprise provision remained at the heart of the policy of the Commission. However, it is important to remember that the powers of the Lunacy Commission were tightly circumscribed. It could publicise shortcomings in its annual reports, it could recommend that new asylum or asylum extension plans be refused by central government where gross inadequacies existed and it could prosecute local authorities and individual asylum personnel where breaches of law were discovered. However, as with the prison inspectors of the same era also pursuing a policy of radical innovation, the reality was that the Lunacy Commission had to negotiate outcomes with formidable and well-entrenched local interests and the central governments of different complexions were exceedingly careful not to alienate local ratepayers and voters by using the letter of the statute in a matter which, like pauper lunacy, won very few votes. The political and social context simply did not allow for ruthless purges of recalcitrant local institutions and any attempt to seize power over and above the minimum allowed by law resulted in intense and orchestrated pressure on the offending body by local members of both houses of parliament and powerful local interest groups. Outcomes had to be secured by negotiation and manoeuvre and it was this context in which every central state board and commission had to operate.

The road of the pauper lunatic to the county asylum always led from the Union officials of the Poor Law, the Guardians, relieving officers, workhouse masters, medical officers and their assistants.[20] The connections between the Poor Law and the disposal of pauper lunatics was clearly an intimate one.[21] Devon's 471 parishes possessed a population of almost half a million when they were reorganised into twenty Unions under the 1834 Poor Law Act to which must be added the two Corporations of the Poor of the boroughs of Exeter and Plymouth.[22] It should be noted that Corporations of the Poor were Unions of urban parishes set up in the late seventeenth and early eighteenth centuries to systematise poor relief across the entire city rather than deliver this parochially as was the norm. These corporations, although small in number, were found in the most prestigious cities and deeply resented the New Poor Law of 1834 from which they claimed their founding legislation gave them immunity. They therefore posed particular difficulties to the new Poor Law regulator under that act and to other central bodies such as the Lunacy Commission whose activities plainly intersected with pauperism. Having regard to the Poor Law generally in Devon, whether rural or urban, most pauper lunatics were certified by the workhouse medical officer and taken from that staging post to the asylum by the relieving officer but a significant minority were taken by the relieving officer direct from their homes certified by the local Poor Law medical officer.

Our interpretation of the nature of 'pauper lunacy' and the designation of 'pauper lunatics' stands in some contrast to that offered by Peter Bartlett's chapter. Almost all of the inmates to the Exminster Asylum were identified as paupers and the responsibility of local Devon Unions, though a detailed analysis of the occupational profile of those admitted to the county asylum indicates that many of those coming through its gates were not destitute within the meaning of the 1834 Poor Law. The Devon evidence indicates that the construction of the pauper lunatic was a complex community process in which the resources and capacities of the individual were calculated by the relatives, neighbours, social superiors and Poor Law authorities who were most usually involved in the certification and dispatch of a person to the Asylum. Far from catering only for the most destitute and deprived of English society, the admissions to the Devon Asylum appear to reflect a wide cross-section of occupational and social classes. The degree to which relieving officers, Guardians and even magistrates colluded in the direction of non-paupers to the county asylum requires detailed research, though initial results indicate that in many instances the Poor Law authorities were willing to allow a certified individual to remain at Exminster provided a contribution to their upkeep was made by relatives or by the estate of the insane person. Very few instances emerge of lunatics with estate being referred to the Lord Chancellor (confirming that wealthy individuals were rarely housed at Exminster), though relatives were sometimes advised that the lunatic should be removed to a private asylum. It would appear that many of the people admitted to the Devon Asylum were not without the means to support themselves but that the onset of insanity usually prevented them from undertaking those responsibilities which their household expected of them. The Poor Law authorities appear to have frequently negotiated with the wider relatives on the maintenance of the individual before the decision was taken to dispatch to the Asylum.

Under the leadership of John Buckmill, its celebrated Medical Superintendant from 1845–1862, there occurred a revolution in provisions for pauper lunatics within the region.[23] It is worth recalling that the numbers of people administered by *both* the Poor Law authorities and the Lunacy Commission were rising steadily throughout our period and indeed the proportion of insane paupers nationally grew rapidly from one in a hundred paupers in 1842 to one in eight paupers by 1910.[24] The main instrument of regulation exercised by the Lunacy Commissioners was the annual visit to the county asylum and the publication of their report in parliamentary papers. Hervey has pointed out that the Commission was not a large body. The salaried personnel comprised initially three full-time Commissioners trained in medicine and three in law, who served together with five unpaid lay members. Their duties were remarkably onerous, for not only had they to visit the occupants of the county asylums each year but also 750 workhouses, 144 private licensed establishments, 13 hospitals, and 20 gaols and private houses where lunatics were kept.[25] Despite their limited resources the Commission was galvanised into determined activity by their hostility to private asylums and to the mechanical restraints which were popularly associated with them. This was reflected in the favourable endorsement of Bucknill's espousal of the moral management thesis of lunacy treatment from his early days at Exminster.[26] Bucknill was cited approvingly as a Superintendent who eschewed mechanical restraint and physical compulsion and who promoted the 'habits of industry, propriety and order' to cultivate the self-control essential to the recovery of the individual's humanity and the withdrawal of surveillance.[27] The Commission clearly believed from the beginning that Bucknill was a pioneer of excellent practice whose pursuit of the best standards would certainly equal those proposed by themselves and they lauded him in their annual reports praising

Exminster as a beacon of excellence and defending Bucknill vigorously when he was attacked.

The impact on Poor Law Guardians of such approving reports, as well as the Commissioners' campaign to raise standards in workhouses, can be gauged from the readiness of such independent Unions as the Exeter Corporation of the Poor to pay the higher rate of 11–12 shillings per week for maintenance of lunatics levied on the Devon boroughs which had not contributed to the original foundation of the Asylum. This compared with the 8–9 shillings charge levied on 'county' Poor Law Unions which had combined to set up the Asylum.[28] Initial optimism amongst the Exeter Guardians soon drained away as pauper numbers and maintenance costs at Exminster rose, prompting the city's Corporation of the Poor to seek the discharge of the uncured back to the workhouse. The dissatisfied borough leaders even entertained the claims of a local mesmerist to provide a more rapid recovery from insanity.[29] Poor Law authorities such as Exeter were clearly anxious to reduce costs and many sought to rebuild their own workhouse accommodation and filter the cases initially sent to the Asylum as a way of retaining the 'harmless' cases in their own hands.[30] It is significant that many such economy drives were blocked after consultations between the Lunacy Commission and the central Poor Law Board.[31]

Plymouth Corporation was likewise pressed by the Lunacy Commission to use Exminster rather than resorting to their workhouse or the notorious private establishment at Plympton House against which establishment the Lunacy Commission conducted an intense campaign. The minutes of the Lunacy Commission reveal recurring complaints against both the 'illegal & improper practices permitted' at Plymouth workhouse and the unsatisfactory conditions at the private establishment used by the borough.[32] The Commission's Report had the intended impact of provoking public interest to such a degree that the Guardians of the Corporation of the Poor at Plymouth decided to send fifty females to the county asylum. Shortage of available beds at Exminster provided the cue for Bucknill's most famous experiment in renting a seaside mansion at Exmouth to add to the accommodation for women, thereby prompting intense and organised resistance amongst the concerned residents of this bathing resort.[33] With the united and very public support of the Asylum Visitors, the Lunacy Commission and the Secretary of State, Bucknill was able to ride out the storm and this seaside therapy was singled out for praise in the Commission's Annual Reports.[34]

Bucknill's skills as a publicist undoubtedly helped him to promote his own institution and to collaborate with the Commission in using the press and official reports to overcome the resistance of economising Poor Law Guardians. Their cause was also greatly assisted by the exposure by Bucknill in the *Journal of Mental Science* and by the Lunacy Commissioners in their annual reports of atrocious cases of neglect and maltreatment within isolated family households in Devon, thereby raising popular anxieties about the secret imprisonment and gross maltreatment of lunatics.[35] Bucknill readily notified the Commission of evidence of neglect or abuse of people arriving from workhouses in such Unions as Okehampton and Totnes which had long traditions of opposition to Exminster. One early consequence of Bucknill's policy was the steady filling up of empty beds at Exminster, which was already showing signs of overcrowding in the late 1850s, though the Asylum continued to receive glowing reports for its work.[36] This was despite signs of some strain in the relations between the Devon institution and the Commissioners as Bucknill attacked the recruitment of non-specialists to their number and opposed proposals to introduce tighter surveillance of medical practice at the county asylums whilst himself treating in cavalier fashion the complaints of the Lunacy Commission that certification procedures were not always strictly followed at Exminster.[37] It is also likely that the Lunacy Commission were very aware of the need to keep on their side a reforming lunacy specialist whose propagandist skills were regularly demonstrated in his editorship of the *Journal of Mental Science*.

Behind the scenes therefore it is no surprise that the seeds of future difficulty were being sown as Bucknill oversaw an institution designed for four hundred quickly fill up and exceed capacity within fifteen years of its opening.[38] By 1861 the Commissioners were covertly writing to the Secretary of State about the 'want of general rules' at Exminster and Bucknill's firm refusal to comply with general regulation.[39] When Commissioners visiting the Devon Asylum found the registration books in a chaotic state (contrary to the requirements of 1853 legislation), the Visitors were privately admonished by the Commission for the blatant falsification of dates by their Asylum Clerk in the returns required by law.[40] Bucknill finally departed for the Chancery in 1862 with his public reputation still intact though leaving a problematic legacy of overcrowding and frayed administration at the Asylum he had overseen for almost two decades. The Lunacy Commission had evidently shifted from their previous policy of unqualified endorsement of the Exminster model as conditions deteriorated, though their alliance with Bucknill in opposition to private madhouses and workhouse care for lunatics hardly faltered. The common problem they faced was the apparent lethargy and hesitancy of the central Poor Law Board when aberrant or truculent behaviour occurred on the part of Unions.[41] The Commissioners' criticisms of neglect and abuse of workhouse lunatics continued in subsequent years, despite the provisions made in 1862 for the retention of certain categories of insane within workhouses which improved their infirmary provision to the satisfaction of the Lunacy Commission and the transparent problems caused by overcrowding under Bucknill's successor.[42]

Decline and fall

The departure of its celebrated mad-doctor proved to be the beginning of a decline of Exminster's reputation as a progressive institution. Bucknill was succeeded by his assistant, Saunders, and relations between the new Superintendent and the Lunacy Commission quickly soured. A radical overhaul of the Devon Asylum was demanded as the Commissioners prosecuted its Clerk in 1863 for failing to make adequate statistical returns and upbraided its Visitors a year later for failing to implement reforms.[43] Thereafter criticisms followed in a steady stream as the care regime was criticised and its staff described as overworked, with the result that cases of patient abuse figured prominently in the reports of annual visitations in the late 1860s.[44]

The magistrates responsible for governing the Asylum were also beginning to express serious disquiet at the rumours of financial and sexual scandal amongst the senior staff and when they brought the Clerk/Steward (the chief culprit) before the Committee in 1869, his 'manner and language' prompted them formally to censure him and record their concern at Saunders' failure to enforce his authority and quash the spirit of insubordination in the institution.[45] The Steward and numerous attendants were dismissed after his apprehension by the Superintendent with stolen Asylum property, provoking a crisis of confidence and the resignation of the Chair of the Visitors.[46] The interesting point is that the justices' subsequent announcement of their detection of fraud and dishonesty that had been rife within the institution for some years brought public criticism not only of the criminal behaviour of the staff but adverse comment on the poor working and living conditions at Exminster by the Lunacy Commission.[47]

Whilst public scandal was in part prompted by the Commission's demand for improvements in both standards of care and administration at the Devon Asylum, the disorders were in part symptomatic of the rapid and uncontrolled growth of the inmate population in its early years, including the acceptance of profitable contracts for accommodating the borough inmates at higher rates. The Commission had promoted the image of Exminster as a model for therapeutic innovation during the Bucknill era and was equally determined to publicise its failings in the Saunders years. Behind the apparent caprice of the annual Reports on the Asylum, we can detect a carefully defined rationale and a deliberate strategy on the part of the Commissioners to force Exeter and Plymouth to make their own provision as required by law whether by upgrading workhouse infirmary lunatic wards under the 1862 Act or providing their own asylums under the terms of the 1845 Lunacy Act. By the early 1870s the Devon Asylum was chronically overcrowded and sought permission to expand. In the mid-1860s the Lunacy Commission had resolved to obstruct not merely the award of a new contract to house Plymouth lunatics in Exminster but also pressed hard for the upgrading of Plymouth workhouse in line with the 1862 legislation enabling workhouses to hold the insane in lunatic wards.[48] The Commissioners ultimately informed the Home Secretary that they would 'oppose any renewal save pending erection of [a] new asylum' by the borough magistrates and threatened the Plymouth magistrates and town council with further advising the Home Office to interfere to secure fit accommodation for the lunatic poor.[49] In 1866 a deputation of Plymouth justices went to London to plead with the Commission for a compromise. The Commission was immovable and warned them that they were about to report the borough to the Home Secretary 'as not having made fit and sufficient provision for its lunatic poor and requiring his interference as authorised by the Statute'.[50]

Their determination to force the boroughs to build specialist institutions remained immovable even though Plymouth pleaded for a fresh contract with the county and offered to finance the building of a new wing to house its lunatics on the Exminster Asylum estate, and by 1869 the Commission was again pressing a reluctant Home Office to prosecute the borough under Lunacy Asylum law.[51] For their part, the Exminster Visitors gloomily reported to the 1870 Quarter Sessions that their only available course of action was to remove the non-county patients with as little inconvenience as possible, though the Exminster governors had themselves been seeking to break their contractual ties with Plymouth (again under pressure from the Lunacy Commission) since 1865.[52]

This strategy appeared remarkably successful when in 1872 the Lunacy Commissioners reported that the Plymouth justices had given a commitment to building their own borough asylum, whilst the Exminster Visitors gave the boroughs notice the following year to remove their patients within six months.[53] The 1875 Report of the

Commission triumphantly announced the removal of Exeter and Plymouth inmates, only to discover to their chagrin that Exeter then resorted to the private asylum at Fisherton.[54] Whilst the compliant Devon Asylum was rewarded with favourable commendations in their annual reports,[55] the Commission now vented its displeasure on the offending boroughs of Devon. Within a decade relations between Fisherton and Exeter had broken down because Fisherton increasingly refused to receive any but tractable pauper lunatics and resented visits of inspection by the Guardians. This, coupled with the high cost, led the borough to opt to build its own asylum and this was duly opened at Digby's Fields in 1886. Plymouth was similarly subjected to the public disapproval of the Commission in 1882 and by 1884 the local justices completed the purchase of the estate near Ivybridge on which the future Moorhaven Asylum would be constructed.[56]

In the face of formidable resistance from two powerful Corporations of the Poor, the Lunacy Commission had been able to achieve its objective of institutional provision by the closing decades of the nineteenth century. Hervey and Bartlett are correct to emphasise the depth of local hostility from magistrates and ratepayers to expenditure programmes but appear seriously to underestimate the shrewd and patient calculation and the determination with which the Lunacy Commission was willing to use the pressures of overcrowding to force its will on recalcitrant representatives.[57] Doubtless Plymouth was particularly visible in its longstanding failure to follow the policy of the Lunacy Commission and represented a public failure of the authority of the Commission. Nevertheless Exeter, which was more receptive, faced similar tactics which were ultimately successful.

A key point in Bartlett's interpretation is his conclusion that the Lunacy Commissioners deferred to the Poor Law Board in their dealings with the local Guardians. The Devon evidence suggests that it was relatively common for local Unions to resist the guidance offered by the Poor Law and Local Government Boards, as when the Axminster Guardians virtually refused to dispatch workhouse lunatics to the Asylum when Lunacy Commissioners recommended their removal.[58] The workhouse medical officers were frequently opposed to the transfer of their charges to the county asylum, whilst the Guardians of Barnstaple and Axminster expressed considerable scepticism when asked to improve workhouse amenities in the mid-1880s.[59] The Poor Law authorities at Okehampton continued to be criticised by the Commission in the 1890s and as late as 1910 for their poor facilities and neglect of pauper lunatics but the Local Government Board was loathe to press the point.[60]

The Lunacy Commission had few powers of compulsion over local Guardians or the central Poor Law regulator and functioned within a strict demarcation of spheres of authority between central boards and commissions. The evidence indicates that the problem lay not so much in a timid approach by the Lunacy Commissioners to matters of interdepartmental concern with the Poor Law regulator but rather in the reluctance of the central Poor Law authorities to enforce a stringent policy on individual Unions when the Lunacy Commission had drawn such matters to the attention of the regulator.[61] As the heroic era of Bucknill gave way to the lassitude of Saunders' early tenure, London Commissioners were swift to manipulate adverse publicity, official censure and even administrative procedures to secure reforms and institutional innovation. The Lunacy Commission appears to have taken the lead in collaboration with the Poor Law (and later Local Government) Board to achieve its policy of creating specialist institutions for the insane, even though there was a growing recognition that 'chronic' and 'harmless' cases might be safely left within a well-provided workhouse ward. The passing of the Local Government Act in 1888 and the Lunacy Act of 1890 changed the terms of central–local relations in respect of the administration of pauper lunacy but the new era again provided the Lunacy Commission with opportunities to exploit institutional crises and secure further reforms within the Devon County Asylum.

From stagnation to standardisation: crisis and reform

A common Lunacy Commission tactic was publicly to praise the Devon County Asylum once the Visitors agreed to do its bidding, as in the case of the long conflict with Plymouth Borough. However the relations between the London officials and Bucknill's successor were never to recover. Saunders made a characteristically contemptuous comment on the departure of two Lunacy Commissioners in late 1890, leaving behind them a 'caustic and choleric report'.[62] After a brief respite period in the 1870s when the Superintendent regained some control of the institution and introduced improvements, the Commission's annual reports again presented a dark account of the Asylum as overcrowding blighted the lives of the patients and the attendants, with medical staff held responsible for the rash of suicides and abuse at Exminster in the 1890s.[63] The Devon Asylum shared with other institutions the pressure of substantial admissions during the 1880s and 1890s, though the ratio of one attendant for almost fifteen patients in 1889 was significantly worse than most comparable asylums in southern England.[64] The severe overcrowding continued to increase despite the opening of the two new borough asylums within the county and the number of inmates rose from just over 900 at the end of the 1880s to 1,200 in 1900 and 1,350 in 1909 before settling just below this peak in the pre-war years.[65]

The criticisms of the Lunacy Commission had damaged Saunders in the 1860s and their adverse reports during the 1890s served to undermine his position once more.[66] Doubts were expressed as to the standards of medical practice and the absence of sufficient post-mortem examinations under Saunders, culminating in severe doubts expressed over his handling of a difficult patient in 1898.[67] Such reservations were a necessary but not a sufficient condition for the crisis which engulfed the institution in the 1890s and secured a revolution in its management. As in the 1860s it was mismanagement and financial impropriety rather than mere brutality or squalor which brought about the downfall of the Exminster Superintendent. The Lunacy Commission could not have secured this outcome without at least the tacit co-operation of the Local Government Board acting through the new administrative and legal structures put in place by the legislation of 1888–1890.

It might at first sight seem that the Local Government Act of 1888 transferred responsibility for local management of Exminster entirely to a new body, Devon County Council. In theory and in law this was certainly the case.[68] In reality, however, three-quarters of the Asylum Visitors appointed by the new county council were justices of the county as well as elected councillors and the dominant figures on the Visitors Sub-Committee (E.A. Sanders, Trehawke Kekewich and Lord Clifford) held both roles. Given the continued presence of magistrates on the County Council Visitors' Committee before 1914, the legislation of 1888 hardly marked a revolutionary break with the personnel of the earlier Quarter Sessions Committee. The chair of new Committee (E.A. Sanders) was also leading the powerful Finance Committee, to which the Asylum Visitors were increasingly answerable.[69]

Nor did the passage of the 1888 Local Government Act and the 1890 Lunacy Act signal a cessation in hostilities between the Devon Visitors and the Lunacy Commission. In their wide-ranging criticism of the management regime at Exminster in 1890, the Lunacy Commission recommended not only regular tours of the wards by the Visitors and improvements in amenities but also the presentation of case books, employment lists and farm accounts at each committee meeting.[70] Such reforms were strengthened by the recommendations of the County auditors who examined the Asylum books after 1889 and the scrutiny of such accounts by the County's Finance Committee.[71] Central officials at the Local Government Board itself uncovered irregularities in the arrangements for building work at the Asylum in the mid-1890s, and it was this central supervision which provoked a crisis which effectively destroyed the autonomy both of Saunders and the Asylum Visitors. The immediate occasion of this was the county council's efforts to raise a major new loan in 1895 to finance Asylum extensions and the serious criticisms subsequently made of expenditure which exceeded estimates which were themselves imperfect.[72] With considerable difficulty, the Finance Committee extracted contractors' estimates from the Asylum Committee as further omissions came to light.[73] Amidst legal actions and mounting criticisms within the county council itself, the Chair of the Asylum Committee was replaced as leader of the Finance Committee.[74] In 1899 events reached crisis point as the estimates for a major new asylum development at a projected cost of more than £45,500 were considered alongside the Local Government Board's criticisms of instances 'of gross carelessness in keeping the Asylum accounts'.[75] The Finance Committee itself sought to deflect criticism by protesting that the Asylum Committee had failed, over many years, to observe the requirements of the 1888 legislation.[76] When the Clerk to the Asylum Committee tried to secure support for additional legal fees for drafting contracts, the Finance Committee saw its opportunity and effectively brought the Visitors under its control by imposing the County Clerk on the Committee.[77]

The reformers in the county council were compelled to break the power of the Asylum Visitors for a number of reasons. Neither the Local Government Board nor Council members were prepared to tolerate estimates for Asylum buildings which were increased from £35,500 to £45,500 within the space of four years, or the consistent excess of expenditure over estimates. Second, the steady growth in patient numbers placed intolerable strains on the water supply and sewerage systems of Exminster, resulting in public controversy and damaging legal actions brought by individuals and rural district councils, further calling into question the legal judgment of the Visitors.[78] A third factor contributing to the sense of crisis in the years 1895–1900 was the strained relationship between the Asylum authorities and the Lunacy Commission, which pressed the Visitors and Superintendent to frame new Rules for the institution in 1897 after a period in which Saunders was criticised for breaches of the 1890 Act in detaining lunatics, and for outbreaks of violence against the patients.[79]

The extent to which the bitter tensions between Saunders and the Lunacy Commissioners informed every aspect of this relationship was revealed when the latter flatly refused in 1895 to approve the plans for the Superintendent's new house unless it were connected by a corridor to the main building.[80] As overcrowding worsened inside the Asylum walls and serious concerns were raised as to the quality of the water supplied to its occupants in 1895–96, the Visitors desperately cast around for an empty house in which to accommodate the overflowing population of the institution.[81] Other boroughs refused readmission of inmates to their workhouses and Plymouth, with the boot now well and truly on the other foot, demanded an extraordinary maintenance fee for taking Exminster patients.[82] The Visitors were reduced to pleading with the Lunacy Commission to recognise their predicament and only the personal intervention and regular journeys to Whitehall by the County Architect, Harbottle, persuaded the Commissioners to relent.[83] As the Asylum Committee became almost completely absorbed with the minutiae of elaborate building, engineering and sewerage projects, the Medical Superintendent was visibly marginalised. Confronted with continuing criticisms from the Lunacy Commission and the Local Government Board, the Visitors abandoned their Superintendent in favour of 'a younger and more active man'.[84]

Dr Arthur Davis appeared much more careful to appease the Lunacy Commission than either Bucknill or Saunders, having seen the consequences of their displeasure. The extensions were successfully completed but by 1903–4 there were again signs of serious overcrowding and a fresh phase of building was undertaken to house the excess. In 1905 the Visitors contemplated a continuation of the lucrative contract to hold Devonport borough patients.[85] Davis was unable to prevent a spate of patient injuries or suspicions of violent attack, even if he avoided imputing responsibility for such incidents to individual staff.[86] His efforts to improve conditions and respond quickly to the Commissioners' annual reports were rewarded by favourable comments in subsequent reviews, though deaths continued to cause concern in Commission correspondence.[87] The impression is generally of a large routinised institution managing a great cohort of pauper lunatics with a low level of aspiration for the human environment at the institution and a high level of concern to prevent any breach of the regulations which had been laid down.

The capacity of Davis and the Visitors to insist on the primacy of asylum care was weakened by the spectre of overcrowding and violence which continued to overshadow Committee discussions in the pre-war years. Davis criticised the provision made for lunatics at Kingsbridge Workhouse after their request to take back some of their pauper lunatics, only to be forced to explain to the Visitors and Lunacy Commissioners the circumstances surrounding the violent death of a

Kingsbridge inmate at the Asylum.[88] The Superintendent himself called for legislation to secure the accommodation of 'quiet and harmless' patients within workhouses with an increase of staff to oversee them.[89] Nor had the legislation of 1890 had the salutary impact on limiting compulsory admissions in all the Poor Law Unions. The Lunacy Commissioner visiting Barnstaple in 1898 was astonished to find that in only one in eight cases were the rigorous procedures to test the evidence of lunacy prior to certification followed, and thirteen years later justices in the same Union were signing sheaves of blank certificates for later completion by relieving officers without any attempt at examination of the individuals to be confined at the Asylum.[90] When the Exminster Visitors requested the Lunacy Commission to amend the magistrates' Reception Orders to include details of the patient's residence, the Commission merely advised a circular to each Union.[91] In responding to the complaint by another Union about the release of a noted lunatic, the Visitors cited not only their legal obligation but the great expense which they had saved the Guardians by his periodic release over many years.[92]

Such evidence confirms the general impression that the Superintendent and Visitors were most successful when they concentrated their energies on the elaboration and improvement of the Asylum estate at Exminster, including the addition of workshops, special wards and physical amenities. Business at the Asylum Committee meetings began with brief and often perfunctory reports from the Medical Superintendent before being immersed in contemplation of the extraordinarily detailed building improvements and financial matters now required by the county council.[93] Davis had even greater difficulty than his predecessor in attracting and retaining medical colleagues.[94] He travelled frequently to London medical schools to lure newly qualified doctors to Exminster but turnover was high and the impression is of an unhappy, stressed medical staff with large numbers of locums. Staffing matters were also routinised under the watchful eye of the Lunacy Commission and even the medical assistants were threatening to unionise before 1914.[95] The medical staff and Visitors at Exminster took their cue from the Lunacy Commission and concerned themselves with running a tight ship, rather than engaging in the wider issues and debates which had featured in Bucknill's tenure at the Asylum. Fresh debates on race and eugenics prompted renewed engagements amongst the county elite. As a prominent landowner, educationalist and leader of the county council, Sir Thomas Dyke Acland pressed the Royal Commission on the Control of the Feebleminded closely to control the procreation of mentally defective females in rural areas, whilst Lord

Clifford (Chair of the Council's Asylum Committee) expressed scepticism at this enthusiasm for certifying 'idiots, imbeciles and epileptics'.[96] The Visitors appear increasingly out of step with the national debate on eugenics whilst the Lunacy Commission itself seemed unable to break out of the comprehensive asylum model formed in the Shaftesbury era and imposed with such hard labour on the Devon boroughs.[97] The Commission itself handed over the supervision of asylums to a new Board of Control established under the Mental Deficiency Act of 1913.

Conclusions

Scholars are now increasingly aware of the complex institutional processes which shaped the admission of individuals to the English county asylum in the nineteenth century. The administration of pauper lunacy in Devon during the Victorian and Edwardian years was defined by the complex and changing relations between the Devon County Asylum and a variety of other institutions. We still know far more about the formative years of the county asylums after the 1845 legislation than the period which immediately preceded and followed the law of 1890. Between these two key measures the relationship between central regulators and local administrators was a critical element in the politics of lunacy provision. As scholars such as Prest and Bellamy have noted, the distribution of state power in the nineteenth century requires a more sophisticated model than the usual acknowledgement of centre–local tensions within the fabric of government. The importance of specific provisions and the changing complexion of the coalitions which supported lunacy reform also indicate the limitations of the Foucauldian grand narrative of institutionalisation and bourgeois rationalism. Recent research has provided a richer understanding of the state's administration of lunacy provisions during the nineteenth century, including the key role of the Poor Law in the transmission of the pauper lunatic to the county asylum. This work has tended to present the Lunacy Commission as a rather weak and conciliatory body which avoided conflict and to emphasise the power of the Poor Law authorities at local and central levels.

This chapter has confirmed the point that the everyday administration of pauper lunacy fell into the hands of magistrates and Poor Law officials far beyond the gaze of the Lunacy Commission. Where we clearly differ from Bartlett's analysis in the present volume is in our emphasis on the capacity of the central state to press reluctant magistrates and Guardians into line where there was some unity of purpose and political will in the regulating agencies. We view Victorian lunacy administration as a contested terrain where distinctive interests and conflicting agencies fought out their visions of governance over the bodies of the pauper lunatics who flowed through the institutional channels towards the county asylum. The experience of counties such as Devon indicate that the coalition of support behind the new lunacy legislation in 1845 included powerful traditional landed groups as well as the wider assembly of humanitarian, professional and religious elements who were also evident in the Welsh movement described by Michael and Hirst, and the Scottish lobby identified by Lorraine Walsh. Such traditionalists and humanitarians were not seeking merely to refashion the New Poor Law in the image of the Old, nor were they enthusiastic advocates of local autonomy against the Lunacy Commission. We need to reconstruct their commitment to the asylum project within the terms of the political and ideological commitments which were developing in this period. There is even a sense in which the creation of a system of specialist lunatic asylums represented a defeat for the New Poor Law and the principles of 1834. Contrary to the impression given in Scull's influential survey, the advocates of commercialisation and free trade were – at least in Devon – aligned behind the primacy of the New Poor Law and firmly opposed to the county asylum project from its inception.[98] We clearly need to tread with care when assigning the new institutions to the camp of modernism and the high ground of liberal ideology. The magistrates who promoted the Devon Asylum most actively and defended Bucknill most steadily were drawn from the Tory county elite. It was the justices, Guardians and ratepayers of the larger boroughs who proved most resistant to the Lunacy Commission's demand that they remove their insane paupers from the workhouse and provide for them in specialist asylums of their own.

The determination of such county elites to engineer the introduction of the county asylum and to control key Poor Law Unions shaped an important part of the political landscape of mid-Victorian England, though by the 1860s intense interest in such institutions was on the wane. What persisted was an extremely complex and laborious administrative system for the dispensing of poor relief which the central authorities sought to manage with a limited bureaucracy. The ability of the Lunacy Commission to impose its will on recalcitrant Guardians of either rural or urban Unions was clearly limited by the reluctance of the Poor Law Board and Local Government Board, at least before the 1890s, to force stubborn representatives into line. Lacking the legal authority of its Whitehall counterpart, the Lunacy Commission pressed

Plymouth and Exeter very hard to follow its preferred course in the 1860s and 1870s, calling on the Home Secretary to prosecute the offending magistrates, with final success in 1886 and 1892. The Lunacy Commission was prepared not only to use its annual reports to feed controversy in the local press, hamper plans to improve workhouse wards and threaten legal sanctions against the offending boroughs, but also to use the potent weapon of overcrowding to prevent the county asylum from meeting the demand of the recalcitrant borough Poor Law Unions for beds. During the overcrowding crises of the 1860s and 1870s, the Commissioners left the Exminster Visitors no option but to expel the inmates of the boroughs whilst permitting other boroughs (such as Devonport) to use the county asylum when it suited the purposes of the Commission.

The reorganisation of local government in 1888, followed by the more stringent Lunacy Act of 1890, altered the terms on which lunatic asylums were administered. These measures gave the Lunacy Commission additional resources to secure the subordination of county and borough asylums to their standards of accommodation and administration. Bucknill's Clerk had been prosecuted for failing to keep adequate patient records and his successor was dismissed (along with attendants) for gross fraud and mismanagement. The determination of the Lunacy Commissioners to force Saunders to fulfil their exacting requirements came not in relation to patient care, where professional incompetence was difficult to demonstrate, but again on grounds of maladministration. Armed with the tacit support of the Local Government Board and the legal requirements of the 1888 Local Government legislation, the Commission consistently rejected and delayed the plans for expansion at the Devon Asylum whilst the probity of the Asylum Clerk was challenged and his resignation forced by the Finance Committee of the County Council. The crisis over the Asylum accounts also prompted the resignation of the leading Asylum Visitor from the chair of the powerful Finance Committee at the Council and the Visitors quickly surrendered almost all autonomy over the financial matters which held the key to the effective administration of the institution itself. This marked the real end of an era as the county council took effective charge of the Asylum and the *ancien régime* of Quarter Sessions' control in Asylum affairs passed away.

The revolution in the administrative control of the Devon County Asylum reached from the closing days of Bucknill until the protracted hostility of Lunacy Commissioners, Local Government Board and county councillors led to the resignation of his successor in 1898. The victory was not a simple triumph of centralisation, for the county council had become an important agent for the administration of social services throughout the region. By that point the Poor Law itself was under intense criticism and the terrain of public debate had shifted from lunacy to mental deficiency and the future education of the race.[99] Acland's own concern with education brought him closer to the spirit of the times than Lord Clifford's long experience as an Asylum Visitor in Devon. The Lunacy Commission itself was preoccupied with the 'total institution' model of asylum care that had been pioneered in the era of Shaftesbury and Bucknill and for all its success appears to have become ultimately imprisoned within the same discourse of institutional specification that dominated discussions of the Devon Asylum Committee in the final pre-war years.

The Devon evidence shows that there was not a simple conflict between central and local forces but a subtle interplay in which local and central elements formed alliances or came into conflict whilst such factors as availability of local resources and agenda of regional interest groups interacted with central bodies and purveyors of professional discourse to bring about outcomes. The Lunacy Commission succeeded in manoeuvring locality into providing asylums by a sustained campaign against recalcitrant Devon authorities after the 1845 Act mandated these to provide asylums. The 1888 Local Government Act and Lunacy Act of 1890 led to further increases in the scope allowed for central state regulation and the setting of national standards for the care of those now increasingly called mental patients. Yet the Devon experience also suggests that practical arrangements for the housing of certified pauper lunatics between workhouse, asylum or community continued to be largely set by local Poor Law officials and that resource constraints blunted the drive of the Lunacy Commission and the legislators of 1890 to ensure more rigourous standards in the certification process.

Acknowledgements

The authors would like to thank Peter Bartlett and Bernard Harris for comments on an earlier draft of this work. We are also grateful to Pamela Michael for suggestions as to sources.

NOTES

1 M. Foucault, *Discipline and Punish: The Birth of the Prison*, Harmondsworth, Peregrine, 1979.

2 O.M. MacDonagh, 'The nineteenth century revolution in government: a reappraisal', *Historical Journal*, 1, 1, 1958, pp. 52–67; D. Roberts, *The Victorian Origins of the British Welfare State*, Connecticut, Archon, 1969; M.

Poovey, *The Making of a Social Body: British Cultural Formation, 1830–1864*, Chicago, University of Chicago Press, 1996, essay on revolution in government provides a recent reappraisal of the thesis.

3 A. Scull, *The Most Solitary of Afflictions: Madness and Society in Britain 1700–1900*, New Haven and London, Yale University Press, 1993, p. 45; P. Corrigan, *Social Forms/Human Capacities: Essays in Authority and Difference*, London, Routledge, 1990.

4 J. Prest, *Liberty and Locality*, Oxford, Clarendon, 1990.

5 C. Bellamy, *Administering Central–Local Relations in its Fiscal and Cultural Context*, Manchester, Manchester University Press, 1988; J. Saunders, 'Institutionalised offenders: a study of the Victorian institution and its inmates with special reference to Warwickshire', University of Warwick, Ph.D., unpublished, 1983.

6 Scull, *The Most Solitary of Afflictions*, p. 45.

7 R. Porter, *Mind Forg'd Manacles: A History of Madness in England from the Restoration to the Regency*, London, Athlone, 1987, p. 278.

8 N. Hervey, 'The Lunacy Commission 1845–1860: with special reference to the implementation of policy in Kent and Surrey', Ph.D., unpublished, University of Bristol, 1987; Bellamy, *Administering Central–Local Relations*; Saunders, 'Institutionalised offenders'. For Lunacy Commission approach to the issue of compulsory treatment see P. Fennell, *Treatment Without Consent: Law, Psychiatry and the Treatment of Mentally Disordered People Since 1845*, London, Routledge, 1996, pp. 14–23.

9 P. Bartlett, 'The Poor Law of Lunacy: the administration of pauper lunatics in mid nineteenth century England with special emphasis on Leicestershire and Rutland', University College, London, Ph.D., unpublished, 1993, pp. 266–7, 294.

10 Hervey, 'The Lunacy Commission 1845–1860', pp. 207–8, 275; Bartlett, 'The Poor Law of Lunacy', pp. 266–7.

11 Bartlett, 'The Poor Law of Lunacy', p. 198.

12 D. Mellett, 'Bureaucracy and mental illness: the commissioners in lunacy 1845–1890', *Medical History*, 25, 1981, p. 243.

13 51 and 52 Vict., cap. 41.

14 53 Vict., cap. 5.

15 W. Forsythe, J. Melling, R. Adair, 'The New Poor Law and the county pauper lunatic asylum: the Devon experience 1834–1884', *Social History of Medicine*, 9, 3, 1996, pp. 335–55; see Scull, *The Most Solitary of Afflictions*, p. 142 for resistance movements elsewhere.

16 Bartlett, 'The Poor Law of Lunacy', pp. 295 and 130.

17 8 and 9 Vict., cap. c; Hervey, 'The Lunacy Commission', p. 457.

18 Ibid., p. 276; W. Parry Jones, *The Trade in Lunacy*, Routledge, 1972, p. 20.

19 W. Bynum, R. Porter, M. Shepherd, eds, Introduction to *The Anatomy of Madness: Essays in the History of Psychiatry. Vol. 3: The Asylum and its Psychiatrists*, London, Routledge, 1988, p. 2.

20 The 1834 Poor Law was nationally administered by the Poor Law Commission until 1849, the Poor Law Board until 1871 and the Local Government Board thereafter.

21 Bartlett, 'The Poor Law of Lunacy', p. 295.

22 *3rd Annual Report of the Poor Law Commission, London*, Parliamentary Papers [hereafter PP] 1837, vol. xxxi, p. 2.

23 J. Bucknill in *Asylum Journal*, 1854, 1, cited L. Brizendine, 'British psychiatric reform: a socio-historical study of Devon County Lunatic

Asylum', M.D. Thesis, Yale University, 1981, unpublished, pp. 35–8; A. Digby, 'Moral treatment at the Retreat 1796–1846', in W. Bynum, R. Porter, M. Shepherd, eds, *The Anatomy of Madness: Essays in the History of Psychiatry. Vol. 2: Institutions and Society*, London and New York, Tavistock, 1985, pp. 57–72.

24 R. Hodgkinson, *The Origins of the National Health Service: The Medical Services of the New Poor Law*, London, Wellcome Historical Series, 1967, p. 590; K. Williams, *From Pauperism to Poverty*, London, Routledge and Kegan Paul, 1981, p. 214.

25 Hervey, 'The Lunacy Commission', p. 165.

26 *Further Report of the Commissioners in Lunacy to The Lord Chamberlain*, London, PP 1847–8, vol. xxxii, pp. 121–2, 197, 216; *Eighth Annual Report Lunacy Commission, London*, PP 1854, vol. xxix, pp. 125–9; N. Tomes, 'The great restraint controversy: a comparative perspective on Anglo-American psychiatry in the nineteenth century', in W. Bynum, R. Porter, M. Shepherd, eds, *The Anatomy of Madness: Essays in the History of Psychiatry. Vol. 3: The Asylum and its Psychiatry*, London, Routledge, 1988, pp. 190–225.

27 *Eighth Annual Report Lunacy Commission*, London, PP 1854, vol. xxix, pp. 125–9; *Eleventh Report*, London, PP 1857, Session 2, vol. xvi, pp. 2–3; *Twelfth Report*, London, PP 1857–8, vol. xxiii, p. 8; *Thirteenth Report*, London, PP 1859 Session 2, vol. xiv, pp. 10–11.

28 Devon Record Office [hereafter DRO], *Corporation of the Poor of Exeter Minute Books*, 5.12.1846; *Lunatic Journal*, report of 4.12.1846, noted 5.12.1846, as rationale for using the county asylum.

29 Ibid., 17.7.1849, 20.8.1850, 5.11.1850, 1.11.1853, 31.7.1855, 10.11.1855, 15.1.1856.

30 Ibid., 24.11.1859.

31 Ibid., 8.9.1863, 26.1.1864.

32 Public Record Office [hereafter PRO], Kew, London, *Minute Books of the Commissioners in Lunacy*, MH50, vol. 8, 27.8.1856, 22.10.1856, 10.10.1860.

33 DRO, *Devon Quarter Sessions Minute Books*, 1/31 1857 Epiphany Sessions; J. Bucknill, 'Description of the New House at the Devon County Lunatic Asylum', *Journal of Mental Science*, April 1858, IV, 25, p. 324.

34 PRO, *Minute Books of the Commissioners in Lunacy*, MH50, vol. 8, 27.8.1856; DRO *Devon County Pauper Lunatic Asylum Visitors Minute Book*, Devon Quarter Sessions, 147/2, 2 June 1857; *Eleventh Annual Report Lunacy Commission*, London, PP 1857, Session 2, vol. xvi, pp. 2–3; *Twelfth Annual Report Lunacy Commission*, London, PP 1857–8, vol. xxiii, p. 8.

35 *Eighth Annual Report Lunacy Commission*, London, PP 1854, vol. xxix, pp. 38–9, for cases of Charles Luxmore and Edward Lancey; J. Bucknill, *Journal of Mental Science*, 1855, no. 15, pp. 116–20.

36 *Eleventh Annual Report Lunacy Commission*, London, PP 1857, Session 2, vol. xvi, p. 2; *Thirteenth Annual Report Lunacy Commission*, London, PP 1859, Session 2, vol. xiv, pp. 10–11.

37 Mellett, 'Bureaucracy and mental illness', p. 228; PRO, *Minute Books of the Commissioners in Lunacy*, MH50, vol. 9, 23.9.1857, 9.6.1858, 17.6.1859, 13.12.1860, for tensions over certification between Bucknill and Commission; Hervey, 'Lunacy Commission', p. 190.

38 *Eighth Annual Report Lunacy Commission*, London, PP 1854, vol. xxix, p. 216; *Fourteenth Annual Report Lunacy Commission*, PP 1860, vol. xxxiv, pp. 104–5. By

January 1859 there were 247 men and 324 women plus 11 criminal lunatics housed in an institution built for 400.

39 PRO, *Minute Books of the Commissioners in Lunacy*, MH50, vol. 11, 20.3.1861.

40 Ibid., vol. 11, 10.7.1861, 8.11.1861, 3.12.1861.

41 Ibid., vols 8–10, 28.12.1855, 4.1.1856. The Commission at 10.10.1860 advised the Poor Law Board of their Commissioners' report on the 'prison like rooms in which Lunatics were confined'.

42 Ibid., vol. 12, 23.9.1863, 26.8.1863, 5.1.1864, for correspondence on provisions of 1862 Act.

43 Ibid., vol. 11, 3.12.1861; *Seventeenth Annual Report Lunacy Commission*, London, PP 1863, vol. xx, p. 35; *Eighteenth Annual Report Lunacy Commission*, London, PP 1864, vol. xxiii, p. 8.

44 *Twenty-first Annual Report Lunacy Commission*, London, PP 1867, vol. xviii, p. 128; *Twenty-second Annual Report Lunacy Commission*, London, PP 1867–8, vol. xxxi, pp. 64–5; *Twenty-fifth Annual Report Lunacy Commission*, London, PP 1871, vol. xxvi, p. 148.

45 DRO, *Devon County Pauper Lunatic Asylum Visitors' Minute Book*, Devon Quarter Sessions 147/ 1, 17.4.1869, 22.5.1869.

46 DRO, *Devon County Pauper Lunatic Asylum Visitors' Book*, Devon Quarter Sessions 147/1, 12.8.1870, 10.1.1871; DRO, *Devon Quarter Sessions Minute Books*, 1/3, Epiphany Sessions, 1871 p. 291.

47 *Trewmans Exeter Flying Post*, 9.8.1871, p. 7, col. e; PRO, *Minute Books of the Commissioners in Lunacy*, MH50, vol. 16, 7.3.1871, decide against demanding explanation from Visitors as to leniency shown to guilty steward.

48 Ibid., vol. 13, 12.12.1864.

49 Ibid., vol. 13, 4.6.1866, 9.4.1866.

50 Ibid., vol. 13, 16.10.1866.

51 Ibid., vol. 15, 21.6.1869; vol. 16, 25.10.1869; DRO, *Devon County Pauper Lunatic Asylum Visitors' Minute Books*, Devon Quarter Sessions, 147/2, 11 January 1870.

52 DRO, *Devon Quarter Sessions Minute Books*, 1/33 Epiphany Sessions, 1870 p. 203; DRO, *Devon County Pauper Lunatic Asylum Visitors Minute Books*, 147/2, 16.7.1866, 4.9.1866, 2.4.1867, 3.12.1867.

53 *26th Annual Report Lunacy Commission*, London, PP 1872, vol. xxvii, p. 28; DRO, *Devon Quarter Sessions Minute Books*,1/33, Epiphany Sessions, 1873, p. 440.

54 *29th Annual Report Lunacy Commission*, London, PP 1875, vol. xxxiii, p. 123.

55 *27th Annual Report Lunacy Commission*, London, PP1873, vol. xxx, p. 144, *28th Annual Report Lunacy Commission*, London, PP 1874, vol. xxvii, p. 146, *29th Annual Report Lunacy Commission*, London, PP 1875, vol. xxxiii, p. 123–4, *31st Annual Report Lunacy Commission*, London, PP 1877, vol. xli, pp. 200–1, *35th Annual Report Lunacy Commission*, London, PP 1881, vol. xlviii, p. 211; *31st Annual Report Lunacy Commission*,London, PP 1877, vol. xli, p. 200.

56 *36th Annual Report Lunacy Commission*, London, PP 1882, vol. xxxii, pp. 114–15.

57 Hervey, 'Lunacy Commission', pp. 207–8, 275; Bartlett, 'Poor Law of Lunacy', pp. 266–7.

58 DRO, *Axminster Guardians of the Poor Minute Books*, 3.9.1885.

59 North Devon Record Office [hereafter NDRO], *Barnstaple Guardians of the Poor Minute Books*, 25.11.1887, 2.12.1887; DRO, *Axminster Guardians of the Poor Minute Books*, 3.9.1885; Bartlett, 'The Poor Law of Lunacy', p. 272, for Lutwidge's castigation of the Barnstaple Guardians in the 1850s.

60 DRO, *Okehampton Guardians of the Poor Minute Books*, 3.9.1898, 25.11.1899; NDRO, *Barnstaple Guardians of the Poor Minute Books*, 26.4.1907; *64th Annual Report of the Lunacy Commission*, London, PP 1910, vol. xli, p. 440.
61 Cf. Bartlett, 'Poor Law of Lunacy', p. 198.
62 DRO, *Annual Report Lunatic Asylum*, DQS 1891, 1037M/SS3/2, Ford of Branscombe, p. 17.
63 *46th Annual Report Lunacy Commission*, London, PP 1892, vol. xl, pp. 58, 171; DRO, *Devon County Pauper Lunatic Asylum Visitors Minute Book*, 174/4, 6 August 1895; *46th Annual Report Lunacy Commission*, London, PP 1892, vol. xl, p. 172.
64 DRO, *Devon County Council/ Quarter Sessions/County Council*, 147/4, 30.4.1889, 2.7.1889.
65 Ibid., 7.8.1900, 7.12.1909, 1.9.1914.
66 Ibid., 5.1.92, 6.9.92, 1.11.92, 28.2.93, 26.9.93, 3.10.93.
67 Ibid., Annual Report 13.4.94 at 5.6.94; 5.4.1898, 3.5.98, for case of Ada W.
68 H. Finer, *English Local Government*, London, Methuen, 1945, p. 226 for obligatory committee of Visitors created under the 1890 Lunacy Act.
69 DRO, *Devon County Council Finance Committee*, 154/4/1/2, 23.3.1894.
70 PRO, *Minute Books of the Commissioners in Lunacy*, MH50, vol. 25, 18.11.1891, for Commission's letter of regret to Devon Asylum Committee at 'finding so many matters unfavourably commented on'; DRO, *Devon County Council/Quarter Sessions/County Council*, 147/4, 7.10.90, 4.8.91, 6.10.91.
71 Ibid., 6.10.1896 for Auditors' suggestion that Saunders keep a proper ledger showing the engagement and discharge of attendants.
72 DRO, *Devon County Council Finance Committee*, 154/4/1/2, 1.3.95, 28.5.97, 2.6.97.
73 Ibid., 27.8.97–10.12.97.
74 Ibid., 25.2.1898, 27.5.1898.
75 Ibid., Letter of H.C. Munro of LGB to DCC 12.10.1899.
76 Ibid., Draft reply of letter at 24.3.1899.
77 Ibid. 23.3.1900, 1.6.1900; DRO *Devon County Council Quarter Sessions/County Council*, 147/4, 6.3.1900, 27.3.1900, 5.6.1900.
78 DRO, *Devon County Council Quarter Sessions/County Council*, 147/4, 22.11.1899, 2.1.1900, 6.2.1900, 3.4.1900, 3.7.1900.
79 Ibid., 5.6.1894, 4.12.1894, 6.8.1895, 5.10.1897.
80 Ibid., 7.5.1895, 2.7.1895, 6.8.1895.
81 Ibid., 7.7.1896, 3.11.1896, 4.5.1897.
82 Ibid., 5.10.1897, 2.11.1897.
83 Ibid., 4.1.1898, 1.2.1898, 1.3.1898.
84 Ibid., 3.5.1898.
85 Ibid., 4.4.1905.
86 Ibid., 7.11.1905, 6.3.1906, 7.8.1906, 5.3.1907, 5.5.1908; PRO, *Minute Books of the Commissioners in Lunacy*, MH50, vol. 33, 23.11.1904, 8.3.1905, 22.11.1905, 6.12.1905; vol. 34, 28.3.1906, 4.7.1906, 25.7.1906, for three cases where further enquiry demanded.
87 DRO, *Devon County Council Quarter Sessions/County Council*, 147/4, 6.4.1909; PRO, *Minute Books of the Commissioners in Lunacy*, MH50, vol. 35, 29.4.1908, 17.2.1909; vol. 36, 11.10.1911; vol. 37, 5.11.1913.
88 DRO, *Devon County Council Quarter Sessions/County Council*, 147/4, 6.2.06, 4.9.06, 7.8.06.
89 Ibid., 7.8.1906.

90 NDRO, *Barnstaple Guardians of the Poor Minute Books*, 19.8.1898, 5.5.1911.
91 DRO, *Devon County Council Quarter Sessions/County Council*, 147/4, 1.4.1913.
92 Ibid., 4.1.1910, case of Elias B.
93 Ibid., 1.7.1913, 2.9.1913.
94 Ibid., 2.11.1914.
95 Ibid., 7.4.1914.
96 Minutes of Evidence to *Royal Commission on the Control of the Feebleminded*, London, PP 1908, vol. xxxvi, pp. 38–9, p. 40.
97 D. Garland, *Punishment and Welfare*, Aldershot, Gower, 1985, for wider context of heriditarian discourse in this period.
98 Forsythe *et al.*, 'New Poor Law', pp. 353–5.
99 M. Thomson, ' "Though ever the subject of psychological medicine": pyschiatrists and the colony solution for mental defectives', in H. Freeman and G.E. Berrios, eds, *150 Years of British Psychiatry. Vol. 2: The Aftermath*, London, Athlone, 1996, pp. 130–43.

5

THE DISCHARGE OF PAUPER LUNATICS FROM COUNTY ASYLUMS IN MID-VICTORIAN ENGLAND

The case of Buckinghamshire, 1853–1872

David Wright

On 15 August 1865, Dr William Hayden wrote to the medical superintendent of the Buckinghamshire County Pauper Lunatic Asylum to report on his evaluation of Sarah Slade, who had been released after spending only six months in the county institution. Sarah, the 32-year-old wife of a shepherd from Wycombe, had been sent to the asylum suffering from 'Mania with Depression'. 'I hereby certify that I have visited Sarah Slade & believe her to be of unsound mind', Hayden testified, adding, 'but the Husband seems anxious to keep her at home'. One month later, Mr J. Poole, a surgeon, reported on the lack of improvement of Mary Ann Foley, also lately a patient of the Bucks Asylum. Mary Ann, a 20-year-old 'chaircaner', had been confined for only two months, suffering from 'Melancholia'. 'I certify that I have this day visited Mr Foley's daughter of Denmark St', Poole concluded, 'and [believe] that she is still suffering from mental disease'. Two days later, William Somerset, another Poor Law medical officer, added his comments to the lamentable state of ex-patients: 'I hereby certify that Esther Howard is still very weak', he asserted', '& that there is no improvement in her health or mind'. Despite these dismal medical evaluations, all three ex-patients, who had been released on one month's probation, were formally discharged by the magistrates of the county, with the consent and signature of the medical superintendent.[1] None of them was readmitted.

These letters of Poor Law medical officers give a rare glimpse into the hitherto neglected area of the discharge of lunatics from public asylums in nineteenth-century England. For it is true, that ever since Michel Foucault's *Histoire de la Folie*, social historians of madness have been fixated on *Le Grand Renfermement* of the insane.[2] Debates have raged over the timing of this great confinement, and over the role of the psychiatric profession in the 'capture' of the mad.[3] John Walton was the first to investigate the movement of lunatics in and out of a pauper asylum, arguing that the principal reason for the 'casting out' of insane family members lay in domestic troubles.[4] Since his pioneering work, a veritable deluge of research on the Victorian pauper asylums has emerged, exploring such topics as the role of prison medical officers in identifying the mentally disabled, the work of Poor Law officials as intermediaries in the process of confinement, and the disparate rates of incarceration from different Poor Law Unions.[5] Moreover, historians are beginning to look at the 'disposal' of sub-groups of the pauper insane, such as women, children and the aged.[6] Case studies of voluntary institutions have also revealed an interdependence of the community and family in the confinement of 'respectable', non-pauper patients.[7] Even the movement of private patients into and out of licensed homes was subject to a delicate negotiation between the family and the proprietor.[8] Notwithstanding the immense importance of this research, most investigation has been overwhelmingly concentrated on the social process of confinement rather than discharge. Walton summed up the attitude of medical historians to the release of patients by stating: 'There is less to say about "bringing back" in this context, largely because there was so little of it.'[9]

This chapter, therefore, hopes to act as a searchlight on this hitherto neglected area of the social history of madness. It will argue that discharge from a county asylum was an important social phenomenon that affected over 65,000 people in England and Wales[10] during the mid-Victorian period. It will show that the release of patients was not age- or gender-specific. Moreover, the criteria for discharge were not solely based on an objective 'medical' evaluation of the patient made by the alienist; rather, it depended on a consideration of the ability and willingness of the inmates' family to receive the person back into the household, the number of unoccupied beds in the asylum, the views of magistrates about public safety, and the financial interests of Poor Law Guardians.

This chapter will begin by surveying the general pattern of patients released from county and borough asylums in England and Wales during the Victorian period, and outline the legal structures enshrined to regulate the discharge of lunatics. It will then explore the length of stay, discharge from, and readmission of, patients to the Buckinghamshire County Pauper Lunatic Asylum in the years 1853–72. Lastly, it will use surviving letters from Poor Law officers to the medical superintendent of the Buckinghamshire Asylum to reveal how the system of probation worked in individual cases. The database study of 1,500 admissions supports the view of Stephen Garton who commented that public asylums, during the period of industrialisation, 'were not merely custodial, they also served as a temporary place of refuge for a significant number of patients each year'.[11] Over one-half of patients admitted to the Buckinghamshire Asylum were discharged from the institution, two-thirds of these within the first year. Moreover, the actual process of discharge was not an arbitrary decision with little consultation. Rather, it was a subtle procedure that took into account the mental state of the patient, the ability and willingness of the family to accommodate the lunatic back into the household, the financial consequences of the patient's continued stay and any potential threat to public safety. Although individual cases of discharge were mediated by local factors and the priorities of Poor Law Unions, this chapter argues that the phenomenon of discharge from public asylums was similar both within and without England and Wales.

Discharging lunatics in mid-Victorian England

Historical perceptions of the Victorian asylum system in England and Wales have undergone profound changes in the last decade, as intense academic scrutiny has been turned to the social history of patients, patterns of confinement, and the history of clinical psychiatry, to name just three very productive areas.[12] Within this emerging new consensus on the social uses of the asylum during the period of industrialisation, researchers have slowly and self-consciously reoriented the asylum from a 'medical' to a 'pauper' institution. In particular, academics have challenged the thesis, proposed by Andrew Scull, that the trajectory of asylumdom was largely the result of a self-conscious effort of the medical profession to expand its own professional domain.[13] Rather, it has been argued recently that the evolution of the county asylums, as pauper institutions, depended greatly on the relationship between Poor Law Guardians (who were required to pay for treatment of their lunatics) and county magistrates (required by law to administer the implementation of the Lunacy Acts) as they both responded to the incessant public demand for secure accommodation for the insane.[14] Although historians may differ about the priority given to the role of Poor Law officials, it is now undeniable that the county asylum system in England and Wales was influenced by the workings of the New Poor Law.

The Poor Law Amendment Act of 1834 reshaped the administration of poor relief in England and Wales. The New Poor Law, as it has come to be known, reorganised over 13,000 parishes into 660 Poor Law Unions, and replaced the Overseers of the Poor with elected Poor Law Guardians. Union Guardians were responsible only for destitute persons who had settlement in parishes within their Union, though financing remained the responsibility of individual parishes until 1865, when funding was transferred to a general Union common fund. According to the 1834 Act, the relief of destitution, directed by the Guardians, was supposed to be centred on the workhouse, and this 'indoor relief' was to be administered on the basis of 'less eligibility' – that is, that relief would be lower than that earned by the poorest able-bodied labourers. The centrepiece of the new system was meant to be the Union workhouse, which acted as the institutional focus of the activities of the local relieving officer and the local medical officer, both hired by, and responsible to, the Union Guardians. As historians have shown, however, the implementation of the New Poor Law was neither straightforward nor systematic. The workhouses themselves did not become occupied by the able-bodied and their families. Rather, these institutions became filled with the sick, disabled, aged and insane. In some cases, these 'non-able-bodied' individuals comprised 80 per cent or more of the workhouse population, and included significant numbers of lunatics, idiots and persons of unsound mind.[15]

The asylum system in nineteenth-century England and Wales was a mix of the new and the old, utilising existing structures of relief whilst establishing novel forms of confinement. The 1808 Asylums Act permitted county magistrates to erect asylums for their pauper insane and charge Overseers of the Poor for the maintenance of lunatics who had settlement in their parishes. Committees of magistrates were responsible for the construction and financing of these new institutions, and, after 1811, for ensuring that all patients admitted to the asylum had been certified as insane by a medical practitioner. Successive amendment acts between 1811 and 1845 extended the remit of magistrates and the system of certification and visiting. Two acts of 1845 – the Lunatics Act and the Asylums Act – enshrined a comprehensive and national system of provision, inspection, certification and licensing. The Asylums Act obliged all counties and boroughs that had not already done so to erect institutions for their pauper insane. A county 'Visiting Committee' of magistrates was responsible for the management of the pauper institution and for quarterly inspections. These two Acts thus gave a great deal of power to magistrates over the confinement process. However, the influence of magistrates was mediated by the Poor Law structures upon which they depended for co-operation. For instance, it was Poor Law relieving officers who were responsible for arranging for the conveyance of lunatics to the county institution, and signing the Reception Orders for new and readmissions. After 1853, Poor Law medical officers did most of the certification. By doing so, relieving officers and medical officers were acting on behalf of Poor Law Guardians, who were responsible for paying the maintenance of all lunatics chargeable to a Union parish.[16]

The administration of county pauper lunatic asylums thus depended on a constant negotiation and co-operation between county magistrates and local Poor Law officials. Unfortunately, unlike the extensive literature on the New Poor Law, little sustained research has been carried out on the operation of the county Visiting Committees.[17] By law, the Visiting Committee was responsible for the establishment and operation of asylums for the insane poor who had settlement in a parish within the boundaries of their respective county or borough. Their duties included the construction of the asylum, its financing, and the hiring of medical officers. The Visiting Committees normally met at their asylums, and discussed matters concerning the operation of the institution with the medical superintendent, who was himself responsible for the hiring and firing of staff, compiling the administrative returns required by the Lunacy Commissioners, and ministering to patients. Despite the authority which resident medical superintendents had within the institution, power over the admission and discharge of all non-criminal and non-Chancery lunatics, however, ultimately remained in the hands of these magistrates.

Magistrates serving on the Visiting Committees, and medical men placed in charge of county asylums, were constrained by a handful of laws regarding the discharge of certified pauper[18] lunatics during the period under study. The 1853 Regulation of Lunatics Act required medical superintendents to give notice to the Visiting Committee that inmates had recovered their wits. If the recovered lunatic had not been discharged within fourteen days, the medical superintendent was also supposed to give notice to the Commissioners in Lunacy explaining why this had not occurred.[19] The medical superintendent thus had a legal duty to report the recovery of one of his patients. The Lunatic Asylums (Amendment) Act of the same year stated clearly that it was lawful, and indeed encouraged, for Visitors or the superintendents to write to the Union Guardians in which the lunatic resided (prior to confinement) to notify them when they intended to discharge a patient back into the community. Standard forms, prescribed by the Lunacy Commissioners, provided the basis for (immediate) discharges, discharges on probation, and discharges after probation.[20] Relatives could also request the discharge of a patient, regardless of whether the patient was deemed to be improved or not. This required a separate form and personal undertaking.[21] The medical superintendent had the right to refuse the request for a discharge if he felt that the patient in question was 'dangerous and unfit to be at large', but the alienist in turn could be overruled by the Visiting Committee.[22]

Discharge could therefore be precipitated by one of two agents: by order of the medical superintendent or by request of the family. The county of Buckinghamshire offers an example of how this worked in practice. John Humphrey, the medical superintendent of the county asylum during this period, reported in his medical journal any patients who were 'so far recovered in their senses' that they were fit enough to be discharged.[23] With the Visiting Committee's approval, the clerk would write to the Poor Law Union in which the insane person resided, to enquire as to the conditions of the inmates' household. Although there is no direct evidence of this, notes in medical case books and letters imply that the Poor Law relieving officer conveyed this news to the inmates' family, who then expressed a willingness, or not, to receive the insane person back into the household. The relieving officer then instructed the clerk of the Union to write back to the Visiting Committee to this effect. Provided members of the Visiting Committee were satisfied all was in order, two magistrates signed the appropriate discharge order with the 'consent' of the medical superintendent, commanding the latter to release the patient either permanently or subject to one month's probation.[24] The magistrates gave an allowance in order to assist a patient's reintegration back into the community. Like the general maintenance of a lunatic in the institution, this allowance was normally charged to the parish of settlement.[25]

The second, and less common, route out of the asylum occurred in cases when the family of insane persons demanded the latter's discharge, regardless of the 'mental' or 'physical' state of the lunatics themselves. Again, this seems to have involved the local relieving officer or clerk of the Union acting as intermediary, though sometimes the family wrote directly to the magistrates or the medical superintendent. Thus Edward Allen, a labourer, petitioned the Buckinghamshire Visiting Committee in 1860 for the discharge of his wife, Elizabeth, who had been admitted five months earlier suffering from 'Mania'. By law, persons requesting the discharge of an insane relative had to sign a declaration that the lunatic would not be 'chargeable to any Union, Parish or County' and, after discharge, 'shall be properly taken care of and shall be prevented from doing injury to (her)self and others'.[26]

Edward signed this declaration, and the justices ordered Elizabeth's release on 22 February 1860. As stated earlier, magistrates could refuse a discharge request. But this situation rarely happened: few families requested the release of a member who was so violent as to be a danger to themselves and the community.[27] Discharges by request, or 'removals' as they were often termed, were infrequent, and constitute fewer than 8 per cent of the total number discharged.[28]

The demographics of discharge from the Buckinghamshire County Pauper Asylum

As stated earlier, the discharge of lunatics has tended to be either ignored or dismissed as a phenomenon affecting relatively few individuals. This lacuna owes much to the characterisation of asylums as 'museums of madness', bins where the refuse of society were dumped or locked away. A brief overview of the returns of the Commissioners in Lunacy shows that this thesis cannot be sustained by empirical scrutiny. Figure 5.1 represents the number of discharges from county and borough asylums in selected years between 1854 and 1872, revealing that 65,124 discharges occurred during this period, a figure in excess of one-half (51.6 per cent) of the total number of admissions. Further, as recent research has shown, the proportion of admissions who were first admissions remained about 85–90 per cent throughout the second half of the nineteenth century.[29] Thus, discharges were not a prelude to readmission and permanent confinement, or to a 'revolving door' syndrome which has characterised most post-war mental health services. Extrapolating from these returns, and assuming an average readmission rate of 20–25 per cent of discharges (10–15 per cent of total admissions), one may estimate that no fewer than 60,000 people in England and Wales were discharged from asylums at least once during the period under study. Discharge from county asylums was thus an important dimension to the social history of madness and to the Victorian asylum system.

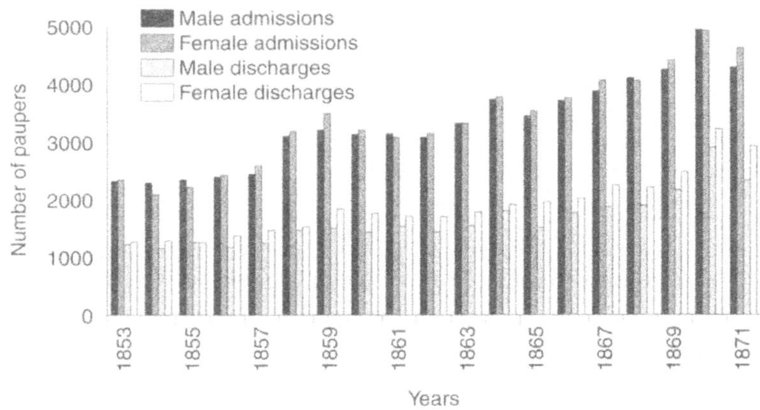

Figure 5.1 Total number of paupers admitted to and discharged from county pauper lunatic asylums, England and Wales, 1853–1872

Source: Annual Reports of the Commissioners in Lunacy, 1854–1873.

A case study of Buckinghamshire reveals this pattern in local detail. The Buckinghamshire County Pauper Lunatic Asylum was established in 1853, some eight years after the 1845 Asylums Act obliged county magistrates to make provision for their indigent insane. Situated in the parish of Stone, just outside the county capital of Aylesbury, the asylum was an unimpressive two-storey building established to accommodate 200–250 patients from this predominantly rural, agrarian county linking the Metropolis and the Midlands.[30] Prior to the erection of the asylum it is clear that Poor Law Guardians of the county had used private licensed homes in Middlesex, as well as unoccupied beds in the Northampton voluntary asylum to house their most troublesome lunatics. The rest of those who were transported to the asylum in the first few months after its completion in 1853 must be assumed to have been housed in one of the seven Union workhouses, or sequestered at home.

An extensive database analysis of the first twenty years of the asylum (n=1,492 patients), based on information taken from the Buckinghamshire Asylum admission registers, elicits a number of immediate and startling findings. First, of the patients admitted to the asylum, 726 (48.6 per cent) were discharged, 705 (47.2 per cent) died there, 56 (3.8 per cent) were transferred to other institutions, and seven lunatics escaped.[31] Since transfers from another institution shortly after admission might artificially deflate the length of stay in the asylum, Figure 5.2 summarises the changing length of stay, by gender, of all non-transfer pauper patients.[32] The median length of stay for male pauper lunatics fluctuated between 10 and 15 months over the period under study; for women there was a dramatic augmentation in the median length of stay in the 1860s to above a median of 20 months before abating and converging to roughly the same levels as male lunatics. The low median length of stay provides further evidence, if further evidence is needed, of the now established phenomenon of short-stay patients to which Laurence Ray alerted us some 20 years ago.[33] Moreover, discharged patients tended to remain in the institution for even shorter periods of time than Figure 5.2 would suggest. Three-quarters of discharged patients resided in the institution under one year, thereby contradicting the suspicion that length of stay appears artificially low because of high

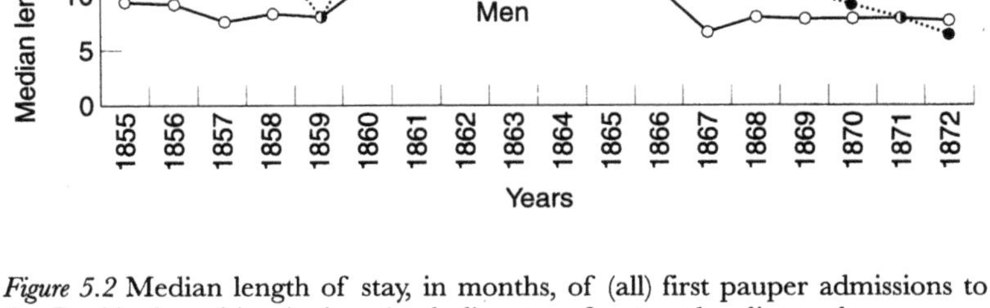

Figure 5.2 Median length of stay, in months, of (all) first pauper admissions to the Buckinghamshire Asylum (excluding transfers to other licensed institutions), in yearly cohorts with a three year moving average, 1853–72 (n= 1,565)

Sources: Medical Registers of Admissions, St John's Hospital (Buckinghamshire Asylum), Buckinghamshire County Record Office (BuRO), AR 100/89/49–53; Alphabetical List of Patients, St John's Hospital, BuRO AR 100/89/64–65; Medical Register of Discharges and Deaths, St John's Hospital, BuRO AR 100/89/69–71.

institutional mortality rates (see Table 5.1). In fact, just the opposite – excluding those who died in the asylum actually lowers the patients' median length of stay considerably.

Table 5.1 Length of stay of paupers discharged from the Buckinghamshire Asylum, first discharges only[34] the first two decadal cohorts (1853–1872)

	Men	%	*Women*	%
<12 months	236	72.6	285	75.0
1–2 years	33	10.2	45	11.8
2–5 years	33	10.2	46	12.1
5–10 years	16	4.9	17	4.5
>10 years	7	2.2	7	1.8
n/a	0	0.0	12	3.2
	325		412	

Sources: Medical Registers of Admissions, St John's Hospital (Buckinghamshire Asylum), Buckinghamshire County Record Office (BuRO), AR 100/89/49–53; Alphabetical List of Patients, St John's Hospital, BuRO AR 100/89/64–65; Medical Register of Discharges and Deaths, St John's Hospital, BuRO AR 100/89/69–71.

Table 5.2 Age (at time of admission) of paupers admitted to, and discharged from, the Buckinghamshire County Asylum, first admissions only, 1853–1872

	Men				*Women*			
	Admitted		*Discharged*		*Admitted*		*Discharged*	
		%		%		%		%
<20	53	7.4	22	9.1	40	5.1	14	4.5
20–29	141	19.8	53	22.0	152	19.2	75	24.0
30–39	140	19.6	46	19.1	172	21.8	75	24.0
40–49	133	18.7	51	21.2	149	18.9	60	19.2
50–59	97	13.6	43	17.8	135	17.1	50	16.0
>59	149	20.9	26	10.8	142	18.0	38	12.2
	713		241		790		312	

Sources: Medical Registers of Admissions, St John's Hospital (Buckinghamshire Asylum), Buckinghamshire County Record Office (BuRO), AR 100/89/49–53; Alphabetical List of Patients, St John's Hospital, BuRO AR 100/89/64–65; Medical Register of Discharges and Deaths, St John's Hospital, BuRO AR 100/89/69–71.

An analysis of the ages of those who were eventually discharged patients defies stereotyping. In fact, these results show that, in the case of Buckinghamshire, anyone admitted under the age of 50 had, *ceteris paribus*, an equal chance of being discharged. Over the age of 50, and especially over the age of 60, the chances of leaving the asylum alive, diminished.[35] Fully one-quarter of all those discharged from the asylum were over the age of 50 (see Table 5.2).

In conclusion, therefore, the quantitative results of the Buckinghamshire case study reveal a diverse group of inmates who were eventually discharged; to generalise, as many as one-third of total admissions stayed fewer than twelve months and then were released back into the community. Moreover, only 159 (24 per cent) of those discharged were ever readmitted to the institution. If this is replicated in other large-scale regional studies based on admission registers, it will be necessary significantly to re-evaluate the asylum and its social uses in the Victorian period.[36]

Returning to the community

The Lunacy Commissioners estimated that the average cost of asylum accommodation in the late 1840s was 8s. per week compared to 3s. per week for workhouse accommodation and less for outdoor relief.[37] By 1856, the *Journal of Mental Science* put the average cost of asylum treatment at 11–12s. per week.[38] Needless to say, successive lunacy laws from 1808 to 1853, which gave magistrates power to order the institutional committal of a lunatic and placed legal obligations on Poor Law officials to report dangerous lunatics, infringed on the prerogative of Poor Law officials. Since asylum accommodation cost three times as much as workhouse provision, and five times as much as outdoor relief, disagreements naturally arose over who actually were persons 'fit to be taken under care and control'. Some Poor Law Unions ignored or evaded the spirit of these laws, whilst others, as Forsythe *et al.* have shown, took different positions as to the necessity of institutional confinement.[39] Despite the apparent differential confinement of lunatics by Unions, few Guardians, it would seem, had any vested interest in seeing their pauper lunatics languish in county institutions *after* they had recovered their senses. Magistrates, on the other hand, were involved in what Peter Bartlett has described as an attempt to reassert control over local governance through the operation of the lunacy laws. They seemed to guard their power jealously, and act conservatively when it came to disputed cases of discharge.[40] Their prime role was to ensure public safety and to act in the interest of the patient concerned. Unless they were Poor Law Guardians as well as magistrates, members of the Visiting Committee did not feel the direct impact of the financial consequences of institutionalisation, leading one historian to suggest that this was one of the reasons for the dramatic growth of resident lunatics in the British Isles compared to elsewhere.[41]

The medical superintendents, it would seem, had a more ambivalent attitude towards the discharge of patients. Andrew Scull has argued that the medical superintendents did not actively prevent the rapid expansion of their asylums, since professional prestige was associated with large public medical establishments.[42] Although the members of the newly formed Association of Medical Officers of Asylums and Hospitals for the Insane, the forerunner to the Royal Medico-Psychological Association, benefited from their administrative control over these new institutions, there seems little evidence to suggest that they acted to retard the discharge of patients. Perhaps if patients were few and far between, medical superintendents may have had an incentive to act conservatively over the release of patients; but the incessant demand for accommodation and the chronic shortage of beds made this unnecessary. Moreover, it is clear from articles in the *Journal of Mental Science*, that medical superintendents were becoming frustrated in the 1850s and 1860s by what they considered to be the confinement of 'incurable' patients in their 'therapeutic' institutions. Discharges reinforced in their minds, and in the minds of the public, the efficacy of institutional treatment. Low cure rates were a source of some embarrassment. On balance, most medical superintendents, like Poor Law authorities, had no vested interest in keeping patients in the institution beyond the point at which their condition made them amenable to release. Indeed Richard Hunter found that, in the case of Colney Hatch, medical superintendents sometimes had to go to great lengths to persuade reluctant magistrates that certain 'dischargeable' inmates had some friend or relative able and willing to take care of them if and when they were released.[43]

The letters from Poor Law medical officers to the medical superintendents, three of which were quoted at the beginning of this chapter, give some insight into the most elusive dimension of discharge: the role and attitudes of the family as they negotiated with Poor Law and Lunacy authorities. Affixed randomly amongst the discharge orders, these letters reveal a consistent policy of consultation between the medical superintendent of the Buckinghamshire Asylum and the Poor Law medical officers of the Buckinghamshire Unions. These same Poor Law medical officers were important in the confinement process itself. Working solely, or in concert with other medical practitioners, they were responsible, after 1853, for certifying most lunatics destined for the county asylum.[44] They often had a knowledge, therefore, of the person and the family involved, and acted as conduits between households and institutional medical authority. Their assessment of the state of an ex-patient was therefore often based on some prior knowledge and experience. Sensitive to the wishes of the family, and the financial considerations of their employers, Poor Law medical officers had to balance a range of interests. An absence of dangerousness, suicidal intentionality or violence towards others, combined with the desire and ability of family members to care for and control an afflicted person, were sufficient conditions to confirm that a discharge was satisfactory. Indeed, some of the letters from local doctors imply that they took it upon themselves to ensure in the first order that the person was being cared for and not 'at large', and only later to express an opinion about the recovery of the person's faculties.[45]

A rather extensive letter shows the range of emotions and priorities of the family as expressed by the Poor Law medical officer, and deserves, for its richness, to be quoted in full:

> Dear Sir, 11 July 1854
>
> I beg to send you the report requested in your letter of the 8th June last relative to the demeanour & state of Ann Clark who has been probationally discharged from the Bucks Lunatic Asylum.
>
> Mr Duke the Medical Officer for the district in which she is residing states that she is much the same as when she came out – perfectly harmless but low & despondingly fanciful. That, for instance, whilst she was in the Asylum a Child of hers died at home of Fever & she fancies she was the cause of its death from not having attended to it herself – that she appears to have a great horror of being sent back – that her attendant daughter thinks her as well mentally as when she left the asylum – that her bodily health is not quite so good. The relieving officer says he considers Ann Clark better mentally & bodily – that she tells him she is better in health – that she says she thinks she shall not have to go back to the Asylum – & that he considers she may well be allowed to stay home.
>
> Clerk to the Buckingham Guardians[46]

Letters are always a problematic source for historians. Unlike the discharge orders and admission papers, which were required for all inmates who ever had the fortune or misfortune to find themselves in a licensed institution, the relative scarcity of letters to the superintendent naturally raises questions of representativeness and selection. Having said that, they do offer a rich qualitative source which provides hints to the subtle negotiations inherent in the discharge process. If the letters from Poor Law medical officers to the Buckinghamshire superintendents do reflect a wider attitude on behalf of local officials, it lends weight to the hypothesis that economic and affective considerations, concerns over social order, and the operation of the local Poor Law, played more of a part than 'medical' evaluations in the movement of lunatics out of and into these controversial institutions.

Conclusions

Andrew Scull, in his influential work on the social organisation of insanity in nineteenth-century England characterised the Buckinghamshire Asylum as typical of most provincial institutions, stating that, after the ascension of Humphrey in 1856, it 'became just another custodial institution'.[47] Scull is half right. Buckinghamshire was typical in many respects of asylums which had been established in the wake of the 1845 Acts. Its founders underestimated the demand for accommodation; it became full shortly after it opened its doors; and the therapeutic optimism of the first medical superintendents gave way to pessimism and acrimony. But he is incorrect in his assertion that it was primarily custodial in function.[48] Over one-half of all those admitted to the Buckinghamshire Asylum between 1853 and 1872 were discharged, the vast majority of them having stayed fewer than twelve months. Since readmission rates were low (fewer than one in four), one must assume that the asylum was but one, albeit, important dimension to patterns of care and control which existed before confinement and after discharge.

The results are very similar to the other studies of the confinement of pauper lunatics in licensed institutions,[49] some of which are represented in this volume; indeed, the revelation that three-quarters of all discharged patients had stayed fewer than twelve months has been replicated in studies of public asylums outside England and Wales for roughly the same period. Mark Finnane and Stephen Garton both discovered that 80 per cent of patients (who were discharged) had stayed for fewer than twelve months in the Omagh County Asylum, Ireland, and the asylum of New South Wales, Australia. Georges Klein and Jacques Gasser computed a figure of 74 per cent for the Swiss Canton of Vaud. Allan Beveridge found between 40 per cent and 60 per cent were discharged from the Royal Edinburgh Asylum within the first six months alone.[50] Other information on South Carolina, Quebec, and other asylums, though not strictly comparable, suggests a very similar pattern of release.[51] Notwithstanding the mediating factors of local decision-making, the remarkable similarities of length of stay, confinement and discharge of lunatics to and from public asylums in different national contexts suggest that the factors shaping these controversial institutions must have been embedded in broader trans-national social, economic and demographic forces.

In his study of the mammoth Middlesex Asylum at Colney Hatch, Richard Hunter concluded that superintendents 'had no control over admissions, never saw patients before they came in, and could only advise when a patient was well enough to be discharged'.[52] Whilst he is correct about the distinct lack of control of alienists over the admission process, this research would suggest that medical men did have a significant role to play in the discharge of lunatics. In the case of Bucks, Humphrey identified patients who had 'recovered their senses', made lists of patients ready to be discharged and brought them to the attention of the Visiting magistrates, and conferred with Poor Law medical officers over the state of probationary discharges. Cross-referencing those people whom he identified in his medical log with the people actually discharged, this researcher could not find any instances where his opinion was over-ruled by the Visiting Committee magistrates. Thus unlike admission, which might, in England and Wales, vary depending upon the priority of Poor Law Unions, and the certification of lunatics, which by law had to be completed by a medical practitioner unassociated with the receiving institution, the process of discharge did involve the medical superintendents in an important and novel way. Indeed, along with the diagnosis of patients, and the direction of treatment, identifying patients for discharge was one of the few areas in which medical superintendents could attempt to establish an expertise in the new field of mental disease.

After leaving the asylum, local Poor Law relieving officers and medical officers were integral to the assessment of the ex-patient. As the letters to the medical superintendents have shown, Poor Law medical officers, many of whom had signed the certificate of insanity for the lunatic about to be admitted to the county institution, were also responsible for confirming his or her safety in the community. Part of the judgement of these local practitioners was based on mental ability, but Poor Law medical officers were also concerned with assessing the ability and willingness of the family to care for the person within the household. Provided there was no threat to public safety, neither Poor Law Guardians nor magistrates had any desire to prolong institutional confinement. And, there is no evidence whatever in the case of Buckinghamshire to support the contention that medical superintendents purposefully prolonged the stay of any patients. It is possible, however, that, as asylums increased in size, medical superintendents became more alienated from their inmates and consequently less efficient and effective at identifying recovered lunatics.

What happened to patients after discharge? It is unlikely that more than a handful of those who were discharged were admitted, at a later date, to a different county institution – the differentially higher cost charged for 'non-county' lunatics made this prohibitive to parishes and Unions. There may, however, have been a proportion of discharges who were readmitted to the local workhouse – although the social implications of this may also have made this option undesirable for some families. Research into the movement of chronic cases back to the Union workhouses, especially when the county asylums reached their capacity in the 1860s, is most needed. Moreover, one cannot assume that care in the household was a benign or beneficial alternative. The period of restraint, seclusion, caring or treatment may well have continued outside the institution in informal ways, and outside the purview, except in extreme cases of abuse or neglect, of the Lunacy Commissioners. Needless to say, a history of this 'care in the community' is beyond the scope of this chapter. Rather, this research underlines the important fact that large numbers of patients were discharged during the Victorian period, families were willing and able to receive ex-patients back into the household, and that this social process represents an important and neglected area in the social history of madness.

Acknowledgements

This essay has been generously supported by a Wellcome Trust University Award.

NOTES

1 Letters of 15 August 1865, 13 October 1865 and 15 October 1865. Discharge Papers of the Buckinghamshire County Pauper Lunatic Asylum [St John's Hospital], Buckinghamshire County Record Office (BuRO) AR 100/89/117.

2 M. Foucault, *Histoire de la folie à l'âge classique*, Paris, Librairie Plon, 1961, chapter two.

3 For three different views of the asylum system in nineteenth-century England, see A. Scull, *The Most Solitary of Afflictions: Madness and Society in Britain, 1700–1900*, London, Yale University Press, 1993; K. Jones, *Asylums and After: A Revised History of the Mental Health Services*, London, Athlone,

1993; D. Mellett, *The Prerogative of Asylumdom: Social, Cultural and Administrative Aspects of the Institutional Treatment of the Insane in Nineteenth Century Britain*, London, Garland, 1982.

4 J. Walton, 'Casting out and bringing back in Victorian England: pauper lunatics, 1840–70', in W. F. Bynum, R. Porter and M. Shepherd, eds, *The Anatomy of Madness: Essays in the History of Psychiatry, vol. 2*, London, Tavistock, 1985, pp. 132–46; Walton, 'Lunacy in the Industrial Revolution: a study of asylum admissions in Lancashire, 1848–1850', *Journal of Social History*, 13, 1979, pp. 1–22; Walton, 'The treatment of pauper lunatics in Victorian England: the case of Lancaster Asylum, 1816–1870', in Scull, ed., *Mad-Houses, Mad-Doctors and Madmen: the Social History of Psychiatry in the Victorian Era*, London, University of Pennsylvania, Press, 1981, pp. 166–97.

5 J. Saunders, 'Institutionalised offenders – a study of the Victorian institution and its inmates, with special reference to late-nineteenth-century Warwickshire', unpublished Ph.D. thesis, University of Warwick, 1983; P. Bartlett, 'The Poor Law of Lunacy: the administration of pauper lunatics in mid-nineteenth-century England with special reference to Leicestershire and Rutland', unpublished Ph.D. thesis, University College, London, 1993; B. Forsythe, J. Melling and R. Adair, 'The New Poor Law and the county pauper lunatic asylum – the Devon experience 1834–1884', *Social History of Medicine*, 9, 1996, pp. 335–55; R. Adair, B. Forsythe and J. Melling, 'A danger to the public? Disposing of pauper lunatics in late-Victorian and Edwardian England: Plympton St Mary Union and the Devon County Asylum, 1867–1914', *Medical History*, 42, 1988, pp. 1–25.

6 For gender and confinement see K. Davies, ' "Sexing the mind?": women, gender and madness in nineteenth-century Welsh asylums', *Llafur – Journal of Welsh Labour History/Cylchgrawn Hanes Llafur Cymru*, 7, 1996, pp. 29–40; For child lunatics, see J. Melling, R. Adair and B.Forsythe, ' "A proper lunatic for two years": pauper lunatic children in Victorian and Edwardian England: child admissions to the Devon County Asylum, 1845–1914', *Journal of Social History*, 31, 1997, pp. 371–405.

7 A. Digby, *Madness, Morality and Medicine: A Study of the York Retreat*, Cambridge, Cambridge University Press, 1985, chapters 8 and 9; D. Wright, 'Families strategies and the institutional committal of idiot children in Victorian England', *Journal of Family History*, 23, 1998, pp. 189–208.

8 C. MacKenzie, 'Social Factors in the admission, discharge, and continuing stay of patients at Ticehurst Asylum, 1845–1917', in Bynum *et al.*, eds, *The Anatomy of Madness. Vol. 2*, pp. 147–74; MacKenzie, 'Psychology for the rich: a history of the private madhouse at Ticehurst in Sussex, 1792–1917', *Psychological Medicine*, 48, 1988, pp. 545–9; MacKenzie, *Psychiatry for the Rich: A History of the Private Ticehurst Asylum, 1792–1917*, London, Routledge, 1992.

9 Walton, 'Casting out and bringing back', p. 141.

10 There is now an overwhelming body of literature on the confinement of the insane in different national contexts, so the remainder of this chapter will concentrate on the history and historiography of the asylum system in England and Wales. A discussion of discharge as it related to other countries is beyond the scope of this chapter, but see concluding remarks.

11 S. Garton, *Medicine and Madness: A Social History of Insanity in New South Wales, 1880–1940*, Kensington, Aus., 1988, p. 36.

12 G. Berrios and H. Freeman, eds, *150 Years of British Psychiatry, 1841–1991*, London, Gaskell, 1991; Berrios and Freeman, eds, *150 Years of British Psychiatry, 1841–1991. Vol. 2: The Aftermath*, London, Athlone, 1996; Berrios and R. Porter, eds, *A History of Clinical Psychiatry: The Origin and History of Psychiatric Disorders*, London, Athlone, 1996; E. Shorter, *A History of Psychiatry: From the Era of the Asylum to the Age of Prozac*, New York, John Wiley, 1997.

13 A. Scull, 'From madness to mental illness: medical men as moral entrepreneurs', *European Journal of Sociology*, 11, 1975, pp. 219–61.

14 Bartlett, 'The Poor Law of Lunacy'; Forsythe *et al.* 'The New Poor Law and the county pauper lunatic asylum', *passim*; and chapters in this volume.

15 'The indoor population of our workhouses has been brought to such a condition' wrote Ernest Hart, 'that in a metropolitan [work]house an average of nine-tenths are chronically infirm and disabled, imbecile, or acutely sick.' E. Hart, 'An account of the condition of the infirmaries of London workhouses' [reprinted from the Fortnightly Review], London, 1866, p. 4. For a survey of literature on the New Poor Law, see A. Digby, *The Poor Law in Nineteenth-Century England*, London, Historical Association, 1982.

16 D. Wright, 'The certification of insanity in nineteenth-century England', *History of Psychiatry*, 9, 1998, in press.

17 K. Fields, 'The visiting committee of magistrates in Oxfordshire', unpublished Oxford M.Phil. thesis, 1994.

18 This chapter will not discuss the process of discharge and removal of criminal lunatics or Chancery lunatics, who were relatively rare in county pauper lunatic asylums, or the discharge of 'private' patients.

19 Fourteen days is consistent with other statutes governing the confinement of lunatics in the Victorian era. For instance, fourteen days was the maximum time allowed for a dangerous lunatic to be detained in workhouses, and the maximum time allowed between the certification of insane persons and their lawful confinement. 16 and 17 Vict., c. 96, 'For the regulation of the care and treatment of lunatics', s. xix.

20 Form No. 2: Probationary Discharge, Form No. 4: Discharge of a Patient after Probation, and Form No. 6: Discharge of a Patient, 16 and 17 Vict., c. 97, s. 79.

21 Form No. 5: Discharge – on undertaking of Relative, 8 and 9 Vict., c. 126, s. 65.

22 16 and 17 Vict., c. 97, Lunatic Asylums (Amendment) Act, 1853, s. 80 and ss. 83–5.

23 Medical Journal, St John's Hospital, BuRO AR 100/89/30.

24 Discharge on one month's probation seems to have been practised widely, see Richard Hunter, *Psychiatry for the Poor. 1851 Colney Hatch Asylum. Friern Hospital 1973: A Medical and Social History*, London, 1974, p. 17.

25 A charge of between 7s. and 10s. per week, depending upon the asylum. The magistrates in Upper Canada also adopted the policy of giving an 'allowance' to recently discharged inmates. See W. Mitchinson, 'The Toronto and Gladesville Asylums: humane alternatives for the insane in Canada and Australia?', *Bulletin of the History of Medicine*, 63, 1989, p. 70.

26 Form No. 5a: Application for Discharge of a Lunatic on Undertaking of Relative.

27 Although sometimes magistrates might investigate the household if they were unconvinced of the ability of the applicant to care for the discharged

person. Two cases occurred in Oxfordshire. In the 1850s a son requested his father's discharge from the Littlemore Asylum and was refused because the visiting justices judged that the boy was incapable of supporting his father 'in a suitable manner'. In another instance, the Oxfordshire magistrates interviewed the family before consenting to a patient's release. Fields, 'Visiting committee', p. 23.

28 Fifty-six total cases. Other secondary works allude to this phenomenon, but do not give any indication how widespread it was in other counties. For Leicestershire and Rutland, see Bartlett, 'Poor Law of Lunacy', p. 214.

29 For a graphic representation of the stability of first admissions from 1845 to 1945, see James Raftery, 'The decline of asylum or the poverty of the concept?', in D. Tomlinson and J. Carrier, eds, *Asylum in the Community*, London, Routledge, 1996, p. 24, Fig. 2.4. See also P. Michael, 'Occupations, gender and insanity in 19th and 20th century Wales', unpublished paper, p. 1.

30 For a survey of the history of the Buckinghamshire Asylum, see J. Crammer, *Asylum History: Buckinghamshire County Pauper Lunatic Asylum-St. John's*, London, Gaskell, 1990.

31 Permanently, that is. Many more escaped but were quickly found and returned to the asylum. For forty-six patients (2.8 per cent) the status was not listed. Transfers often represent individuals who were committed first to the Buckinghamshire Asylum, and then were transferred to another county or borough institution when it was established that their parish of settlement lay outside the county.

32 W. Parry-Jones, *The Trade in Lunacy: A Study of Private Madhouses in England in the Eighteenth and Nineteenth Centuries*, London, Heinemann, 1972, p. 207; Hunter, *Psychiatry for the Poor*, p. 53. L. Ray, 'Models of madness in Victorian asylum practice', *European Journal of Sociology*, 22, 1981, pp. 231; C. MacKenzie, 'Social factors in the admission, discharge, and continuous stay of patients at Ticehurst Asylum', Table 8.3 and 8.4; A. Digby, *Madness, Morality and Medicine*, p. 219, Table 9.2; A. Beveridge, 'Madness in Victorian Edinburgh: a study of patients admitted to the Royal Edinburgh Asylum under Thomas Clouston, 1873–1908 (part I)', *History of Psychiatry*, 6, 1995, pp. 22–54.

33 Ray, 'Models of madness in Victorian asylum practice'. Compare the findings for the Denbigh Asylum, Wales, which found an average length of stay of 498 days (16.5 months) for women and an average length of 471 (15.6 months) for men. P. Michael, 'Occupations, gender and insanity in 19th and 20th century Wales', unpublished paper, p. 3.

34 The numbers of second and subsequent discharges are quite few. For second discharges, 16 of 25 women (64 per cent) were discharged within a year, and 22 of 36 men (61 per cent). A small handful of people were readmitted several times for short periods of time. Twenty-three women were admitted three times, seven of those for four or more times; fourteen men were admitted three times, four of those for four or more times.

35 Of course, life expectancy (inside and outside the asylum) also decreased for over 60s, thereby making the decline of the proportion discharged less dramatic than it might at first appear. See R. Woods, 'Mortality patterns in the nineteenth century', in Woods and J. Woodward, eds, *Urban Disease and Mortality in the Nineteenth Century*, London, 1984, p. 43, Table 2.1.

36 There is already fragmentary evidence to suggest that this level of discharges was widespread. See for instance, Hunter's analysis of Colney Hatch for 1861 (in which he found 50 per cent of patients recovered their senses within one year), Hunter, *Psychiatry for the Poor*, p. 53.
37 Further to the Second Report of the Commissioners in Lunacy, p. 436.
38 *Journal of Mental Science*, 1856, vol. 2, p. 260.
39 Forsythe *et al.*, 'The New Poor Law and the county pauper lunatic asylum', p. 341.
40 See n. 28 above.
41 Walton, 'Casting out', p. 133.
42 Scull, *The Most Solitary of Afflictions*, p. 263.
43 Hunter, *Psychiatry for the Poor*, p. 64.
44 Wright, 'The certification of lunatics'.
45 'I do not consider that she [Mary Price of North Marston] has recovered but from the report of her relatives, consider that she has improved since she left the asylum and is safe to be this much at large.' Letter to the Buckinghamshire Superintendent, 11 October 1866. Discharge Papers of the Buckinghamshire County Pauper Lunatic Asylum, BuRO AR 100/89/117.
46 Ibid., Letter to the Buckinghamshire Superintendent, 11 July 1854.
47 Scull, *The Most Solitary of Afflictions*, p. 312.
48 Scull does address the then limited literature showing the short-stay of patients in his revised and expanded version of *Museums of Madness* – Scull, *The Most Solitary of Afflictions*, pp.271–2 and ff. 10–16 – but refers to short-stay patients as existing 'at the margin' of the asylum world. By contrast, he continues, 'a very substantial proportion of the admissions remained behind to swell the population of chronic long-stay patients'. This research suggests that the 'very substantial proportion of chronic long-stay patients' admitted to these asylums was, in fact, smaller than the proportion of short-stay (i.e. less than 1 year) admissions.
49 See Ray, 'Models of madness', pp. 233, 161–2.
50 M. Finnane, *Insanity and the Insane in Post-Famine Ireland*, London, Croom Helm, 1981, p. 175; Garton, *Medicine and Madness*, p. 181; G. Klein et J. Gasser, 'L'évolution de la psychiatrie à travers les dossiers de patients: l'exemple de l'Hôpital psychiatrique de Cery, 1873–1959', *Revue Historique Vaudoise*, 103, 1995, p. 67; Beveridge, 'Madness in Victorian Edinburgh: a study of patients admitted to the Royal Edinburgh Asylum under Thomas Clouston, 1873–1908 (part I)', *History of Psychiatry*, 6, 1995, p. 43 and Tables 15–16.
51 P. McCandless does not give comparable figures, but states that between 1835 and 1860, the cure rate for the South Carolina state asylum was 45 per cent, a rate broadly comparable to the other asylums mentioned above. McCandless, ' "A House of Cure": the Antebellum South Carolina Lunatic Asylum', *Bulletin of the History of Medicine*, 44, 1990, p. 241; P. Keating, *La Science du Mal: l'institution de la psychiatrie au Québec, 1800–1914*, Québec, Boreal, 1993.
52 Hunter, *Psychiatry for the Poor*, p. 17.

Part II

THERAPEUTIC REGIMES IN THE NINETEENTH CENTURY

6

FRAMING PSYCHIATRIC SUBJECTIVITY

Doctor, patient and record-keeping at Bethlem in the nineteenth century

Akihito Suzuki

Introduction

In November 1859, Sarah Rebecca Thorley, a 28-year-old governess, was admitted to the Middlesex County Asylum at Colney Hatch. A letter, written by one Dr Fraser, accompanied her, which stated some extra information about the cause of her disease:

> Yesterday I signed a certificate of insanity in the case of Miss S.R. Thorley, previous to her removal to Colney Hatch – There is one circumstance connected with her condition which you ought to know, as it will guide you in adopting the treatment most likely to be beneficial – The fact was hinted to me by Mr Heally, in consequence of which I questioned Miss Thorley's sister, and learnt from her that at an early age (9 or 10 years) the patient, being under the evil influence of the worthless maid servant, contracted vicious habits of self-indulgence which have increased with her years. An operation (probably excision of part of the clitoris) was performed, but without any apparent benefit. You will probably have a visit from the sister, who can give you further information respecting your patient's antecedents, the family are strangers to me, but I promised the sister (a rather superior young lady, but straitened in circumstances) that I should write to you on the subject, as she might otherwise feel indelicacy in alluding to it.[1]

This is a graphic example of how complex and delicate a task a psychiatric practitioner needed to perform when he attempted to identify the cause of madness a patient of his was suffering from: the aetiology of insanity, as well as the disease itself, was often located in an intensely private realm of family secret, hard to tell and harder to ask. Sheer technical difficulty aside, negotiating one's way to the true cause of the disease, through the intricate web of secrecy, etiquette and protocols was obviously a daunting piece of detective work. Besides with the stigma associated with mental disease and the sense of shame the family felt over the madness of its member, one of the major reasons for the complication lay in the distinctive characteristic of psychiatric clinical encounter. Dr Fraser's letter exemplifies the fact that the psychiatric doctor–patient relationship was normally a triangular one: the patients did not typically report their illness to the doctor, the accounts of the disease being normally given to the doctor by the third party, who did not experience the disease subjectively but knew the patient and their illness well enough – usually members of the patients' family, or their relatives, neighbours and so on. (For the sake of convenience and historical correctness, below I shall refer to the third party in general as 'friends'.)

The doctor–patient relationship, especially in an institutional setting, has attracted the keen interest of historians of medicine in general, many of them utilising the rich resource of hospital case records.[2] These studies have paid special attention to the power structure of the clinical encounter in charitable settings and showed that complex power relations were going on, between the doctor and the patient, between lay governors and medical staff, and so on. Between the patient and the doctor, there existed a contest for interpretative authority over the act of decoding and defining disease, or what Katherine Hunter has called 'a silent tug-of-war over the possession of the story of illness'.[3] Moreover, the relationship at the bedside was affected in crucial ways by the pattern of control of the whole institution, often characterised by the doctors' quest for medical hegemony over the charitable institutions and their bypassing lay governors' power.[4] Historians of medicine have found that such power relationships were embodied in hospital case records. The most famous and important among historical investigations of the role of case record is that of Michel Foucault. In his *Discipline and Punish*, Foucault famously observed that the practice of keeping case records was not merely record-keeping but the cornerstone of modern human science: 'The examination, surrounded by all its documentary techniques, makes each individual a "case": a case which at one and the same time constitutes an object for a branch of knowledge and a hold for a branch of power.'[5] So far, however, relatively little attention has been paid to the structure of the psychiatric bedside and its embodiment in case records by historians of British psychiatry, and this chapter aims to show that careful scrutiny of the shifting ways in which case records were kept yields unique insights into the nature of psychiatric enterprise in the past and to examine whether Foucault's characterisation of case record as a vehicle of objectification of patients is an accurate one.[6]

With such historiographical concerns in mind, this chapter attempts to investigate changing practice of keeping patient's case records at Bethlem in the nineteenth century and shifting patterns of the distribution of power in the triangular relationship between the doctor, patient and friends. To put it briefly, my argument is that a quiet but definitive change took place in 1852, the year of an important reform of Bethlem. Before 1852, the friends of the patient had relatively unchallenged authority over identifying the cause of the attack. After 1852, their authority was routinely impugned not only by the doctor, but also by the patient. At the core of this shift was the struggle over the power to define the identity of the patient. What kind of life had he or she really led? What had really driven him or her to madness? Who knew the best about his or her private secret, and who could best identify him or her? I shall argue that after 1852, the patients were increasingly defined in the light of what the doctor observed in the institution, and, more interestingly and importantly, what the doctor heard from the patients. Put in another way, the doctor framed the patient's subjectivity into their attempt to understand the real identity of the patient, hidden by or unknown to his or her family members.

Charitable narrative: Bethlem under the old regime

In Bethlem, the practice of keeping patients' case records seems to have started in 1815, no doubt in response to the Parliamentary inquiry in the year before.[7] After 1815, there were two visiting physicians, Edward Thomas Monro from that year up to 1852 and Sir George Tuthill, who was in 1835 replaced by Sir Alexander Morison who remained until 1852. They visited the hospital two or three times a week, each visit lasting about two hours.[8] At first, they were nominally responsible for filling in the case books with the information provided at the admission, but the actual business of putting in entries was increasingly performed by one resident apothecary.[9] The format of each case is an ordinary one. At the beginning of each record, there is a long paragraph including information taken at the admission of the patient, consisting of the patient's mini-biography and pathography: patient's name, sex, age, occupation(s), place(s) of residence, marriage status, number of children and the progress of the disease from its beginning up to the point of admission. From around 1832 there came into use a hand-written standardised format with fixed sections to be filled in, and in 1837 there appeared its printed version.[10] Information gathered at the admission is followed by subsequent entries about treatment, remarkable changes, general observation, major events such as attacks on other patients and so on.[11] There is therefore a neat division of each case record into two parts, one containing information about the patient's pre-institutional life, taken at the admission, the other recording episodes after the institutionalisation of the patient. This chronological division overlaps with the different sources of the account in the case book. The doctors usually obtained the pre-admission information from those who brought the patient to the hospital, or the 'friends' of the patient. Whereas the events recorded in the post-admission entries were normally observed first-hand by them.

The admission procedure, in which the doctors obtained information about pre-institutional episodes, was essentially a process of petition and charity-giving.[12] The decision over admission was one of the duties of the so-called Bethlem sub-committee, which consisted in seven, mostly lay, governors who met weekly. At the sub-committee meetings, the patients were brought in by their friends, who made formal petition to the governors, explaining the distressed situation of the patient.[13] Since Bethlem was very choosy about the suitable subject for admission on the basis of the patient's medical condition, the visiting physicians were asked to attend the committee to offer advice. But their function was explicitly stated as that of *assistance*, and their opinions were sometimes overruled by governors.[14]

Surviving evidence suggests that the petitioner's presentation of the case prevailed over the ideal of medical interview at the admission committee. It seems that doctors filled in a sheet called 'Memorandum upon admission of patients into Bethlem Hospital'. Many surviving memoranda were inserted into the relevant pages of the case books, into which was transcribed the information in the memoranda. Its format shows the doctors' aspiration for the ideal of systematic information-taking, with printed columns, specifying the type of information to be put in. The actual practice of taking notes was, however, messier. Take, the example of the memorandum for John Bool, admitted on 10 March 1825. The entry into the section 'when this attack commenced' reads as follows:

> Caught cold working in a Hothouse at Montacute in Somersetshire when exposing himself to the cold air in the garden 2 months ago, then about 5 weeks ago his mind became affected. being then restless melancholy, violent towards his wife, wandering about the country leaving his work & crying 'lost man'. Then refused his food, would have destroyed his wife and himself; confined by the parish at home. [15]

The important point is that this entry not only contains much surplus information about the cause, symptoms and other episodes which should not be put here, but also physically spills over the two sections below, unrestrained by the printed format. This seems to suggest that the medical staff of Bethlem were incapable of imposing the pre-established order on what they heard at the admission of a patient, unable to process and neatly pigeonhole the data they received. I shall later come back to this point and explore its wider implications: here suffice it to say that the doctors, in practice, did not possess the power to reconstruct the individual as a 'case', which, as I have mentioned above, Foucault believed, was exercised in prisons, schools and hospitals in the nineteenth-century West.[16]

The entry in the memorandum was unbroken not only because of the doctor's lack of control over the material presented by the friends of John Bool, but also because of its internal integrity. The story of his mental disease is well told: major episodes are arranged chronologically, the cause of the disease is implied at the beginning, and symptoms are described clearly, with emphasis on a piece of eye-catching stereotypical mad behaviour ('crying "lost man" ').[17] Indeed, the case books of Bethlem contain numerous very well-told narrative of madness. One of the best is the entry made by Tuthill in the case note for Sarah Hartley, a 36-year-old wife of a picture-frame maker in London:

> Her present disorder is reported to have begun in August last and to show itself on the death of one of her children. She positively refused to suffer the body to be buried and continued in a distracted state persisting in her refusal till at the end of a fortnight the parish officers were obliged to remove her to the Workhouse in order to make the family to proceed with the funeral. She has remained in Whitechapel Workhouse to the present time and when she first went thither she raved in search of her lost child and could only be removed without very great violence by suffering her to carry with a pillow which she nursed and caressed and called it her child. Since that time she

> has remained tolerably quiet but her manners and observations have been very constantly irrational.[18]

Again arranged chronologically, this story traces the disease of the mad mother to its origin and cause and narrates the symptoms of her mad grief, culminating in the intensely dramatic delusion about her lost child – a literary and visual topos being established at that time.[19] The story of Sarah Hartley is a gripping mini-biography of a mad mother, written with highly effective dramaturgy which seems to have compelled the reader/listener into charitable sympathy.[20] Small wonder, Tuthill put down the entire story in one breath.

The obvious question is: who was the author of this story? Almost certainty Tuthill exercised some editing on the story told by the friends. All the material for the entry, however, must have come from the presentation of the case given by the friends at the admission procedure, for obviously Tuthill was not able to witness any episode contained there. Without running the risk of speculating on the extent of medical editing process, one can certainly say that lay people did provide extremely rich and commanding raw material.

Numerous other entries testify to lay people's ability to make sense of the madness of those whom they knew well and to tell dramatic stories about their downfall into madness. Particularly remarkable was their readiness to provide causal explanation: *why* did this man or woman become insane? The majority of the cases include the attributed causes of the present attack of madness of the patient, usually explicitly stated as given by the patient's friends. In some cases there is evidence which suggests that the lay people conducted somewhat elaborate enquiry about possible causes.[21] The friends gave their own causal explanation partly because the doctors and the governors expressed their desire to know the cause, but also because there existed strong lay cultural frameworks which enabled them to detect and understand the origin of the madness. There is a plenty of evidence from other types of material such as private correspondence which show that people were ready to search for causes when their family members or relatives became insane, without being asked or helped by doctors.[22] Rather than seeing it as a mysterious visit or an esoteric and technical question, lay people frequently expressed their own opinions about the causes of the mental diseases of their acquaintances. Entries for 'cause' section were dominated by this kind of lay cultural understanding of madness rather than medicalised aetiology.

The most striking feature of the lay observation is that it understood madness in relation to the life events and their psychological impact on the patients in question. The events that were regarded as having prompted insanity are usually acute and painful ones. Perhaps reflecting so-called affective individualism, the death of a family member was believed to have driven many into insanity. Influenced by romanticism in general and by the 'Crazy Kate' figure in particular, disappointed love was one of very common attributions made by the friends of insane women as the cause of their insanity.[23] For men, anxiety and stress over business and economic-related matters loomed large. The ideology of self-help and respectability came into play here. Sometimes the petitioning party showed elaborate observation and causal speculation, exercising some empathic reasoning and seeing things from the patient's view. Mary Solomon, for instance, gave birth to an illegitimate child and fell insane soon after. The parish officers reported that 'it is believed that the pregnancy and consequent loss of character have so dwelt upon her mind as to increase her present disease'.[24]

The lay narrative at the Bethlem was, therefore, centred around well-articulated and more or less clearly defined incidents, and their psychological effects, mainly painful emotions such as grief, anxiety, shame, etc. The attribution of madness to drastic and emotion-shattering life events made the madness of the patient *understandable*, something with which one could feel empathy and sympathy. Little doubt the sympathetic framing of madness of the patients was due to the protocol of asking for charity and the strategy of petitioners to present the case as one deserving charity. By representing the disease of a patient as a result of misfortune over which the patient had little control, the friends could depict him or her as a victim. Moreover, there was a striking absence of cases in which the blame was put on the patient, which is abundant in other types of sources.[25] The Bethlem case records presented more or less a sanitised version, putting the patient in a favourable or at least neutral light.

The important question is: what was the doctors' attitude to these lay accounts of the cause of the attack of madness? Of course, the doctors were not nodding their approval to everything presented at the admission committee. Knowing the 'causes' of madness, however, involved a tricky epistemological problem: by reason of chronology, the doctors were denied direct access to observing the patient's transition from sanity to insanity. The family members, relatives, neighbours and Poor Law officers of the patients had a clear epistemological advantage over the doctors, because they usually observed the crucial transitional process first-hand. Take, for example, a letter written by Mr James Ogle, of the Oxford Asylum, accompanying the admission document for Ann Sparkes who was admitted as Morison's patient:

> I was requested to visit Mrs Ann Sparkes about a month time and found her labouring under a paroxysms of mania....There did not appear any very evident cause of the paroxysm but her neighbours said she had long suffered considerable anxiety respecting her domestic affairs and did not hesitate to ascribe her malady to that origin.[26]

This is a very graphic example of psychiatric inability *vis-à-vis* lay ability to identify a cause of insanity. The neighbours, who were familiar with her personal situation, had no problem in finding why she became insane, while the doctor was clueless about the cause. The crucial point here is that the doctor could not offer his own opinion. He seems to have been aware that he should not trust the lay practice of aetiological reasoning, but he did not possess a lever to overturn the confidently expressed lay opinion.

This pattern dominates the entries of 'causes' in Bethlem case books. The doctors were aware that they had learned the causes from 'dubious sources'. Some accounts in the case books indicate that the doctors were aware of the indirect or second-hand nature of the information they had: the phrases 'it appears', 'it seems', 'the cause is attributed', etc. abound, showing the reservation tacitly expressed by the doctors. Occasionally, they expressed explicit doubt, but they rarely attempt to correct lay attributions and offer alternatives. The case books of Bethlem under the visiting physicians do not reveal any systematic undertaking to appropriate the power to decode the cause of a patient from his or her lay friends into the hands of the medical profession.

The reasons for this lenient attitude to lay interpretation of madness are manifold. Apart from the built-in structural obstacle of chronology and epistemology and the sheer lack of technical sophistication, there are signs that the doctors were often convinced by the powerful, cogent and poignant representation of the madness of the patient narrated by the friends. The friends were playing the game with very strong cards, capitalising on the resourceful and compelling ideologies of romanticism, self-help and affective individualism. One could safely argue that the lay decoding of the aetiology of madness, capitalising on the current cultural understanding of human emotional life, made its way into Bethlem case books, relatively unblocked and often sanctioned by the doctors. This paradigm essentially continued up to 1852, when William Charles Hood assumed the responsibility of resident physician. In the next section, I shall examine the new game started by him.

Voyeurism or empowerment of the patient?

In 1852, due to pressure from the Commissioners in Lunacy, Bethlem went through a large-scale reform.[27] The Commissioners finally secured a right to inspect items in Bethlem: the patients, the staff, the building, devices for restraint and, most importantly, for the purpose of this chapter, the case books. Although stated as one of the duties of physicians or apothecary, keeping case books before 1852 was not always taken seriously and performed attentively. As early as the beginning of the 1820s, the business of record-keeping was rather irregular. For some years around 1822, case books were entered by a person who was obviously not up to the task: entries were written in an extremely clumsy hand, and the author often missed or misspelled medical terms and occasionally did not understand what he was putting down.[28] In the 1830s, the committee inquiring into the misconduct of Edward Wright, the apothecary to the hospital from 1819, learned from him that he could not produce recent case books and the cases of the patients had not been regularly entered.[29] While the 1830 insider committee was not particularly concerned about Wright's failure to keep case books, the 1852 inquiry by the Commissioners in Lunacy repeatedly pointed out the unsatisfactory state of the hospital's record-keeping.[30] The case books of Bethlem now became public record, to be scrutinised by the central government's inspectors. Second, they succeeded in convincing the governors of Bethlem to get rid of the Byzantine system of line-management with two visiting physicians at the nominal top and with day-to-day management left to the apothecary and matron. The new system installed by the end of 1852 was one that had already become the norm for county asylums, centring around one all-powerful resident medical superintendent. The visiting physicians, Monro aged 62 and Morison 73, made a rather ignoble exit, and the superintendentship was taken by William Hood, a 28-year-old Dublin MD, fresh from the job of the resident physician of the Middlesex County Asylum at Colney Hatch.[31]

It appears that there were not great changes in the basics of the admission procedure. Neither was there a drastic change in the format of the case book, although they were kept more regularly, reflecting the fact they were now inspected by the Lunacy Commissioners. On closer scrutiny, however, it turns out that Hood utilised the old formula for a different strategy. One can detect this by looking at how he filled in the 'causes' sections. A hand different from Hood's, perhaps that of the clerk, filled in all sections except 'causes', which were entered by Hood himself. Internal evidences suggest that the 'causes' sections were systematically left open at the time of admission, to be filled in later by Hood. From what Hood wrote in the monthly observation pages, it is clear that he spent a few weeks or a month in observing, examining and interviewing the patient and comparing the result with the information presented at the admission, trying to discover the real cause of the disease. Sometimes Hood deleted earlier 'causes' entries written in a different hand by strikeout double lines, making new ones by himself. For instance, the initial 'exciting cause' entry in the case note of Angus Mackay's was 'disappointment and drink'. About three weeks later, Hood recorded additional and crucial information:

> Since he has been a patient at this hospital it has been stated that he is a man of most temperate habits and that he has not indulged at all lately in that respect, but the cause of this illness can be traced to anxiety of mind and over study, he having made music his ruling thought lately, endeavouring to set to written notes music adapted for the pipes.

Accordingly, he deleted the former entry and replaced it with 'overstudy of music'.[32] For Hood, the 'causes' sections were not something to be simply filled in at admission: rather, they should be completed only after observation of the institutionalised patient. In other words, he made retroactive use of his own institutional observation: reasoning backward from the direct observation of the patient to the causes of disease, which he could not witness first hand.[33] There was no sign that his predecessors ever did this. Even if one makes concession to the possibility of their retroactive inferring of the cause of the disease without recording it in the case books, one can still argue that Hood made an innovation, by *systematically* using post-institutional data to infer pre-institutional events as causes of madness. Hood made it a *routine* work to infer the unobservable from the observable.

This involved a more critical attitude to lay report on the causes of the disease: now the lay aetiology presented to the doctor was systematically suspended until it was confirmed or rejected by him. Hood exercised elaborate detective work in the case of Emma Riches, a 25-year-old wife of a broker. The 'exciting cause' entry was 'grief at loss of the eldest child', a typically acceptable lay aetiological representation asking for charity. Hood did not entirely deny this attribution, but his further inquiry led him to downplay the role played by the event. Learning that 'there is no particular distressing occurrence about the death of her child that could account for this attack', he emphasised a more important part played by hereditary nature of the disease.[34]

Rather than being content with the cause given by the friends of Mrs Riches, Hood inquired into details and found that the explanation was not convincing.

This systematic discredit of the lay aetiology and illness narrative certainly involved the imposition of professional and scientific authority, which has been the major historiographical focus for the last twenty years.[35] In the case of Emma Riches, Hood was medicalising and somaticising aetiological identification in a rather straightforward way, refuting lay attribution with his negative finding and somatic aetiology of heredity. Simple dichotomy of the physical and the moral and one-sided emphasis on the former was, however, obviously an untenable attitude in the context of day-to-day practice at Bethlem, given the lack of zeal for scientific and somatic psychiatry in Hood. Sophia Sell's case, in which Hood wrote '[this] case may be fairly considered one of puerperal mania, though the circumstance of the child being illegitimate would probably increase the liability to mental disturbance', is a typical mixture and compromise of the moral and the physical.[36]

Hood's critical attitude to lay narrative of disease is in itself not surprising to any medical historian studying the nineteenth century, when the combination of physical examination and pathological anatomy was making doctors less dependent on what patients told them. What is interesting here is the means he utilised to discredit the lay aetiology and the ramification of the new strategy on the psychiatric doctor–patient relationship.

An obvious lever for Hood to counter the lay narrative of the cause of madness was *the patient*, which had been a relatively unexploited resource before. It is not that medical staff at Bethlem before Hood had not listened to the inmates. The entries in the case books reveal, however, that they had been more concerned to detect fraud in terms of the duration of the disease from the conversation with the patients. Five months after the admission of Jeffrey Muggridge, whose derangement had been reported to have lasted for 'five or six months', Tuthill wrote: '[he] is certainly more quiet and tranquil. He will converse freely on the nature of his disorder and from that conversation it has manifestly existed for years.'[37] Another prominent concern of theirs is to record 'interesting' delusions.[38] Light-hearted interest in the content of amusing delusions had long been established in medical and lay culture, and given the occasion to travel in the exotic terrain of numerous insane minds, Bethlem doctors during the old regime assumed the attitude of armchair ethnographer collecting curious stories.[39]

Hood made more active use of the patient. He introduced the patient into the scene, hitting a new balance in the triangular relationship of doctor–patient–friends, increasing the power of the former two parties, at the cost of the friends. A most striking example is that of Mary Ann Musard. Before Hood was appointed, she was admitted first as Monro's patient on 31 July 1851, at the age of 23. The 'cause' entry says that the disease was caused by 'anxiety and distress of mind on account off some supposed frivolous misunderstanding between her self, her mother and her husband'. In December 1853, she was readmitted, this time under Hood. The 'cause' section was apparently left empty at the admission. Two weeks after the admission, Hood thought he had discovered the real cause:

> There are quite sufficient causes for this attack. Her husband is a [skirmish] and not only beats her but keeps another woman. He excuses his conduct by accusing her of forming intimacies with other men, and declares he will never live with her again, but it is not considered that his tale is worthy of credence and if it is the weakness of mind induced by his cruelty, is a sufficient excuse and cause for a crime she may have committed.

Perhaps at this time, he entered 'ill-treatment of husband' in the 'exciting cause' section. In February next year, he recorded in his monthly observation in a similar vein: 'If her story is true her husband is one of the most unmitigated brutes that ever lived.'[40]

The crucial thing about Mary Ann Musard's case is that Hood listened to the patient's own narrative about her domestic situation (she was 'very fond of talking'), and in effect discredited the husband's story of her adultery, which had probably been told at the admission. Note that he preferred the insane wife's version to that of her sane husband. The same pattern repeated itself in the case of Fanny Tebay, whose column for cause was apparently kept blank at admission. Less than a month later, Hood apparently thought he had discovered the true cause, both by listening to her story and observing the husband: 'Her husband has all the appearance of being a bully, and ill-treating her as she represent to be the case she declared now she will not live with him again, and that his brutality has been the cause of these attacks.'[41]

A crucial aspect about Musard's and Tebay's cases is that Hood was aware that domestic disagreement, dispute and cruelty could cause the madness of a family member, and he was fond of detecting domestic cruelty as the cause. It is true that the domestic conflict or cruelty had been recognised as a cause of insanity by the physicians of the previous regime, their reports occasionally listing 'familial troubles', 'domestic unhappiness', 'unkindness of the mother', 'father's misconduct', as the cause of the disease.[42] Hood's innovation again lay in his active and systematic attempt to reveal domestic problems as the cause of the disease, which were likely to be hidden or suppressed by the family, for they were trying to represent the case as one deserving sympathy and charity. The other members of the family thus became a suspect and biased source.

The case of Emma Nichols, a single 26-year-old waistcoat maker, graphically tells how different the two versions could be. Soon after she was admitted to Bethlem, Hood wrote in his monthly entry that 'her family have to strive hard for a living and she has exerted herself to the utmost to maintain a respectable appearance'. Then she started to recover and started to talk, and Hood learned from her that the situation was more complex than this sanitised version. He recorded: '[it] appears, in addition to the privations she has had to undergo...a brother has on several occasions behaved in a very brutal manner to her and her mother has thrown obstacles on two or three occasions in her way to prevent her marrying when she had the opportunity for fear she should thus lose the labour of her daughter who supported her'.[43] The pattern is the same in the case note for William Day, a 56-year-old widower and infant school master. Hood learned from Day himself that he had to break off an engagement against his will due to his family's objection, and 'this preyed much on his mind'.[44]

The mode of the patients' narrative listened to and recorded by Hood is that of confession. The patients told their own life histories, riddled with calamity and psychological agony, and sense of guilt and shame. They were often centred around the innermost secret of their private life. Hood was, of course, not the first medical figure who started to take the confessional story of the mad seriously. One Mr George Harcourt, who had attended Michael Walker before he was admitted to Bethlem in 1830, wrote a letter to the governors of Bethlem about Walker, in very similar language to Hood:

> At the request of his friends I continued my visits in consequence of the great depression of his nervous energies and by degrees draw from him the cause of his sufferings. He had been living for some years in a gentleman's family and had engaged to marry a young woman but...had connection with a female and caught a gonorrhoea. His mother being a very religious character & it coming to her knowledge, lectured him on...the punishment that would surely await him. This he took so much to heart that he soon fancied himself a ruined man (altho' the disease had long ceased to exist) and incapable of

> performing the matrimonial duties. He therefore broke off the engagement and thereby added much to his disease.[45]

The secret sense of shame and guilt of getting gonorrhoea from a prostitute while engaged to a woman, the fear of the punishment for the sin preached by the mother, the anxiety of transmitting it to his future wife – all these private agonies were confessed to the doctor. The remarkable thing about Hood was, as I mentioned above, that he made this a routine aspect of his duties.

Another avenue which he used to explore the secret life of the family and patient was his investigation of masturbation, which was gaining greater importance in contemporary explanations of insanity. William Mason, aged 30 was admitted on 9 October 1854, apparently with the 'exciting cause' column left empty. On 26 October, Hood triumphantly wrote that '[there] is no cause stated by his friends or known to them at all to account for the present attack. He has told an attendant that from a very early age he has practised masturbation and not even given up the habit since his marriage' and entered 'masturbation' in the section. (Note the crucial use of the information provided by the patient.) The case note of Thomas Burgess indicates that Hood was bold enough to ask his father whether the son practised onanism: 'He is thin and unhealthy looking and has the appearance of a person emaciated from masturbation, but his father considers he has not indulged in such practices.'[46]

Conclusion

It is rather difficult to tell how typical Hood was – whether he was just an isolated figure with voyeuristic curiosity about other people's secrets or whether he represented a new culture in psychiatry. Certainly it is highly unlikely that medical superintendents of country asylums, overburdened with bureaucratic paperwork and demoralised with low cure rate, shared Hood's vigorous interest in identifying the 'true' cause of the disease, and the case books of Colney Hatch Asylum, which Hood himself was responsible for keeping, are no exception in their minimal account.[47] Nevertheless, I would like to extend my argument and maintain that Hood's new practice signals the coming of modernity in psychiatry, in three aspects, all related with each other: 1) disfranchisement of the family as a proper component of psychiatric discourse, 2) the penetration of psychiatry into the private realm, and 3) the framing of individual psychiatric patient as subject.

It is fairly obvious that Hood entertained an *a priori* distrust for the narrative of the friends of a patient, especially about the cause of the disease. Although he did not entirely abandon the information given by the family, he did not let their aetiology make an easy way into case books. The aetiological judgement and report made by the family was systematically suspended until the medical superintendent detected the real cause. This built-in suspicion against the family might be a remote echo of the concern against wrongful confinement, stereotypically represented as a conspiracy between scheming family members of the alleged lunatic and an unscrupulous doctor.[48] Or his powerful status as the single head of the hospital boosted his confidence into conducting detective work by his own initiative. Whatever the reason, Hood represents a doctor with modernised professional ethos, who was relatively independent from his client's view when making his judgement. This was achieved at the cost of the family, or lay people who had known the patient much more closely than the doctor. Their long, personal and intimate knowledge of the patient, especially at the crucial time of the beginning of the disease, no longer gained them the status of the best judge about the cause of the disease. The direct access to the innermost privacies of the institutionalised patients, Hood seems to have believed, enabled the psychiatrist to 'discover' the secret life of the patient in the past, hidden even to his or her family. About James Aransolo, a 15-year-old youth, Hood wrote '[he] probably practised masturbation a considerable time though his father has only recently become aware of the fact, for although during the last two years his parents have tried him in several trades yet he would not take to either but on each trial ran away and refused to continue in that or any other occupation'.[49]

The family, Hood thought, were not only unaware of the true cause of insanity; they actively concealed the key information. The friends most typically framed the cases as cultural stereotypes of madness commanding sympathy. In the process, they sanitised their representation, exonerating both the patient and themselves, consciously and unconsciously suppressing data which would put either party in an unfavourable light. A mother who became mad because of her grief over her dead child, young women seduced and discarded, and a failed businessman were all *presentable* figures for their family. The extensive use of interview with the patient enabled Hood to go beyond these façades and make voyeuristic penetration into the domestic and private secret. Hood discovered people who had become insane from causes which were secret, indecent and embarrassing to tell: a husband who masturbated after marriage, a wife abused by a cruel husband who carried on adultery, a daughter ill-treated by the exploitative mother and so on. In so doing, Hood often assumed the role of a patrolman of domestic harmony and propriety. About Emmanuel Caronel, Hood found that 'the fact appears to be that he was a bad husband and his wife an indifferent woman, and consequently he drank and then beat her. He had suspicions too of her faithfulness to him, and he certainly did not confine his attentions to her.'[50]

Probably Hood's concern to uncover domestic problems was due to the rise of public health as an attempt to uncover vices in the private realm. It seems significant that this systematic attempt to penetrate into the private and domestic sphere of the patient started when the Bethlem case books became, like other asylum records, public documents under the scrutiny of government inspectors. George Robinson, a public health activist and an owner of a private asylum summarised the view in his *On the Prevention and Treatment of Mental Disorders*, published in 1859. Using analogies with public health, he maintained that:

> the physician must look beyond the precincts of the asylum. He must not rest content with there observing the various forms of insanity, recording their progress and searching for their effects...the veil of conventionalism and routine must be drawn aside, and the light of truth and reason allowed to penetrate into the darker recesses of civilised existence.[51]

The asylum inmates thus became an important window through which the doctor penetrated into the private realm, or the Englishman's castle. There had to be some anomaly or irregularities, or deviancy from the ideal domestic situation, in order for the third party to intervene into the guarded private sphere – for example, marital discord or sexually transmitted disease.[52] Madness could be another justification of assault on domestic privacy and secret.

In his persistent attempt to present domestic cruelty or violence and 'vices' related to sexuality as the prime objects of psychiatric investigation, Hood preceded more 'scientifically' oriented psychiatrists of the early twentieth century.[53] Hood's practice could be interpreted as a signal to psychiatric modernity, or what Elizabeth Lunbeck has called 'the enlightened antithesis to Victorianism', in which allegiance to science and endeavour to find 'truth' were accompanied by frankness on matters related to sexuality and attacks on outmoded propriety.[54] Hood's practice at Bethlem however, did not lead to systematic or scientific research combined with quantification and definition of normalcy. Hood spoke in the language of reform framed around the issue of class and respectability rather than the language of science. His practice resonated with the contemporary concern for the hidden vices practised in the private realm of the families of the lower orders.

To achieve this goal – and this is my third point – Hood relied on the patient's own story, elicited through interview. He thus created a new pattern of the institutional psychiatric bedside, in which the patient told their life story and were listened to by the doctor, replacing the old pattern that consisted in the doctors listening to other people's story about the patient's past. Hood introduced a new scheme where the patient was not only the object of their friends' report, but also a subject who could and did refute the narrative about him or her, by telling his or her own stories. The patient, in collaboration with the doctor, became a legitimate storyteller about their own life.

This seems to compel us to rethink the way in which we should interpret the development of psychiatric power from the mid-nineteenth century. Historians of English psychiatry, most notably Thomas Szasz and Elaine Showalter, have generally assumed that the development of modern institutional psychiatry silenced the voice of the mad, highlighting the role of psychiatry as a prohibiting power, patrolling the patient's morality and labelling social or morally undesirable or disturbing behaviour as pathological.[55] My findings about the Bethlem under Hood shows that this model of, so to speak, 'tug-of-the-war' between the alienist and the patient is grossly simplistic. It was under the modernised, rationalised and bureaucratic regime of the new Bethlem, with more inquisitive power exercised by the doctor, that the voice of the mad started to be heard. One can certainly say that Hood's new practice represented a new culture, which aimed at more medical power and, *at the same time*, put premium on the stories told by the mentally diseased patient.[56]

Unfortunately, there is no way to tell how authentic the voice of the patient recorded by Hood was. First of all, we do not know how the patients responded to Hood's probe into their privacy. Although Hood naturally did not record any instance of hostile reaction to his investigation, that does not mean his relationship with the patients were entirely a benign one. There is little doubt that Hood made his own use of the patient's report and perhaps sometimes put what he wanted to hear in the patient's mouth – he was so fond of identifying domestic cruelty against the patient as the true cause of the disease and he must have derived satisfaction by fashioning himself as the guardian of the patient against the abuse of the family.

It seems, however, too cynical and simplistic to regard Hood's search for cause as an invention to massage his professional self-image. His use of the subjectivity of the patient is best understood as the new scheme of psychiatric power described in Foucault's later works. In the light of the new practice of Hood at Bethlem, where the patient could challenge and alter the content of the record about himself or herself, the role assigned by Foucault to the patient in *Discipline and Punish* seems too passive. The case book was a far more dynamic and fluid space than Foucault's account suggests, ripe with struggle for the status of legitimate storyteller between the patient, the doctor and family. Foucault's concept of 'confessional technology', put forward in his *History of Sexuality*, captures the complex dynamics of Hood's practice.[57] Instead of repressing the patient's self, Hood regulated his or her subjectivity, encouraging (perhaps occasionally forcing) inmates to narrate their stories to be incorporated into the case book entries, which now became public property. In that sense, Hood's patients signalled modern individual subjectivity constructed by 'psy' professions, 'in which all the "private" effects of psychological interiority are constituted by our linkage into "public" languages, practices, techniques and artefacts.'[58] We should recognise that psychiatry often regulated patient's subjectivity, rather than simply prohibiting it. Michael MacDonald has succinctly stated that 'insanity has been defined by experts but discovered by laymen'.[59] My findings at Bethlem seem to show that between the definition and discovery there existed a complex process of struggle for the appropriation of power/knowledge and the patient's own voice was a vital component for psychiatric modernity.

Acknowledgements

The research on which this paper is based was conducted while I was a visiting research fellow at the Wellcome Institute for History of Medicine. I would like to thank the hospitality of the staff of the Institute, particularly Roy Porter and Michael Neve, who gave invaluable comments and suggestions. Patricia Alleridge, the archivist of Bethlem was invariably helpful. The generosity of the Japan Society for the Promotion of Science, who funded my extended stay at the Wellcome Institute during 1993–5 as well as my trip to Lausanne was truly remarkable. I also benefited from the comments and encouragement of Clark Lawlor, my colleague at the Thomas Reid Institute at the University of Aberdeen in 1995–6, and those of attendants of the conference held at Lausanne, as well as seminars and workshops held at the Universities of Glasgow and Exeter.

NOTES

1 Greater London Record Office, H12/CH/B11/5 Case Book Females no. 7, a letter inserted at p. 331.
2 For a standard overview of the history of doctor–patient relationship in general, see Stanley Joel Reiser, *Medicine and the Reign of Technology*, Cambridge, Cambridge University Press, 1978; Edward Shorter, *Doctors and Their Patients: A Social History*, 2nd edn, Brunswick, NJ, Transaction Publishers, 1991; Guenter B. Risse and John Harley Warner, 'Reconstructing clinical activities: patient records in medical history', *Social History of Medicine*, 5, 1992, pp. 183–205; Mary E. Fissell, 'The disappearance of the patient's narrative and the invention of hospital medicine', in Roger French and Andrew Wear, eds, *British Medicine in an Age of Reform*, London, Routledge, 1991, pp. 92–109; Fissell, *Patient, Power, and the Poor in Eighteenth-Century Bristol*, Cambridge, Cambridge University Press, 1991.
3 Kathryn Montgomery Hunter, *Doctors' Stories: The Narrative Structure of Medical Knowledge*, Princeton, NJ, Princeton University Press, 1991, p. 13.
4 Fissell, *Patient, Power, and the Poor*, pp.110–70.
5 Michel Foucault, *Discipline and Punish: the Birth of the Prison*, Harmondsworth, Penguin, 1979, p. 191. See also Ruth Leys, 'Types of one: Adolf Meyer's Life Chart and the representation of individuality', *Representation*, 34, 1991, pp. 1–28.
6 See, however, Peter Bartlett, 'The Poor Law of Lunacy: the administration of pauper lunatics in mid-nineteenth century England with special emphasis on Leicestershire and Rutland', University of London, Ph.D., 1993. Sally Swartz, 'Colonising the insane: causes of insanity in the Cape, 1891–1920', *History of the Human Sciences*, 8, 1995, pp. 39–57.
7 Jonathan Andrews, Asa Briggs, Roy Porter, Penny Tucker and Keir Waddington, *The History of Bethlem*, London, Routledge, 1997.
8 Ibid., p. 441.
9 *Standing Rules and Orders for the Government of the Royal Hospitals of Bridewell and Bethlem*..., London, by H. Bryer, 1818, pp. 62–3.
10 Case Books (CB) from 1815 are now kept at the archive of Royal Bethlem Hospital. CB/19 curable patient Monro; CB/22 Curable patients Morison.
11 In theory they should be entered at least once a month, but in practice the entries were extremely irregular.
12 Fissell, *Patient, Power, and the Poor*, pp. 74–93. See also the chapter by Lorraine Walsh in this volume.
13 Andrews *et al.*, *History of Bethlem*, pp. 436–63.
14 *Standing Rules*, 1818 states at p. 63 that one of physicians' duties is 'To attend the sub-committee, at Bethlem Hospital, every meeting, to assist the committee with their advice in taking in and discharging patients'.
15 Memorandum upon admission of patients into Bethlem Hospital for John Bool, inserted in CB/11.
16 Michel Foucault, *Discipline and Punish*, pp. 184–94.
17 See Mary Fissell, 'Readers, texts, and contexts: vernacular medical works in early modern England', in Roy Porter, ed., *The Popularisation of Medicine 1650–1850*, London, Routledge, 1992, pp. 72–96.
18 CB/8, p. 229.

19 Sander Gilman, *Seeing the Insane*, New York, John Wiley and Sons, 1982, pp. 138–9.
20 For powerful linguistic analysis of discourse of charity, see Thomas Laqueur, 'Bodies, details, and the humanitarian narrative', in Lynn Hunt, ed., *The New Cultural History*, Berkeley, University of California Press, 1989, pp. 176–204.
21 In the case of Amelia Lawrence, at CB/2, pp. 97–9, it is stated that the family asked her about the cause of the disease. See also, for example, CB/1, pp. 167–8, 239–40.
22 See American examples in Nancy Tomes, *The Art of Asylum-Keeping: Thomas Story Kirkbride and the Origin of American Psychiatry*, Cambridge, Cambridge University Press, 1894; paperback reprint with new introduction, Philadelphia, University of Pennsylvania Press, 1994, pp. 92–103.
23 For the literary topos of love-sick woman, see Elaine Showalter, *The Female Malady: Women, Madness and English Culture, 1830–1980*, London, Virago, 1987, pp. 11–14; Helen Small, *Love's Madness: Medicine, the Novel, and Female Insanity, 1800–1865*, Oxford, Oxford University Press, 1996.
24 CB/2, pp. 177–8.
25 See, for example, Alexander Morison, MSS Reports and Notes of Cases, Royal College of Physicians of London, SR/471, 'The case of Miss Mary M – by her sister'.
26 CB/20, p. 3.
27 Commissioners in Lunacy, *The Report of the Commissioners in Lunacy to the Secretary of the State on Bethlem Hospital*, London, Spottiswoodes and Shaw, 1852. About the 1852 investigation and the new regime of Hood in general, see *History of Bethlem*, pp. 464–511.
28 The case book numbered CB/12 (Admissions curable male and female) holds inserted admission memorandum sheets, from which the entries seem to have been transcribed with numerous errors. In a single entry for William Adams, the author missed two terms 'insensible' and 'Rheumatic fever' and wrote 'health week' for 'health weak'. CB/12, p. 33.
29 Bethlem Hospital, *Minutes of Evidence Taken by the Committee, appointed to inquire into the charges preferred against Dr. Wright*, London, by Mills, Jowett, and Mills, 1830, p. 36.
30 Commissioners in Lunacy, *The Report*, 1852, pp. 6, 15, 17, 28, 34 etc.
31 For the Colney Hatch Asylum, see Richard Hunter, and Ida Macalpine, *Psychiatry for the Poor: 1851 Colney Hatch Asylum. Friern Hospital 1973*, London, Dawsons, 1974.
32 CB/64, pp. 45–8.
33 For the retroactive nature of medical reasoning, see Hunter, *Doctors' Stories*, esp. pp. 51–82.
34 CB/61, p. 49.
35 The most forceful and sophisticated proponents of this model are Andrew Scull, *The Most Solitary of Afflictions: Madness and Society in Britain, 1700–1900*, New Haven, Yale University Press, 1993; W.F. Bynum, 'Rationales for therapy in British psychiatry: 1780–1835', *Medical History*, 18, 1974, pp. 317–34; L.S. Jacyna, 'Somatic theories of mind and the interests of medicine in Britain, 1850–1879', *Medical History*, 26, 1982, pp. 233–58.
36 CB/61, p. 54. In any way, since heredity belonged to 'predisposing' cause and moral ones largely to 'exciting' one, Hood's concern for the hereditary

nature of insanity and his desire to find moral cause were *not* mutually exclusive.

37 CB/1 (Tuthill), pp. 99–102, entry on 1 April 1817.

38 See for example, CB/1 (Tuthill), pp. 151–3.

39 Tuthill, for example, once faithfully recorded the popular expression ('according to the expression of a petitioner') 'addiky', perhaps a corrupted form of 'addictive'. CB/1, the entry for Joseph Aves pp. 231–3.

40 CB/63, p. 33.

41 CB/62, p. 5.

42 *The Royal Hospital of Bethlem. The Physician's Report for the Year 1845*, London, G.J. Palmer, 1846, pp. 29–30.

43 CB/62, p. 24.

44 CB/64, pp. 129–31.

45 CB/14, p. 14.

46 CB/64, pp. 213–15.

47 GLRO H12/CH/B/11/1/A, Middlesex County Lunatic Asylum Colney Hatch, Case Book Female Side No. 2.

48 Peter McCandless, 'Liberty and lunacy: the Victorians and wrongful confinement', in Andrew Scull, ed., *Madhouses, Mad-Doctors, and Madmen: the Social History of Psychiatry in the Victorian Era*, London, The Athlone Press, 1981, pp. 339–62.

49 CB/64, pp. 209–11.

50 CB/64, pp. 81–3.

51 George Robinson, *On the Prevention and Treatment of Mental Disorders*, London, Longman, Brown, Green, Longmans, and Roberts, 1859, p. 5.

52 A. James Hammerton, *Cruelty and Companionship: Conflict in Nineteenth-Century Married Life*, London, Routledge, 1992, p. 18. Elizabeth Lunbeck, *The Psychiatric Persuasion: Knowledge, Gender and Power in Modern America*, Princeton, Princeton University Press, 1994, pp. 52ff.

53 Lunbeck, however, observed that psychiatrists at the Boston Psychopathic Hospital failed to 'frame domestic violence as an issue in its own right' (Lunbeck, *Psychiatric Persuasion*, pp. 102–3). The contrast between Hood and Boston psychiatrists is perhaps due to the latter's self-conscious pursuit of 'science', whereas the former tended to use the language of reform.

54 Lunbeck, *Psychiatric Persuasion*, p. 52.

55 Thomas Szasz, *The Myth of Mental Illness*, New York, Dell, 1961; Showalter, *Female Malady*, pp. 121–64.

56 The result of Hood's practice could amount to a free-flowing narrative of enormous scale by the patient. See Forbes Winslow, *On Obscure Diseases of the Brain and Disorders of the Mind*, Philadelphia, Blanchard and Lea, 1860, pp. 69–113.

57 Michel Foucault, *Histoire de la sexualité 1. La volonté de savoir*, Paris, Gallimard, 1976. For the centrality of the 'confession' of the object of study or punishment in the modern power, see Michel Foucault, 'The dangerous individual', in Michel Foucault, *Politics, Philosophy, Culture: Interviews and Other Writings 1977–1984*, ed. by Lawrence Kritzman, London, Routledge, 1988, pp. 125–51.

58 Nikolas Rose, 'Assembling the modern self', in Roy Porter, ed., *Rewriting the Self: Histories from the Renaissance to the Present*, London, Routledge, 1997, pp. 224–48, 226.

59 Michael MacDonald, 'Popular belief about mental disorder in early modern Europe', in W. Eckart and J. Geyer-Kordesch, eds, *Heilberufe und Kranke im 17. und 18. Jahrhundert*, Münster, Burgverlag, 1982, pp. 148–73, 148.

7

'DESTINED TO A PERFECT RECOVERY'

The confinement of puerperal insanity in the nineteenth century

Hilary Marland

'Cases of puerperal insanity appear to afford a better prospect of recovery than any other' (John Conolly, 1846).[1] 'Puerperal patients should always be treated as though they were destined to a perfect recovery' (William Tyler Smith, 1856).[2] 'Many of the cases with the worst symptoms, bodily and mental, made good recoveries' (Thomas Clouston, 1887).[3] Unlike the dreary prognosis for many 'insane' patients during the nineteenth century, the condition which came to be known as 'puerperal insanity' or 'insanity of childbirth' was treated by contemporaries as a temporary, albeit often very serious, aberration, likely to be curable. Hard-pressed superintendents of asylums greeted the disorder, which accounted for large and growing numbers of female admissions during the century, as a potential boost to rates of recovery and discharge. Yet at the same time, there was a striking discrepancy between the number of women said to have been suffering from puerperal insanity and asylum intake under this category. The advocacy of domestic management of such cases, particularly by obstetric practitioners, seems responsible for filling the gap between occurrence and asylum admissions.

Childbirth and puerperal insanity

The phenomenon of erratic, crazy, even violent behaviour on the part of pregnant women or new mothers had been described long before the nineteenth century. A small number of largely uninfluential continental works on the subject had been published from early in the eighteenth century, particularly a run of German dissertations,[4] while various authors on midwifery had made mention of the condition. There was nothing to compare, however, with the massive upsurge in interest in puerperal conditions which occurred during the 1820s and 1830s, and beyond. It could be argued[5] that puerperal insanity was 'classified into existence' during this period, to become one of the most clearly recognised disease entities of nineteenth-century psychiatry, one of the few disorders which doctors could point to and label with some degree of confidence, with its roots firmly embedded in the childbearing experience. Across Europe and North America treatises, articles and correspondence to medical journals on the identification and treatment of puerperal insanity proliferated.[6]

Puerperal insanity burst forth onto the medical stage then in a quite spectacular way and was seized upon as a condition following hard upon the heels of childbirth, which was also being redefined around the same period as abnormal and full of risk.[7] Puerperal insanity was spectacular for the speed with which it was propelled into the medical literature and also because it appeared to become part of the medical dialogue of a wide range of practitioners.[8] It was also spectacular in the way it was described, as an abrupt and devastating disorder, which could just as well strike poor women, debilitated by want and hardship, as upper-class ladies, cushioned by luxury and attended in childbirth by the 'best' medical men available.

Concerned to identify and label emotional responses to childbirth – and in a sense to separate out the abnormal but expected from more extreme forms of the disorder – the medical profession divided puerperal insanity into two categories, melancholia, characterised by depression and not considered a particularly odd accompaniment of childbirth, and mania, distinguished by overexcited, disruptive and deviant behaviour, the condition most dangerous and most likely to be brought into the asylum. Though mental disorders could also develop during pregnancy and lactation, it was the insanity following hard upon the heels of delivery which attracted most commentary and which was considered to be most prolific. The eminent French psychiatrist, L.-V. Marcé, in a 400-page monograph on disorders of pregnancy, birth and lactation, defined the 'puerperal period', marking the time during which the disorder could originate, as lasting up to six weeks after childbirth, with mania occurring three times as often as melancholia.[9]

It was mania which violated nineteenth-century norms and captured most interest, although as childbirth became defined as ever more risky and pathological, and women, locked into their 'biological straitjackets',[10] ever more subject to bouts of insanity, there is often a powerful sense in writings on the subject that this kind of condition was only to be expected amongst women too feeble to give birth naturally and without major disruption to their reproductive organs and nervous systems. Mary Poovey has declared that doctor–female patient relationships in the nineteenth century were governed by a set of assumptions: 'that woman's reproductive function defines her character, position and value, that this function influences and is influenced by an array of nervous disorders'.[11] The conclusions of Poovey's article, published in 1986, have since been modified and revised according to particular periods, locations, responses and conditions. In the case of puerperal mania it is true that understandings of it were shaped by notions of women's reproductive function, but doctors also saw the condition in a sense as *betraying* women's character, position and values, letting them down briefly but not irrevocably.

Despite (or perhaps because of) the feeling of risk linked to women's shaky reproductive systems, great concern was expressed about the more florid symptoms of puerperal mania, the self-neglect, restlessness, promiscuity, violence and intense aversion to husband and children, particularly the new-born.[12] Robert Gooch referred to the rumbustious behaviour which could go with the condition: 'the patient swears, bellows, recites poetry, talks bawdry, and kicks up such a row that there is the devil to play in the house; it is odd that women who have been delicately brought up, and chastely educated, should have such rubbish in their minds'.[13] Another authority, writing in what would become typical terms, described the obscenity of puerperal patients, which 'constantly turns upon sexual matters, the movements of the body and actions being such as to indicate a nymphomaniacal condition. Delicate ladies will use language which it would be thought impossible they could ever have had the opportunity of hearing.'[14] Puerperal mania rocked prevailing Victorian mores and notions of maternal affection and feminine behaviour. Yet because it was seen predominantly as a temporary disorder, its darker aspects were judged too to be passing phenomena; women sufferers needed to be closely guarded whilst ill, but were likely to recover their faculties fully.

Not all doctors writing on the condition chose to stress the more flamboyant and disturbing symptoms of puerperal insanity; for many it was as much bound up with the after-effects of giving birth as the potential to fall ill from childbed fever or other physical disorders. Yet even when authors on the disorder stressed its more shocking features, we need to place their remarks in context, and not forget that they were attempting to write up and attract attention to a 'new' condition, and portray its significance, particularly as a threat to domestic contentment and maternal well-being, and the happy undertaking of women's 'natural duties'. The rhetoric did of course also reflect elements of competition on the part of those seeking to treat the condition and claim expertise. Described by most commentators as a pre-eminently 'curable' condition, there was a good deal at stake in terms of claiming patients who would make either good testimonial material when building up a private practice (often including midwifery), or would make significant improvements in asylum statistics.

Territories of puerperal insanity

The fact that interest in the condition tracked the formation of the profession of psychiatry, the building of vast asylums to house the insane, and the continued proliferation of private asylums is of significance but perhaps less than we might first assume. Alienists wrote on the subject of puerperal insanity, but their hands-on involvement was deferred by practitioners of midwifery, who were keen to keep patients suffering from this condition out of the asylum. The earliest publications on the topic – and the majority up until the mid-nineteenth century – were written by obstetricians rather than alienists. Dr Robert Gooch, an eminent London obstetrician, physician to the Westminster Lying-in Hospital and lecturer on midwifery at St Bartholomew's Hospital, was the first to write a treatise in English on the subject in 1820.[15] Despite Gooch's premature death before the treatise was published, he came to be recognised posthumously as an important authority on the condition.[16] Gooch's work was followed up by a number of publications by, often eminent, specialists in obstetrics and the diseases of women: Fleetwood Churchill, James Reid, Robert Lee, William Tyler Smith and J.Y. Simpson. Aside from the adepts, no nineteenth-century textbook on the 'diseases of women', of which there were vast numbers, would be complete without a section on puerperal insanity. Up to the middle of the century it was by and large obstetricians who presented themselves as *the* authorities on the condition and its treatment.

In doing so obstetricians were offering one more piece of testimony to show precisely why they, and not midwives, should deliver babies. By the 1860s and 1870s there was growing enmity between midwives and accoucheurs, and efforts were stepped up to keep midwives out of well-paid practice.[17] More and more the claim was advanced that civilised women were likely to undergo many forms of trauma during pregnancy, birth and breast-feeding, as their comfortable lives and tendency toward nervous behaviour had ill-prepared them for strain and physical effort. Michael Ryan summed up the dangers of childbirth thus in 1867:

> Happily for humanity, the process of labour, in a vast majority of cases, is safe and free from danger, especially when women live according to nature's laws; but among the higher and middle, indeed all classes in civilised society in which these laws are frequently violated or forgotten, or when the constitution is impaired by the luxury or dissipation of modern times, the process of child-bearing is attended with more or less danger, both before and after it is completed....It is, however, fortunate for suffering humanity, that the process of parturition may now be greatly accelerated, and the greatest of mortal suffering relieved by the advice and skilful exertions of the obstetrician or medical attendant, and with the most perfect safety to the parent and offspring...there are few intelligent women who do not prefer medical attendance during labour, to that of midwives.[18]

Ryan warned too of the dangers of puerperal mania which could occur soon after delivery or during lactation when the system was 'exhausted', but believed it 'rarely incurable'.[19] Like other authors, Ryan stressed mild treatment, careful handling and removal of the patient from her home and its associated distress; preventative action took the form of the employment of a doctor trained in obstetrics.

As part of their claim to expertise, the incidence of puerperal insanity was tied in closely by male practitioners of midwifery to the method of delivery and immediate after-care, and it was also linked to difficult, lengthy and excessively painful confinements. William Tyler Smith described how the transient form of mania, which occurred at the moment of birth itself, could be triggered by the use of forceps, it was more apt to occur in first labours than in multiparae, and if the head of the child was larger than usual. When the infant's head passes through the *os uteri* or *os externum*, women can, wrote Smith, 'sometimes lose their self-consciousness, or self-control, and commit, if allowed, extravagant acts, in these brief intervals of insanity'.[20] Both Smith and James Young Simpson believed the danger of harm during labour either to the mother, the infant or birth attendants, expressed in this highly transient form, could be prevented by the use of chloroform, which would prevent the pain becoming so great that it made the patient frantic.

In his *Clinical Lectures* published in 1872 J.Y. Simpson related the story of Christina S. who had been admitted to the Edinburgh Royal Infirmary in a sorry state in March 1860, with an 'acute attack of puerperal mania', and also suffering from a vesico-vaginal fistula.

> Eight weeks before admission she was confined, in the country, for the first time, of an illegitimate child; and was in labour for three days. The pains, according to her own account, were so severe that she was constrained to keep her bed throughout the entire period. The child was still-born; although she stated that she was sensible of its movements not long before its delivery. There was no medical man in attendance, and no instrumental or other artificial aid was afforded her, the whole process having been conducted by a midwife.

The links with ideas about who should be attending women in childbirth and the necessity of pain relief and instrumental intervention are obvious. Simpson emphasised that the patient was slovenly and dirty, and he also referred to her as becoming noisy and troublesome but did not dwell on this. Christina was moved to the ward for the insane within the hospital, 'where she lay for three days with the mental faculties completely in abeyance, being sometimes slightly excited, but usually quiet and unimpressionable'. On 1 April she sank and died; it is not clear what of. But her feeble-mindedness, hopelessness, dirt, poverty *and* the way she had been failed by her childbirth attendant are woven into her story.[21]

Where did this leave the alienists? It is tempting to see the cornering of puerperal insanity in terms of a sub-plot, reflecting the vested interests of two ambitious groups of emerging medical specialists, both laying claims to expertise. There is something in this, but it is too simple an explanation. One way of thinking about this relationship is to see puerperal insanity as a 'bridge' between the two specialties, connecting the strains of reproduction to the potential for female insanity, and thus directly linking the specialties of obstetrics and gynaecology and psychiatry. By the mid-nineteenth century the struggle to take this bridge was on, and there is increased evidence of grappling between the two specialties. By the end of the century the bridge had been largely seized by the psychiatric profession, evidenced by rising rates of admission to asylums of women suffering from puerperal mania. Many more alienists were writing on the subject, particularly those in charge of the larger English and Scottish asylums who had more such cases passing under their care – John Conolly, J.B. Tuke and D.H. Tuke, Thomas Clouston and A. Campbell Clark – and we can see a slippage in terms of the bulk of publications away from obstetric specialists towards alienists.

More significant than any links with building institutions to house the insane was the firming of the link between 'moral insanity' and insanity of childbirth. Dr James Cowles Prichard introduced the concept of 'moral insanity' in 1835, defining it as 'a morbid perversion of the natural feelings, affections, inclinations, temper, habits, moral dispositions, and natural impulses, without any remarkable disorder or defect of the intellect, of knowing and reasoning faculties, and particularly without any insane illusion or hallucination'.[22] Moral insanity redefined madness, not as loss of reason, but as deviance from socially accepted behaviour, a failure to cope with poverty, the temptations of drink, domestic crises, disappointments in love, cruelty, mis-applied religiosity, or, in the case of puerperal insanity, the strains of childbearing. The purpose of moral management of the insane was restoration through close supervision and paternal care, based largely on the 'moral management' outlined by the Tukes at the York Retreat.[23] Puerperal insanity was in many respects a 'perfected' example of moral insanity, in the descriptions of its causality, symptoms, prognosis, and the strong thread of recovery and redemption running through largely optimistic accounts which stress its curability. It involved a temporary lapse of acceptable norms into extremely bad and disruptive behaviour, particularly the dereliction of maternal duty and upsetting of the domestic environment and order. Yet it was also accepted as being a condition likely to be redeemable and in a relatively short space of time.

Confinement of puerperal insanity

As alienists became more actively involved in claiming and treating cases of puerperal insanity, asylum admissions under this category stepped up. Statements concerning the extent, the timing and causality of puerperal insanity vary enormously, and the number of female asylum cases attributed to puerperal insanity also show great discrepancies. In 1858 Bucknill and Tuke gave a range of 5 to 25 per cent (for insanity of pregnancy, childbirth and lactation aggregated); many asylums claimed around 10 per cent of their female patients as cases of puerperal insanity.[24] This is the estimate given in 1872 by James Young Simpson for all female lunatic asylum admissions, and by the time Simpson was writing it appeared to be rising.[25] In Bucknill's own institution, the Devon County Asylum at Exminster, however, less than 2 per cent of female admission certificates indicated puerperal insanity between 1845 and 1914.[26]

There are several problems relating to the classification of puerperal insanity. While some authors were rigorous in separating off puerperal mania from other conditions following on from childbirth, particularly puerperal fever, others presented a confused, blurred picture. Fleetwood

Churchill pointed to this lack of precision in discussing the work of Marshall Hall, an early authority on puerperal disorders, writing in the 1820s and 1830s. Hall claimed that puerperal insanity resulted 'from all the circumstances following parturition combined, but chiefly from the united influences of intestinal irritation and loss of blood'. Failing to be clear about its distinctiveness from puerperal phrenitis, Hall recommended puerperal insanity be treated as a mixed case of intestinal irritation and exhaustion, an assumption which Churchill clearly found difficult to take on board.[27] This lack of clarity may often have been carried over into asylum admissions, and it is likely that some cases of puerperal mania were in fact women suffering from puerperal fever and in a state of delirium. Some of the small number of deaths from puerperal mania were likely to have been misdiagnosed fever cases. Irvine Loudon refers to a case cited by Simpson in 1873, where a post-natal patient with a fever of 103°F attempted to jump out of the window. She was restrained, but died later in delirium and her death was ascribed to puerperal mania. A post-mortem revealed pus in the peritoneal cavity, a clear indication of puerperal sepsis.[28]

The other cause of potential confusion relates to labelling; although puerperal insanity has been described as one of the most clearly defined psychiatric conditions of the century, it is clear that many asylum record keepers simply did not know what to call it. Cause and category were often confused, and many asylum reports demonstrated abrupt shifts in attribution between insanity of childbirth and insanity of lactation; the break-off point between the two conditions was not clear, as most women developing puerperal mania would be breast-feeding their infants. Definitions of the period within which puerperal insanity could begin were also ambiguous; most authorities saw the puerperal period as lasting six weeks, but cases were cited where the 'puerperal mania' had begun several years after the delivery. Leaving details of classification aside, however, it suffices to know, as we do, that large numbers of women were admitted to asylums because they were thought to suffer from puerperal insanity, or because it was a convenient label. Even J.B. Tuke, an authority on the subject, talked in terms of the 155 cases admitted to the Royal Edinburgh Asylum, Morningside, as cases of 'so-called puerperal mania'. On the distinctions between insanity of pregnancy, puerperal insanity and insanity of lactation, Tuke stressed that 'no series of cases has as yet been recorded in such a way as to bring out prominently the characteristics of each group distinctively'.[29]

'Confinement' takes on a poignant double meaning in the context of puerperal mania. The happy event of being confined in childbirth became tainted by the illness of the mother and the disruption of family life. And it is in such terms that medical men describing the condition write. While paying service to the idea that such a follow-up to birth was not entirely unexpected given women's intrinsic vulnerability, at the same time puerperal mania is also seen as a cruel twist of fate, often unaccountable given the mother's previous medical, moral and family history, and the result in some sense of an unlucky combination of events. It is also described as a terribly sad occurrence, marring what should be a scene of joy to the mother and her family and connections: 'It is a very distressing malady in itself, but doubly so from occurring at a moment ordinarily so joyful'.[30]

Once diagnosed, fairly rapid decisions needed to be made about what to do with the patient and how she should be treated. Although large numbers of patients suffering from puerperal insanity were placed in asylums, many remained under domestic management. One, admittedly high, estimate suggested that as many as one-quarter of female confinements were associated with puerperal insanity in some form, while only one in fourteen female asylum admissions were accounted for by this condition.[31] The gap between these two figures suggests that many women, and not just the well-to-do whose families could afford to have them boarded out at a private house with a nurse in attendance, were treated in a domestic setting of some kind. It is not clear whether being assisted by a doctor at the delivery rather than a midwife would slow or speed the process of asylum admission; it would depend on the family circumstances and the view of the practitioner involved, but it would seem likely that poorer women attended by midwives would have fewer buffers delaying their removal to an institution of some kind. In the first instance, this could be the workhouse. Many women delivered in workhouses appear to have remained there even when they became disturbed after giving birth, unless they became particularly disorderly and unmanageable. The distressing case of Elizabeth A., who accompanied by several children, arrived at the Plympton St Mary Workhouse in Devon on a number of occasions in desperate circumstances between 1868 and 1872 has been described by Adair *et al.* Moving in and out of the workhouse, ill and destitute, she was finally removed to the Exminster Asylum, when, following the birth of a new baby in 1872, she became very disturbed, calling out the names of imaginary people, and trying to burn herself in the fire. She remained there until her death in 1894.[32]

Domestic management of cases was commonly advocated, with reference to the specificity of the condition – it not being like other forms of madness – and its generally good prognosis. Treatment, many argued, should not be linked to incarceration, but to separation from the specific domestic circumstances which so distressed the patient. As in the above case, women in most cases were only admitted to the asylum once they had become dangerous, suicidal, reckless or excessively troublesome. This could occur soon after the delivery or with a delay of many weeks, when the practitioner attending the patient at home clearly found it impossible to continue to manage the case himself. Mrs Q., a 26-year-old housewife, was admitted to the Glasgow District Asylum in June 1881 after being insane for two weeks, the medical certificate declaring her as 'violent in word and action: never asks after her child; incessant talking, most absurdly singing, &c.'.[33]

But many physicians were firm in their belief that even such difficult cases were best kept out of institutions. Obstetric doctors appear to have been, if not unanimous, then fairly certain in expressing their opposition to asylum treatment, advocating instead private seclusion and good nursing, or keeping the patient in the labour ward or lying-in charity if the insanity had begun there. Many alienists too stuck to the view that in mild cases the asylum was no place for the puerperal maniac. James Reid, one of the foremost authorities on puerperal disorders, physician to London's General Lying-in Hospital, maintained that the 'general opinion' was against the removal of patients labouring under puerperal insanity to the asylum, unless the case lapsed into a 'chronic and lingering form':

> If change of scene be deemed requisite, it is better that the patient should be removed at first to a quiet country village, or to the sea-side, under the care of an experienced nurse, but the frequent visits of the medical attendant will here be advisable.... The friends of the patient should also pay occasional visits, to examine into the domestic arrangements and comforts of the place, without, however, seeing the patient herself...[34]

William Tyler Smith, Physician-Accoucheur to St Mary's Hospital, Lecturer at St Mary's Hospital Medical School and President of the Obstetrical Society of London, opposed institutionalisation on the grounds that women suffering from puerperal mania were not like other insane patients, and should be protected from the stigma of the asylum; such cases should always be treated as if they would recover fully. He cited the example of Bethlem, where some of the women incarcerated had killed children while suffering from puerperal mania:

> Some of these poor creatures have passed the childbearing age, are perfectly clear in intellect, conscious of what they have done, and suffer intense misery therefrom, while they have their desolation enhanced by mixing constantly with confirmed lunatics.[35]

Many women who fell ill after giving birth in a lying-in hospital remained in these institutions where they were treated by the hospital physicians. Thomas More Madden, physician to the Rotunda Lying-in Hospital in Dublin, reported how he had extensive opportunities to study puerperal mania in the Rotunda. Indeed, Madden stressed that doctors were far more likely to meet this condition in hospital obstetric practice than privately, where 'patients were generally in better circumstances and social condition, having less mental anxiety and physical privation'.[36] A major part of the doctors' brief in such institutions was to guard against the dangers of the women harming their infants.

If it seemed that early recovery was not likely then Rotunda patients were transferred to an asylum, such as a woman delivered in June 1868. This was a case of a primipara, aged 20, married a year previously to a man of greatly inferior station to her own, a familiar trope in cases of puerperal mania, and one which confirmed the need to keep the woman isolated from more troublesome or threatening classes of lunatic, as individuals facing not only temporary insanity but also some slippage in social standing. The woman had passed from a condition of affluence and comfort to one of poverty and privation. Constipated and sleepless, expressing intense dislike of her child and husband, ten days after giving birth she became 'exceedingly loquacious and excited'. She had given 'the child who had incautiously been left with her "a right good smacking" ' which had, she reported, made her feel much better. Two days later she was removed to the Richmond Lunatic Asylum, where she remained for six weeks, when she was discharged 'perfectly well'. She later returned to see Madden, and a year later it was recorded that her circumstances had improved, her husband being employed in a good situation in England. Before she joined him, Madden attended her second confinement which passed off well, without any return of the mania. A success thus for asylum and lying-in hospital.[37] Another bad case was Mrs B., confined in 1869, violent, suffering from delusions, and suicidal, who was saved from jumping from the window to the paved area below by the ward maid grabbing her hair. She was put into a straight waistcoat, and removed the same day to Richmond Asylum.[38] Other cases, less violent and troublesome, were retained and treated in the Rotunda Hospital, until they were discharged together with their infants. Out of 26 cases of puerperal mania following on from delivery in the Rotunda between 1847 and 1854 (out of 13,748 deliveries, so not so many as Madden implied), 18 recovered, 5 were removed and 3 died.[39]

Even as considerable and rising numbers of women were admitted into asylums suffering from 'puerperal conditions', asylum superintendents were expressing ambivalence about this development. Thomas Clouston, reporting on the activities of the Cumberland and Westmorland Lunatic Asylum which he superintended in the 1860s, remarked that cases of insanity occurring after childbirth helped 'keep up the standard of curability', at the same time suggesting that when symptoms were mild and manageable, there was really no need for such women to be in the asylum at all.[40] John B. Tuke, writing up cases treated in the Royal Edinburgh Asylum, Morningside, again in the 1860s, referred to puerperal mania as '*the* most curable form of insanity', to be placed under asylum treatment 'as a *dernier ressort*'.[41] Yet of course the *dernier ressort* patients would also be those most likely to lapse into incurability, dementia, imbecility, or be liable to attempt suicide. And while alienists professed that milder cases need not be admitted to asylums, at the same time stress was placed on treating puerperal insanity quickly, on catching cases before they became serious and entrenched. Cases which developed slowly or some weeks after delivery could become the most intractable, such as the extreme example cited by Campbell Clark of a woman who had become insane three months after the birth of her first child, who was finally, after four years of insanity, admitted to the asylum.[42]

As to treatment, the majority of therapeutic regimes were gentle, with many physicians supporting sleep, peace and quiet, gentle purgatives and tonics, nutritious food, stressing the need to sooth and encourage the patient, to separate her from her domestic responsibilities and her family. There is often a powerful sense of the patient being offered and achieving respite. Powerful drug regimes, including the use of opiates, excessive bleeding and other radical therapies were derided for the most part. Yet, again, we can detect a change toward the second half of the century, with some authorities advocating powerful drugs, including opiates, forced feeding, and even surgical intervention. This coincides with the shift to asylum treatment and while many aspects of the earlier gentle therapeutic methods were retained, the slow, almost painstaking, regimes, emphasising moral as much as physical remedies, and endless patience, began to be lost in the institutional context. The use of gentle laxatives, warm hip baths, mild stimulants, occasional application of leeches, and good food advocated by Conolly in 1846, were bolstered by more rigorous therapeutics; in 1883 Campbell describes frequent resort to feeding with a pump, the administration of morphine and the use of powerful emetics.[43] It is important to stress that in the first half of the nineteenth century mild regimes were advocated even for the most violent and resistant cases.[44]

Many authors related puerperal mania to strain, usually the strains of childbearing, combined with some other debilitating factors, domestic troubles and, for the poor, hard physical labour, poverty, miserable conditions, poor diet, or indeed the disappointment associated with women marrying beneath themselves or who found themselves living with a bully, inebriate or poor provider. Shock or fright, as with other forms of moral insanity, was often cited as a trigger, the immediate cause. At Hanwell Asylum a total of 88 females were admitted in 1840, and in 70 cases the cause of insanity could be ascertained. Four were attributed to 'childbirth', 3 to milk fever, and 3 more resulted from pregnancy or alarm in pregnancy. Some 25 cases were attributed to the combination of 'fright and childbirth', so more than a third of the total of all female cases where causes were identified.[45] J.E.D. Ésquirol, who rather than providing case notes, set out to provide life histories of his patients dating back to childhood or puberty, emphasised disappointments and domestic crises, but also hunger and weariness as predisposing causes of puerperal mania.[46] Rather than stressing the neglect of maternal responsibility which followed on from the condition, many authors blamed overly maternal tendencies, particulary prolonged breast-feeding when the mother herself was malnourished, as a precipitating cause.

Puerperal mania was linked on the one hand to excessive luxury with its enfeebling effects on women, but poverty and want were also cited as causal factors. It was associated closely with the crime of infanticide. Descriptions abound of the poor, semi-starved, haggard, and desperate women – often deserted and alone – who fell victim to the condition or committed the crime, or both. As with infanticide, puerperal mania was reputedly far more likely to afflict single mothers; Thomas More Madden put the figure at 12 out of 20 cases;[47] a sixth of Tuke's cases were unmarried.[48] Cold and chills are often described as triggering the condition. Hunger is frequently mentioned, and the restorative diet and tonics which formed an important part of the therapeutic regime also take on a practical, directly curative aspect, the woman's mental powers being linked directly to her physical well-being.

Though family members interact in the treatment of the case, their role is minimised, at least until the implications of heredity began increasingly to be explored towards the end of the century. Husbands, often the butt of hatred on the part of the women sufferers, come out badly in case notes and reports. The wealthy variant is rarely criticised but he is decisively pushed out of the therapeutic regime, his wife being removed from his presence and authority, taken from her home and separated from her 'dearest' connections, with the authority of the physician replacing that of the husband. In poor families, if the husband is mentioned at all, he is often blamed for the woman's condition; he was a poor provider, the woman had married 'beneath her', he was violent, a drinker, or a womaniser. Behind every infanticidal woman lay a blackguard, according at least to many doctors acting as trial witnesses, and blame was firmly apportioned with the husband or lover who ill-treated or deserted the woman, making her insane. When the condition began to be linked to insanity in the family, it was the father who was the most likely culprit.[49]

Redemption from puerperal insanity

Most patients were recorded as recovering quickly, within a few months. Discharge rates from asylums confirm the good expectations, even as accounts of treatment regimes become more depressing to read. Haslem reported cure rates of 50 to 85 per cent at Bethlem, most during the fourth month; Ésquirol two-thirds within six months.[50] Thomas More Madden cited several sources, all of whom claimed reasonable or good rates of cure: Gooch in private practice and Johnston and Sinclair at the Rotunda both had rates of almost 70 per cent.[51] J.B. Tuke declared 54 out of 73 patients (74 per cent) as cured within six months. Such cases contrasted starkly with other categories of insanity with expected stays in the asylum running into several years, and who fed into the silting up of such institutions. However, expressing a widely held view, Tuke emphasised that the chances of cure diminished rapidly as time passed: 'if the mania is prolonged more than a month, or at the outside six weeks after confinement, the probabilities of ultimate cure are very faint'.[52] Insanity of lactation was in general considered more difficult to treat, as were melancholic cases, which tended to set in rather later than mania.

The discussion about who should be treating puerperal insanity and where lasted many decades. In a series of articles published in the *Lancet* in 1883, A. Campbell Clark, medical superintendent of the Glasgow District Asylum at Bothwell was still explaining how puerperal insanity called for the attention of the general practitioner as well as the asylum physician. He also saw the need to maintain the link between the specialties, to make puerperal insanity the 'common cause' of the obstetrician and 'psychological physician' alike.[53]

> For various reasons many patients of this class are not sent to an asylum; and where home conditions are favourable it is well that this should be so, for two reasons: first because puerperal insanity is mainly an evolution of a bodily state, an insanity by sympathy, and frequently implies potential insanity only under extraordinary physical conditions; secondly, because the stigma of lunacy is considerably minimised, if not entirely obliterated, by private treatment.[54]

By the close of the century, however, authority over the condition was increasingly claimed and captured by psychiatrists. Some were sceptical about the existence of 'puerperal insanity' as a distinct form of mental trouble. In making claims of mis-diagnosis and stressing the inadvisability of cases being called puerperal because the women 'chanced to be pregnant' or had recently given birth, changes in therapeutic practices become evident, particularly a move to the asylum and to harsher therapeutic regimes.[55] At the same time as some doctors were expressing scepticism about the existence of puerperal insanity, increasingly elaborate classification schemes were being developed, and the numbers admitted under this category were increasing; at the Warwick County Lunatic Asylum from 11 per cent in the 1850s to 18 per cent in the late 1880s.[56]

W.F. Menzies, senior assistant physician to the Lancashire County Asylum at Rainhill, Liverpool, reported in 1893 on 140 cases of puerperal insanity in the *American Journal of Insanity*.[57] Between 1889 and 1891 968 female patients were admitted to the Rainhill Asylum. Because of the want of room, restrictions were imposed on numbers, but every endeavour was made to accommodate acute cases, and 'probably no well-established puerperal case was refused'.[58] These women were drawn from the poorer classes and from an estimated female population of about 455,000. The births in this population were 98,065, meaning that the 140 cases of puerperal insanity admitted represented one case in every 700 deliveries (excluding twins). Menzies' article was rigorous in its effort to recategorise puerperal insanity into 'puerperal established types', expressed by delirious excitement, suicidal impulses, delirium and melancholia. Puerperal cases had the potential to pass through a maximum of six stages: prodromal disturbance, early delirium, melancholia, stupor, mania and dementia. While many patients passed through the first five stages and still recovered, Menzies surmised that in general the fewer the stages, the better the prognosis. Menzies also defined three different types of mania which could occur. He broke down the aetiology of the disease according to age, number of pregnancies, previous attacks, heredity, the sex of the child, and other causes, including drink, domestic worry, difficult labour, and a variety of medical conditions, ranging from rheumatism to syphilis. His use of his patients to come up with detailed statistics of insanity represents a striking shift from the rather more romanticised, anecdotal reports which typify the earlier part of the century, with case histories detailing stories of slow, but steady progress towards recovery. Menzies' linkage of the condition to hereditary is especially striking. Some 25 per cent of puerperal cases had a history of insanity (compared with 28.2 for female asylum admissions as a whole), with the father being the relative most commonly insane, then the sister and mother.[59]

By the second half of the century the increase in asylum admissions under the category of puerperal insanity represented a shift away from treatment by individual practitioners, the family doctor or obstetrician who had attended the delivery, to therapies catering for large groups of institutionalised insane, and cases of puerperal insanity were more likely to be subsumed into general asylum regimes and therapeutics. The kind of analysis and ways of thinking about insanity encapsulated in Menzies' article – with its breakdown into typologies, causal factors, and prognosis – only became possible with larger groups of patients. Earlier in the century it is not unreasonable to envisage a different picture of interaction and alliance between doctor and patient; cases were much more likely to be presented individually as narratives of fall, redemption and recovery.[60]

In or out of the asylum, however, most women were recorded as making 'full' recoveries, within the space of a few months. Redemption is a persistent motif. The women are not always but often depicted as 'respectable', such as the domestic servant, K.C., described by Thomas Clouston. Though of a respectable family, she was a 'fallen woman' who had borne an illegitimate child at a maternity hospital. Under treatment the patient did well; she was put on nourishing food and taken out for airings. Sleep became regular once more, but K.C. remained boisterous. A return to work – the usual token of successful treatment and a requirement of the asylum regime – got rid of this excess energy:

> in three months she was fattening, quieting, and working hard. In four months after admission she was stout, sensible, and well in mind and body, menstruation having begun, and she was

> then sent back to her situation, which had been kept open for her in consideration of her previous good conduct.[61]

Clouston described recovery from puerperal mania – and therefore redemption – thus:

> In a month she will be knitting a stocking, and will know her friends when they come to see her. Within three months she is well – a joyous mother, in her right mind, clasping her child, the whole of the disturbed mental period seeming like a dream to her, that is very soon altogether forgotten in her new duties and delights...few things are more pleasant than to see the restoration of the mother back to all that makes her life worth having.[62]

The given causes of puerperal insanity, its symptoms, its classification, its incidence, the recommended therapeutics and place of treatment all remained highly ambiguous throughout the nineteenth century. The condition was associated with both poverty and excess. It was linked closely to both women's life cycle and at the same time to anxieties about the domestic sphere. It was depicted as a terrible, alarming, 'unexpected', follow-up to childbirth, but at the same time one to be anticipated. Even as there was an increasing tendency to lump puerperal insanity patients with other categories of the insane towards the end of the century, at the same time admissions to asylums under this heading were rising. While puerperal insanity was seen as having its strongest associations with difficult deliveries, it was triggered, contemporaries believed, by the act of giving birth, not by a particular gynaecological disorder or disease. Its danger was not in its long-term impact, or even its dramatic manifestations, but the fact that it could potentially affect so many women. Perhaps most significantly, claims to expertise on the condition and the best methods of dealing with it were made strongly by obstetric specialists and alienists well into the closing decades of the century. The ambiguities of the condition were in part the product of the claims made upon puerperal insanity by those seeking to treat it.

Acknowledgements

This research was carried out as a Wellcome University Award Holder, and I am grateful to the Wellcome Trust for their support. My thanks to the participants at the Exeter Conference for their feedback, and particularly to the editors for their detailed commentary on earlier drafts of this article.

NOTES

1 J. Conolly, 'Clinical lectures on the principal forms of insanity, delivered in the Middlesex Lunatic-Asylum at Hanwell', Lecture XIII: 'Description and treatment of puerperal insanity', *Lancet*, 28 March 1846, pp. 349–54, on p. 350.
2 W. Tyler Smith, 'Puerperal mania', Lecture XXXIX: 'Lectures on the theory and practice of obstetrics', *Lancet*, 18 October 1856, pp. 423–5, on p. 424.
3 T.S. Clouston, *Clinical Lectures on Mental Diseases*, London, J. and A. Churchill, 1887, p. 517.
4 See S. Day, 'Puerperal insanity: the historical sociology of a disease', unpublished Ph.D. thesis, University of Cambridge, 1985, esp. p. 154.
5 As suggested by I. Loudon, 'Puerperal insanity in the 19th century', *Journal of the Royal Society of Medicine*, 81, February 1988, pp. 76–9.
6 Very few historical studies have dealt with puerperal insanity, with the important exceptions of Day, 'Puerperal insanity' and N. Theriot, 'Diagnosing unnatural motherhood: nineteenth-century physicians and "puerperal insanity" ', *American Studies*, 26, 1990, pp. 69–88.
7 See, for example, O. Moscucci, *The Science of Woman: Gynaecology and Gender in England 1800–1929*, Cambridge, Cambridge University Press, 1990; J.W. Leavitt, *Brought to Bed: Childbearing in America, 1750–1950*, New York and Oxford, Oxford University Press, 1986.
8 In evidence presented at infanticide trials the medical witnesses were often surgeons or general practitioners, who, while presumably coming across few cases of puerperal mania in their practices, declared knowledge of the condition and were content to apply the label in order to explain the actions of the women accused: see, for example, J.P. Eigen, *Witnessing Insanity: Madness and Mad-Doctors in the English Court*, New Haven and London, Yale University Press, 1995, esp. pp. 142, 147–9.
9 L.-V. Marcé, *Traité de la folie des femmes enceintes des nouvelles accouchées et des nourrices et considérations médico-légales qui se rattachent à ce sujet*, Paris, J.B. Bailièrre, 1858.
10 See Anne Digby's essay, 'Women's biological straitjacket', in S. Mendus and J. Rendell, eds, *Sexuality and Subordination: Interdisciplinary Studies of Gender in the Nineteenth Century*, London and New York, Routledge, 1989, pp. 192–220.
11 M. Poovey, ' "Scenes of an indelicate character": the medical "treatment" of Victorian women', *Representations*, 14, 1986, pp. 137–68, on p. 146.
12 For the relationship between puerperal insanity and infanticide, see Day, 'Puerperal insanity', and Hilary Marland, 'Murdering mothers revisited: infanticide, responsibility and puerperal insanity in nineteenth-century Britain', unpub. paper, 1997.
13 Robert Gooch, *A Practical Compendium of Midwifery, Being the Course of Lectures on Midwifery, and on Diseases of Women and Infants, Delivered at St. Bartholomew's Hospital*, London, Longman, Rees, Orme, Brown and Green, 1831, p. 290.
14 Smith, 'Puerperal mania', p. 424.

15 Robert Gooch, *Observations on Puerperal Insanity*, London, 1820 (extracted from 6th volume of Medical Transactions, Royal College of Physicians, read at the College, 16 December 1819).
16 See also Gooch, *Practical Compendium* and *On Some of the Most Important Diseases Peculiar to Women*, London, New Sydenham Society, 1831.
17 See Moscucci, *The Science of Woman*, pp. 70–1.
18 M. Ryan, *A Manual of Midwifery and Diseases of Women and Children*, 4th edn, London, pub. by the author, 1841, p. 167.
19 Ibid., p. 334.
20 Smith, 'Puerperal mania', p. 423.
21 J.Y. Simpson, *Clinical Lectures on the Diseases of Women*, Edinburgh, Adam and Charles Black, 1872, pp. 555–6.
22 Cited E. Showalter, *The Female Malady: Women, Madness and English Culture, 1830–1980*, New York, Pantheon, 1985, p. 29. See also V. Skultans, *Madness and Morals: Ideas on Insanity in the Nineteenth Century*, London and Boston, Routledge and Kegan Paul, 1975, esp. the extracts in Part Two.
23 A. Digby, *Madness, Morality and Medicine: A Study of the York Retreat*, Cambridge, Cambridge University Press, 1985.
24 J.C. Bucknill and D.H. Tuke, *A Manual of Psychological Medicine*, London, J. and A. Churchill, 1858, pp. 236–7. Cited Digby, 'Women's biological straitjacket', p. 206.
25 Simpson, *Clinical Lectures*, p. 556.
26 J. Melling and B. Forsythe, 'Madness, marriage and mortality: gender and admission to the pauper lunatic asylum in Victorian and Edwardian England. The Devon Country Asylum, 1845–1914', forthcoming, p. 9. With thanks to the authors for allowing me access to their findings prior to publication.
27 M. Hall, *Commentaries on Some of the More Important of the Diseases of Females*, London, Longman, Rees, Orme, Brown and Green, 1827, pp. 251–2; F. Churchill, *On the Diseases of Women; Including those of Pregnancy and Childbed* (4th edn), Dublin, Fannin and Co., 1857, p. 744.
28 I. Loudon, *Death in Childbirth: An International Study of Maternal Care and Maternal Mortality 1800–1950*, Oxford, Clarendon, 1992, p. 145.
29 J.B. Tuke, 'On the statistics of puerperal insanity as observed in the Royal Edinburgh Asylum, Morningside', *Edinburgh Medical Journal*, 19, 1865, pp. 1,013–28, on pp. 1,013, 1,014.
30 Churchill, *On the Diseases of Women*, p. 737.
31 C. Mercier, *A Textbook of Insanity*, London, Macmillan, 1902, p. 155. Cited Digby, 'Women's biological straitjacket', p. 206.
32 R. Adair, B. Forsythe and J. Melling, 'A danger to the public? Disposing of pauper lunatics in late-Victorian and Edwardian England: Plympton St. Mary Union and the Devon County Asylum, 1867–1914', *Medical History*, 42, 1998, pp. 1–25, on pp. 18–19.
33 A. Campbell Clark, 'Clinical illustrations of puerperal insanity', *Lancet*, 21 July 1883, pp. 97–9, 180–1, 277–9, on p. 98.
34 J. Reid, 'On the causes, symptoms, and treatment of puerperal insanity', *Journal of Psychological Medicine*, 1, 1858, pp. 128–51, 284–94, on p. 290.
35 Smith, 'Puerperal mania', p. 424.
36 In contrast to Reid who stated that this condition was rarely met with in lying-in institutions: Reid, 'On the causes', p. 128. T.M. Madden, 'On

puerperal mania', *British and Foreign Medico-Chirurgical Review*, XLVIII, 1871, pp. 477–95, on p. 477.

37 Ibid., pp. 489–90.

38 Ibid., p. 492.

39 E.B. Sinclair and G. Johnston, *Practical Midwifery: Comprising an Account of 13,748 Deliveries Which Occurred in the Dublin Lying-in Hospital, During a Period of Seven Years, Commencing November 1847*, London, John Churchill, 1858, pp. 528–31.

40 *Annual Reports of the Cumberland and Westmorland Lunatic Asylum, 1863–1870.*

41 J.B. Tuke, 'Cases illustrative of the insanity of pregnancy, puerperal mania, and insanity of lactation', *Edinburgh Medical Journal*, XII, 1866–7, pp. 1,083–101, on p. 1,092. Many interested parties in Scotland were anxious to keep asylums as a last resort for many categories of insanity, and the notion of moral treatment was more pervasive and long-standing than in England; this may well have influenced the reports of the Scottish authorities on puerperal mania. See the essays of Lorraine Walsh and Jonathan Andrews in this volume.

42 Campbell Clark, 'Clinical illustrations', p. 180.

43 Conolly, 'Clinical lectures', pp. 350–1; Campbell Clark, 'Clinical illustrations'.

44 See Hilary Marland, 'At home with puerperal mania: the domestic management of the insanity of childbirth in the nineteenth century', forthcoming in P. Bartlett and D. Wright, eds, *Outside the Walls of the Asylum: Historical Perspectives on 'Care in the Community' in Modern Britain and Ireland*, London, Athlone, 1999.

45 *The Report of the Resident Physician of the Hanwell Lunatic Asylum presented to the Court of Quarter Sessions for Middlesex, at the Michaelmas Sessions, 1840.*

46 J.E.D. Ésquirol, *Mental Maladies. A Treatise on Insanity*, 1845 (English edn), London, Hafner, 1965.

47 Madden, 'On puerperal mania', p. 478.

48 Tuke, 'On the statistics of puerperal insanity', p. 1,019.

49 For different takes on the relationship between insanity and the family, see the essays of David Wright and Akihito Suzuki in this volume.

50 Bucknill and Tuke, *A Manual of Psychological Medicine*, p. 239.

51 Madden, 'On puerperal mania', p. 485.

52 Tuke, 'On the statistics of puerperal insanity', pp. 1,028, 1,019.

53 Campbell Clark, 'Clinical illustrations', p. 97.

54 Ibid., p. 97.

55 See, for example, E.B. Lane, 'Puerperal insanity', *Boston Medical and Surgical Journal*, CXLIV, 1901, pp. 606–9.

56 Loudon, 'Puerperal insanity in the 19th century', p. 77.

57 W.F. Menzies, 'Puerperal insanity: an analysis of one hundred and forty consecutive cases', *American Journal of Insanity*, 50, 1893–4, pp. 147–85.

58 Ibid., p. 148.

59 Ibid., pp. 160–1.

60 See Marland, 'At home with puerperal mania', which deals with the period dominated by midwifery practitioners.

61 Clouston, *Clinical Lectures*, p. 505.

62 Ibid., pp. 503, 502.

Part III

ON THE EDGE

The English model and national peripheries

8

ESTABLISHING THE 'RULE OF KINDNESS'

The foundation of the North Wales Lunatic Asylum, Denbigh

Pamela Michael and David Hirst

It has been suggested that at the end of the eighteenth century the British state appeared to the public 'only as the power that enlisted men and levied taxes...central government did nothing to secure the public safety, provided no schools, made no roads, gave no relief to the poor'.[1] If this was true of England, it was more so of Wales. Literature on eighteenth-century social policy has concentrated on English governance, to the neglect of significant differences between the four nations.[2] Implementation of English laws regarding poverty and vagrancy and adoption of a standardised system for the collection of poor rates came but slowly to Wales. Similarly the 1808 County Asylums Act had little impact in Wales, despite the prominent role played by Charles Watkyn Williams Wynn, MP for Montgomeryshire, in introducing the legislation, and notwithstanding an early response by some local magistrates.[3] An advertisement placed in the Chester Chronicle gave notice of a meeting to be held in Ruthin in January 1811 to consider 'the expediency and propriety of providing a LUNATIC ASYLUM...or, to treat with anyone or more of the adjacent counties to unite for that purpose...'[4] This led to further meetings, including one held in February 1811 where a Committee of Magistrates of Denbighshire and Flintshire were to treat with the County of Merioneth regarding the proposal to build a joint lunatic asylum. In response to an advertisement for this gathering Charles Watkyn Williams Wynn wrote to the Clerk of Denbighshire Quarter Sessions, to inform them that Montgomeryshire magistrates had likewise appointed a committee to treat with adjoining counties for the same purpose. 'I should apprehend', wrote Wynn,

> that it might be highly desirable that the union should embrace as many of the Counties of North Wales as are disposed to unite for the purpose as it has been found from experience that the greater the number of patients may be which is assembled together (provided it does not exceed 300) the smaller will be the expense of the care and maintenance of each individual.[5]

However, alongside competing demands on county expenditure to fulfil the increasing duties of the state, the difficulties of achieving a satisfactory agreement proved insurmountable.[6] It was another thirty years before a successful attempt was launched which finally united five counties of North Wales, omitting Montgomeryshire, which had by this time entered an agreement with Shropshire.[7] Only the heavily populated southern industrial counties were able to afford asylums of their own, Monmouthshire's being opened at Abergavenny in 1851 and Glamorganshire's, at Bridgend, in 1864.[8] The remaining counties of Wales negotiated alliances to run joint establishments, with the North Wales Lunatic Asylum, opened in 1848, being the first of these collaborative ventures. The joint counties asylum for south-west Wales was only opened in 1865 in Carmarthen, and not until 1903 was an asylum opened at Talgarth to serve Brecon and Radnor.[9]

There were no private madhouses in North Wales and no lively indigenous debate concerning rival methods of institutional treatment. Ideas concerning 'progressive' methods of treatment had necessarily to be 'imported'.[10] As Scull has observed, even by the middle of the nineteenth century, the standards of the reformers were not universally shared, and this was one reason why 'local power centres resisted efforts to set up a system of nationally supervised, publicly supported asylums'. And as he further points out 'the constitution and consummation of the reformers' project was dependent upon...a profound shift in the cultural understanding of madness. That metamorphosis proved vital in creating and sustaining the moral outrage which drove the whole process forward.'[11] Wales was a seat of resistance to the system of public asylums, as it was to the New Poor Law.

The establishment of the first joint public asylum in Wales was achieved by means of a moralising campaign, led by a tightly knit social group of landowners, magistrates, solicitors and medical men. This study serves to emphasise the paternalistic thrust of the movement to institutionalise the insane, and the extent to which investigation, surveillance and enforcement were essential to achieve the ascendancy of institutional treatment in a country wedded to a pattern of domestic arrangements. Our research has revealed the tensions between the magistrates who controlled the county asylum and the local administrators of the Poor Law. By illustrating the complexity of the situation, it suggests the need for caution before labelling the asylum as simply a 'poor law institution'.[12] The narrative highlights the unique factor of the Welsh language, indicating how the debate over the insane fits into a wider mid-nineteenth century discourse concerning the position of the language, and portrayals of 'the Welch', and forms part of that fascinating dialogue between 'the observers and the observed'.[13] The outsider as observer plays a critical role in the narrative. Indeed, this aspect was remarked upon at the time: 'a stranger, an Englishman, came amongst us, and in a visit of 3 or 4 weeks, saw for us, that which we, who always here, had never before known', wrote 'A Poor Welshman' in 1843.[14]

Despite growing interest in the subject at the beginning of the nineteenth century, a piecemeal system of local arrangements, combined with an inadequate system of recording, rendered estimates of the incidence of presumed insanity unreliable. Sir Andrew Halliday visited Wales to gather evidence for his report which he presented to Lord Seymour in 1829. He found in the counties of North Wales only 111 males and 138 females recorded as insane, and observed 'that a very large proportion of the insane persons in Wales are idiots', a situation which he noted to be similar to that in Scotland.[15] In Anglesey he found that 'of the 24 males and 27 females, only 2 males and 5 females were said to be dangerous, the rest being for the most part harmless idiots'. Not one was confined in an asylum, but rather 'the whole number are taken care of by their relations'.[16] Halliday speculated upon the cause of this seeming preponderance of idiots as opposed to lunatics in Wales. He considered the influence of climate and topography, but focused on what he regarded as a particular evil:

> one great cause of the increase of this species of insanity has arisen from our careless inattention in suffering female, as also male, idiots to procreate their species. The Cretins of the Alps, and the idiots of Scotland and Wales, have become numerous from this cause alone.[17]

Halliday had complained of the difficulty of obtaining information from the clerks of magistrates to whom he placed his enquiries.[18] Under the Asylums Act of 1828 it became obligatory for magistrates to make a return of the number of pauper lunatics and idiots maintained in each county. The ensuing returns are notorious for their inadequacy. Yet whilst, as a quantitative indicator, they are misleading, they can provide a useful index of the pattern of arrangements within each county.

A run of surviving Lunacy Returns for Denbighshire[19] for the years 1828–1858 has been analysed by the authors, with 572 individual detailed cases identified in a total of 1,926 entries. This analysis indicates that whilst some cases recur frequently in the returns, more than half of the cases appeared only once or twice. These returns for Denbighshire also confirm the overwhelming importance of close family in the care of idiots (as opposed to lunatics), outside of institutions. The original forms differentiate between 'lunatic' and 'idiot', making it possible to analyse the changing pattern of care. The results point to a clearly emerging division, following the opening of the Denbigh Asylum, between institutional care for the lunatic, and the continuance of outdoor care for those defined as idiots.

The previous arrangements often retained even the most difficult cases in the community, as a longitudinal reconstruction of the case of one lunatic, Evan Lewis, over a period of thirty years shows. It gives some insight into the problems and expense of organising care for a lunatic of long standing. Lewis appears to have been first presumed a lunatic in the 1820s, on his return from soldiering in India, and the Abergele Vestry at first sought to care for him in the community, transferring responsibility to the family where possible. Thus, in September 1823, it was ordered that the 8s. then being paid for Lewis should be discontinued, and that his father was to maintain him thereafter.[20] The following year, he was again the subject of arrangements, and of an agreement with Edward Roberts to 'look after' and feed Evan Lewis for 2s.6d. weekly.[21] For the next two years, Lewis appeared only in the Overseer's Accounts, where small grants for clothing and footwear were paid.[22] Subsequently he was sent to the subscription Asylum in Liverpool, a rather more expensive solution, since in 1830 the Overseers Accounts record a payment of £63.17s.3d. to the Liverpool Asylum for his treatment, just over two years costs at the rate of 12s. weekly.[23] Lewis was then returned to Abergele, where he was kept in some restraint. It was here that he came to the attention of Assistant Poor Law Commissioner, William Day, who wrote to the Guardians, stating that 'The Commissioners have received complaint that a Lunatic Pauper at Abergele in the St Asaph Union is brought out to bask in the sun, chained'.[24] This interesting complaint, which suggests a mixture of compassion and cruelty, was, from the evidence of Day's letter, not the first time Lewis had been the subject of correspondence, and Day wrote that he 'had imagined [Lewis] had long since been sent to the Chester Asylum'.[25] After threatening the Guardians with legal sanctions if they failed to act, Day wrote to George Cornewall Lewis, stating that he knew about this 'insane pauper of Abergele Union' personally, for he:

> came to my notice in consequence of having following Mrs. Day into a shop in that town, and abused her exceedingly. Great objection was made to the *Parish* Guardians to sending him to the Chester Asylum in consequence of the increased expense which would attend such a step but at length the Guardians at large overruled it, and an order was made to have him taken before the magistrates for the purpose of placing him there. The man is at all times insane and periodically violent at *known* intervals....I sent a letter to the Clerk of the Union on the subject, but if it were to come officially from you instead of myself it would have more effect.[26]

It appears that the Dean of St Asaph, Charles Scott Luxmoore, had actively intervened, and following receipt of this letter Lewis was sent to Chester Asylum, being removed to the North Wales Lunatic Asylum in Denbigh, when that opened in 1848.

The heavy dependence on outdoor care of the insane, and the late adoption of any form of institutional care, was associated with the rather different nature of social care under both the Old and New Poor Law in Wales. There was generally a preponderance of outdoor relief, and almost everywhere the biggest item was the payment of cottagers' rents, with some help for food and clothing. In North Wales there was an almost complete absence of anything akin to either the 'Speenhamland system' or the 'roundsmen's system'.[27] Care for the insane was heavily dependent on family arrangements, and on the boarding of idiots and lunatics for small sums of remuneration, a pattern of care more akin to that of Scotland, than to the asylum-based model already evolving in England and Ireland.[28]

Where families failed to provide care the alternative arrangements could be somewhat casual. In 1844 the Visiting Metropolitan Commissioners remarked on the slow erosion of customs, noting that in the Ffestiniog Union, for instance, 'the practice of rambling about begging had not been so common of late'. Yet it was not uncommon for the Guardians of some Unions, in fixing the amounts of weekly payments to: 'take into account the casual relief which the poor Lunatics and idiots may obtain by begging'.[29]

Some explanation of the foregoing can be found in the fact that the imposition of the New Poor Law had encountered difficulties peculiar to Wales. Assistant Poor Law Commissioner William Day was given responsibility for supervising the setting up of Poor Law Unions in North Wales, finding it, as he wrote to Chadwick in 1837, 'a devilish queer country to have to do business in'.[30] Although half Welsh himself, he did not have a working knowledge of the language, which was a source of difficulty when 'There are whole districts where hardly the parson himself can read English.'[31] The language, the religion, and above all the poverty, set Wales apart. The different standard of living, and in particular the diet, created a serious problem for a Commissioner trying to establish a workhouse regime based upon the principle of 'less eligibility'. 'The scale of living is so low', he wrote to the Commissioners in London,

> that no table yet issued by you would be at all safe either in practice or in principle....It would actually disagree with the paupers...the common diet here being the coarsest brown bread, and red herring and potatoes...and in principle it would place the pauper in a far better position than the labourer.[32]

The low level of money incomes and the lack of capital, which was a perennial problem for small farmers, extended to the parish funds. The increased demand for relief in the early 1840s had forced a general crisis, and in October 1841 only three of the North Wales Unions were not overdrawn on their account. Banks refused to extend their overdrafts, and in January 1843 the relieving officer had insufficient money to distribute to paupers in Ffestiniog, and in Pwllheli paupers had received no payments, other than credit notes, for the whole of the last quarter. The problem in North Wales was not so much one of pauperism, Day exclaimed, as of 'mendicity!'[33]

There was widespread Welsh opposition to the New Poor Law system. Day had a particularly rough reception at Dolgellau, where two of 'the most violent' of the Guardians assured their colleagues that the 'corner stones of the system were starvation and infanticide'.[34] Throughout the western counties opposition simmered, and in August 1840 Day wrote in exasperation:

> You cannot know the miseries of forty Welsh Guardians who *won't* build a Workhouse, and consequently meet in the parlour of a pothouse twelve feet by fourteen and keep all the windows shut and spit tobacco on your shoes – to say nothing of know-

> ing not a word of what they are talking of in an unknown tongue.[35]

In these circumstances the successful campaign to found a lunatic asylum for North Wales, revived in the 1840s, is in some ways remarkable. Certainly it was part of an ongoing process of modernisation, during which commerce and central government united to undermine local difference, although the apparently inevitable progression to a unified system may obscure a brief bureaucratic power struggle over the nature and direction of change.

The 1845 Act and the establishment of the Lunacy Commission gave increased power to central government to monitor and inspect asylums. It required local authorities to provide asylum care for pauper lunatics. However, their maintenance was to be paid for by the Poor Law Guardians, thereby counterbalancing the power of the magistrates. Thus, as other writers have noted, the history of the pauper lunatic occupies an uncertain space between the history of the hospitals and medicine, the history of the Poor Law, and the medico-legal framework. The early 1840s witnessed a struggle for jurisdiction over the pauper lunatic between the Poor Law Commissioners and the Metropolitan Commissioners in Lunacy.[36] The Poor Law and Lunacy Commissioners were vying with each other to map out the territory of insanity, and to identify and quantify the extent of lunacy as a social problem. As a result various inquiries were instigated.

Samuel Hitch, the Superintendent of the Gloucester Asylum, was sent by the Home Secretary to investigate the counties of North Wales, in 1842. He discovered that in the six counties there were 664 insane persons chargeable to the different parishes within those counties as 'lunatic paupers'; but as he pointed out, there was no way of ascertaining the number not counted as paupers, though in all likelihood it was a figure of similar proportion, 'making a frightful exhibition of the demented amongst our Welsh neighbours'.[37] Of the 664 pauper lunatics in North Wales, he reported, 'only 19 are placed in lunatic asylums, and those English ones', and of the remaining 654 only 32 'enjoy that comparative mental repose and limited care and solace which Union workhouses can supply; whilst no less than 303 are left with relatives to undergo all that injudicious fondness, injurious if well intentioned'. For Hitch, as a leading exponent of asylum treatment, even the workhouse was preferable to family care of the insane.

Central government concern over the situation in Wales was growing, for it was found that 'imperfect as the provision for lunatic poor may be in England, it is beyond all comparison more defective in

Wales'.[38] The Poor Law Commissioners knew of 'No county asylum and no licensed house for lunatics…in the whole principality of Wales.' They expressed regret at the deficiency, and contrasted the situation in Wales with that in England, demonstrating that whereas in England 42.2 per cent of lunatics chargeable in 1843 were receiving medical treatment in either asylums or licensed houses, the figure in Wales was only 6.5 per cent. They suggested that one asylum for South Wales and another for North Wales would 'probably answer every purpose', but acknowledged 'the practical difficulties in bringing about such a voluntary junction', and suggested that if the matter was not speedily resolved 'some legislative interference should take place' in order to secure for the lunatic poor of Wales the advantages of treatment which they ought to receive.[39]

Meanwhile the Metropolitan Lunacy Commissioners, who were preparing a General Report on the Condition of the Insane, extended their enquiries to make a special investigation in Wales. Thus, on 25 July 1844, the Metropolitan Commissioners in Lunacy entered North Wales 'for the purpose of inquiring into the condition and treatment of the Insane in that part of the Principality'.[40] They were to explore the arrangements and provisions for six counties, covering an area of 3,204 square miles, for which there was 'not, at present…a single Lunatic Asylum, public or private'.They began their tour at St Asaph where, being welcomed by the Dean, they were taken on a visit of the workhouse, followed by an inspection of the proposed site for the asylum in Denbigh. From their detailed investigations, which included discussions with 'Several Medical Gentlemen of eminence…the Surgeons of the various Unions…the Clerks of the several Boards of Guardians, and the Relieving Officers, the latter of whom accompanied us, in some cases, upon our visits', they were able to produce a well-documented report.[41] This included a number of exemplary cases, such as that of Mary Jones of Llanrhaiadr, who had been confined in the loft over a blacksmith's forge for some fifteen to eighteen years.[42] In summing up their enquiries the Commissioners wrote:

> We have found, generally, that, in disposing of their Insane Poor, the leading consideration with Boards of Guardians, is the cost of their maintenance – that in many cases their safe custody, and the security of the public, are lamentably neglected – that little provision is made for the cleanliness and comfort of this most helpless class; and that medical treatment, with a view to the cure or alleviation of their mental disease, is almost wholly lost sight of.[43]

They showed that the majority of pauper lunatics were boarded out, citing as an example that 'out of 207 Lunatics and idiots, belonging to seven Unions, nine only were in Asylums, twenty-four in Workhouses, and 174 boarded out...with their friends and elsewhere'.[44]

The findings received considerable publicity, especially when Lord Ashley referred to them in the House of Commons:

> If they went to the Principality, they would find that they were too often treated as no man of feeling would treat his dog; that they were kept in outhouses – chained – wallowing in filth, and without firing, for years.[45]

The Commissioners Report appeared in the same year as the Commission of Inquiry for South Wales, appointed in the wake of the Rebecca Riots to investigate the effects of the 1834 Poor Law Amendment Act. The concern regarding the widespread use of the Welsh language, particularly in districts where 'the lower orders speak almost universally a language unknown to the educated classes' articulated in that report, did not find an echo in the Report on the Condition of the Insane. The Report did not attribute the condition of the insane in Wales to use of the Welsh language in the way that the highly contentious Reports of the Commissioners of Inquiry into the State of Education in Wales were soon to link the low standard of educational provision to the obstacle represented by the Welsh language.[46] Thus, whilst representing a fairly damning indictment, the 1844 Report on the Condition of the Insane was not hailed as 'treasonous' within Wales. None the less the Report on the Insane still contributed to that mid-nineteenth century discourse which represented the 'superiority' of English mores and values, and the 'inferiority' of Welsh customs and practices, and thereby reinforced the hegemony of the dominant culture.[47]

The 1844 Report gave impetus to the efforts to establish the North Wales Lunatic Asylum, with which it was in some ways enmeshed.[48] In Parliament Lord Ashley quoted the view of one of the campaigners, Dr Lloyd Williams, that 'the greatest of all cruelties was to send the wretched pauper to a people whose language he could not understand'.[49]

Certainly, the issue of the use of the Welsh language in the treatment of the insane in Wales was central to the campaign for the asylum. In a letter to *The Times*, Samuel Hitch, an early supporter of the foundation of a North Wales asylum at Denbigh, drew attention to the plight of Welsh-speaking lunatics:

> So few of the lower class of the Welch…speak English…whilst both the officers and servants of our English Asylums, and the English public too, are equally ignorant of the Welsh language – that when the poor Welchman is sent to an English Asylum he is submitted to the most refined of cruelties, by being doomed to an imprisonment amongst strange people, and an association with his fellow-men, whom he is prohibited from holding communion with. Nothing can exceed his misery: himself unable to communicate, or to receive communication; harassed by wants which he cannot make known, and appealed to by sounds which he cannot comprehend, he becomes irritable and irritated; and it is proverbial in our English Asylums that the 'Welchman is the most turbulent patient wherever he happens to become an inmate'.[50]

Hitch spoke from direct personal experience, since a number of Welsh patients had been treated by him at the Gloucester Asylum, where the Welsh Chaplain, Mr Evans, had volunteered his services as translator.[51] Thus Hitch had proof of the effectiveness of moral therapy upon the Welshman, if only he could be communicated with in his native tongue:

> the effectiveness of the use of his own language on the Welch lunatic I had lately an opportunity of observing in two cases, neither of whom spoke or understood English, and who derived more comfort and made more progress towards recovery through an occasional conversation with a Welch clergyman, who conveyed to them what were my wishes towards them, than by all the other means which are placed at my command.[52]

The impropriety of sending Welsh patients to an English asylum was claimed to be one reason why so many were still lodged with relatives.[53] The editorial columns of the *Carnarvon and Denbigh Herald* proclaimed that:

> In addition to this general argument in favour of lunatic asylums, the institution of such an asylum for Welsh patients, is rendered necessary by the consideration that if sent to any English Hospital the patient is precluded from every curative tendency which conversation and mental solaces can supply.[54]

The rules of the North Wales Lunatic Asylum were to include the stipulation that all staff must be fully conversant in the Welsh language. Soon after it had opened the Revd W.H. Owen wrote in his report as Visitor of the benefits to the patients of the use of the Welsh language in the asylum, remarking on:

> the soothing results of being spoken to in their own language, and the great comfort and happiness it seemed to afford them. I saw none of that fear and exasperation which was so distressing a symptom among the Welsh patients I have seen in the Asylums in England.[55]

The asylum for North Wales was unique. The founding members launched a subscription account in 1842, and joined with magistrates for the counties of Denbigh and Flint. Subsequent to the 1845 Act three other counties, Anglesey, Carnarvon and Merioneth, joined the Union. The group of influential magistrates, churchmen and medical men who initiated the foundation had a wide network of connections based on religious affiliations, family ties, educational background and cultural interests. The Chairman of the Subscribers was John Heaton of Plas Heaton, Chairman of the Denbighshire Quarter Sessions for twenty years, and a staunch Whig in politics.[56] A fellow landowner donated twenty acres of land, a mile or so from the town of Denbigh. The Commissioners visiting in 1844 warmly approved of the site, on which it was proposed to build an asylum 'for 160 patients, of whom ten or twelve are to be Private Patients of the first class, fifty of the second class, and the remainder Paupers'.[57] The location conformed to important criteria,[58] yet the decisive factor in the location of the North Wales asylum was the enthusiasm of a cohesive circle of subscribers in the Vale of Denbigh, who had influence on the local Quarter Sessions.

The founding of the asylum coincided with a period in the history of Denbigh when the corporation was dominated by a group of solicitors, doctors and squires, with shopkeepers in the minority.[59] In 1848, when the asylum was opened, six of the twelve members were doctors or surgeons. A prominent part was played in the founding of the asylum by Richard Lloyd Williams, a medical practitioner in Denbigh, and brother-in-law to John Heaton. Dr Lloyd Williams was re-elected mayor to hold a second term of office during 1848, it being regarded as fitting that the doctor should preside as mayor in the year that the asylum was opened.[60] Subsequently Dr Lloyd Williams served as Visiting Physician, until shortly before his death in 1864. When he relinquished the post of campaign secretary in 1843, it was assumed by J.H. Clough of Denbigh, cousin of A.H. Clough, whose Oxford connections may account for some of the subscriptions from that source.[61]

The church connection was strongly represented on the lists of early subscribers. The Dean of St Asaph, Charles Scott Luxmoore, was an influential figure amongst the small group of men who initiated the fund-raising campaign. As Dean of Hereford, his father had been Chairman of the Governors of Hereford Infirmary, when that hospital had decided to establish an asylum for lunatic patients, in 1791. Charles Scott Luxmoore was a member of the governing body of the Denbigh Infirmary, where the first meetings of the subscribers were held.[62] He had first-hand experience of the problems of an asylum visitor, being one of the visiting justices who petitioned parliament for an enquiry into the management of the Hereford Asylum. The Dean's knowledge of the problems of such a venture was therefore intimate, and may from the outset have influenced the very tight control which the committee exercised over the management of the North Wales Lunatic Asylum. He took an active interest in ideas on lunacy and in 1839 had written to his old friend Charles Bathurst, Chairman of Visitors of the Gloucester Asylum, enquiring about methods of treatment. In December 1840 he and the High Sheriff of Herefordshire had visited the Gloucester Asylum and 'expressed their unqualified admiration'.[63]

Anglicans were by this time in the minority in North Wales, most parts of which were overwhelmingly nonconformist in religion. In an attempt to widen their basis of support, the committee of subscribers approached Thomas Gee of Denbigh, the prominent Welsh publisher, and 'other influential persons resident in this town and connected with the different Congregations of Dissenters' to seek their active support in the campaign for the asylum. Mr Gee undertook to recruit 'persons who collect for the Bible Society' to conduct a general house-to-house collection.[64]

A prominent role was played by Dr O.O. Roberts in obtaining the support of the western counties for the planned asylum at Denbigh. He had fought for the Whigs in the 1835 election, was a prominent anti-tither, vociferous in his criticism of landlords and stewards, and during these years an outspoken critic of the New Poor Law. He took a petition to Parliament to call for an enquiry into the conduct of the Haydock Lodge Asylum, and his exposure of events there finally led the three western counties of North Wales to support the establishment of a joint public asylum at Denbigh. He gave valuable testimony to the Commissioners in Lunacy, but when the Blue Books on Education were published in 1847, O.O. Roberts rushed into print with an attack on Johnson's report on North Wales.[65]

Much of the early financial support for the asylum came from wealthy donors, though innkeepers and the new shopocracy feature in the subscription lists, published regularly in the North Wales newspapers. The more substantial supporters were members of the landed elite, such as Lord Mostyn, Sir Henry Browne and Lord Clive, who had vehemently opposed the introduction of the New Poor Law. This lends support to Scull's contention that amidst the threat of Chartism, the impact of the industrial capitalism and the New Poor Law 'the Victorian governing classes could at least find a source of pride in the generous and kindly treatment now accorded to the mad'.[66] In their active promotion of lunacy reform the gentry and magistrates of Denbighshire were valuable friends of the reformers in central government.

A management structure was established which gave considerable power to the magistrates and subscribers, who were to determine policy through their quarterly meetings, and supervise the operational side of the asylum through sub-committees. In establishing an institution run on strict bureaucratic lines they performed a role similar to that played by Middlesex magistrates in the reform of the Hanwell Asylum.[67] Familiar with his writings on moral restraint, Dr Lloyd Williams wrote to Dr Conolly, asking him to nominate a suitable candidate for the post of Medical Superintendent.[68] Conolly's nominee declined, and when in 1847 a medical superintendent, matron and steward were appointed some months before the hospital was opened, they were sent to the Gloucester Asylum for a period of training.[69]

The operational philosophy of the asylum was based on the 'rule of kindness'.[70] As patients were admitted to the asylum, it became evident that amongst them were some who had suffered years of neglect and ill-treatment, such as Mary Lloyd, the wife of a small farmer, who had for some years been tied to the bed with a cart-rope. When Mary was subsequently removed from the asylum by her husband, the House Committee wrote to the relieving officer of the Ruthin Union, calling attention to his legal duties under the Act of 8 and 9 Victoria, c. 126, s. 49, and requesting that he monitor the case.[71] Surveillance was an important function of the legislative process, and it served the interests of the reform movement to enforce these powers.

The networks of clergymen, doctors and solicitors who had been active in founding the asylum were assiduous in pursuing cases of neglect and maltreatment of lunatics in the community for some years after the asylum had been opened. They remained in close correspondence with the Lunacy Commissioners. The Reverend J. Williams Ellis, son-in-law to J.H. Clough, drew their attention to cases of neglect and unfair treatment in Carnarvonshire and Merionethshire.[72] In these, and in other cases, the Commissioners, who were rarely keen to prosecute, referred the complainant to the legal responsibilities of the Relieving Officer. However in May 1853 the Lunacy Commissioners decided to involve themselves directly in the case of a single lunatic, Evan Roberts, who was 'alleged to be confined and chained to the leg in a dirty and neglected condition at a Farmhouse occupied by his younger brother and sister at Llanfairfechan'. After consultations it was resolved that immediate application be made to the Lord Chancellor for an order under the 112th Section, to be directed to a medical man in the neighbourhood authorising him to enquire and report upon the case. This order was issued to Dr Lloyd Williams and his son, who found the lunatic confined in an outhouse and chained and riveted to the bed. After considering their report the Commissioners decided that 'the offence was of so aggravated and disgraceful a kind, that we had no alternative left but to institute a prosecution'. A bill of indictment was preferred against William Roberts for 'unlawfully confining and imprisoning his brother, Evan Roberts, in an improper, excessive, and cruel manner', and was tried before Lord Chief Justice Campbell at the Carnarvonshire Summer Assizes in 1853. The defendant was found guilty and sentenced to one calendar month's imprisonment. The Commissioners regarded the sentence as 'excessively lenient' and noted that the sentencing decision:

> had proceeded on a strong recommendation of the defendant to mercy by the jury, on the ground that he had acted through want of judgement, and not from malice, and perhaps also, in some measure, on the ground of its appearing that the mode of treatment adopted by the defendant had been previously sanctioned by the Lunatic's father, and was regarded as the usual course in North Wales in similar cases.[73]

This *cause célèbre* highlighted the strong sense of familial responsibility in Welsh society; for it was claimed that the father had left the farm, a small-holding of some five acres, to his second son 'in trust for the support of Evan Roberts and his mother for life'.[74] The legal intervention of the Commissioners demonstrated a clear fracture between the new, modern standards represented by asylum care, but requiring state intervention and control, and the older familistic patterns of domestic solutions.

Clearly the inquisitorial role of doctors, solicitors and clergymen was crucial in establishing a new code of conduct which contributed to the acceptance amongst popular opinion that the asylum was the correct place for the treatment of the insane. The concurrence of both church and nonconformist opinion helped to establish this as the consensus view. Shortly after the asylum was opened it was visited by Samuel Roberts of Llanbrynmair, the celebrated writer and Independent minister, who spoke warmly and approvingly of the benevolent care which he observed. The influence of doctors on some local Boards of Guardians hastened the medicalisation of lunacy, by encouraging relieving officers to refer cases for medical examination. However the transition was slow and the balance between the proportion of pauper lunatics and idiots in the community and those in the asylum was only fully reversed after many decades. In the longer term it was the acceptance by families that the asylum offered a period of respite or a solution to their domestic problems, to periods of crises arising from violence or suicidal attempts of relatives, or the disruption caused by household members who could never sleep or refused to eat, which ultimately determined the increased use of the asylum. The perception that asylum care was a preferred solution to these manifold problems gradually broadened out from being the view of an elite group and gained generalised acceptance.

This was not achieved without some coaxing, and further policing of the system. In order to establish their ascendancy and enforce new treatment standards the magistrates and the Lunacy Commissioners persisted in drawing public attention to cases which failed to conform to their criteria. In April 1855, the Committee of Visitors to the asylum drew the attention of the clerk to the Anglesey Union, to the cases of three separate women in the Llanerchymedd District, 'it appearing to the Visitors assembled at this meeting that Lunatics "requiring to be restrained" are not in a fit state to be at large'. They also wrote to the clerk of the Bangor and Beaumaris Union, pointing out, with regard to a boarded out female in their area, that 'a Lunatic requiring to be "occasionally restrained with a strait waistcoat" is not in a fit State to be at large'.[75]

The central inspectorate reinforced the efforts of the magistrates. A Visiting Lunacy Commissioner in 1864 reported on a visit to a single pauper lunatic L.J., who lived with his sister in Bala. When there, he said:

> I found his bedding in a most discreditable state. It consisted of loose straw, saturated with urine, over which was cast a wet

> sheet, and he had, for bed coverlets, merely an old dirty quilt and a tattered great coat. He was dressed in a ragged and filthy set of clothes.

The same Commissioner stated his belief that in some Unions 'idiotic inmates are most improperly sent out and made Single Pauper Patients merely from economical motives'. He referred to the example of 'an idiotic young woman' who had been sent out of the workhouse, and 'was allowed to ramble about almost in a state of nudity'.[76]

Thus both visiting magistrates and the Lunacy Inspectorate brought a considerable degree of influence to bear on local Poor Law officers and Boards of Guardians in an attempt to get them to comply with requirements. None the less, for some twenty to thirty years after the North Wales Asylum opened there was still, even by the recorded annual returns, as large a group of lunatics and idiots outside of the asylum as there were housed inside. Indeed for the first twenty years the numbers entering the asylum were not matched by any diminution in the numbers recorded as being 'in lodgings or with relatives'. The gradual shift in the pattern of care is illustrated in Table 8.1 for the five North Wales counties affiliated to the asylum.

Table 8.1 Placement of lunatics and idiots in North Wales

Year	*Asylum*	*Licensed houses*	*Workhouses*	*In lodgings; with friends*	*Total*
1847	6	33	38	341	418
1867	303	1	86	391	781
1877	376	0	153	319	854
1897	631	24	216	271	1,142
1907	813	1	173	231	1,217

Source: Annual Reports, North Wales Asylum

Some parishes were slower than others to consign patients to the asylum, and on the whole the more westerly areas showed least enthusiasm for the asylum. This table confirms the limited use of the workhouse for housing the insane in North Wales prior to the last quarter of the nineteenth century, and the continued emphasis on 'outdoor care'. In the 1860s over 50 per cent of pauper lunatics and idiots in North Wales were boarded out with relatives or in lodgings compared to only 19 per cent for England and Wales as a whole. In

North Wales the rise of 'asylumdom' was neither immediate nor assured. Whilst the Welsh language was undoubtedly of key importance in differentiating the Welsh situation from that in England, though not necessarily that in Scotland and Ireland, it was clearly not the only factor and should be seen as part of a larger set of dynamics. Family ties and the pattern of family care and domestic arrangements operating through the community and the Poor Law itself had perpetuated a network of non-institutional provisions for the insane. The fears of an asylum using an alien language probably deterred the dispatch of Welsh lunatics to English asylums, as well as the distance and costs incurred by families and parishes with very limited resources. The practical experience of dispatching patients to such institutions as Gloucester Asylum, Haydock Lodge, Chester and Liverpool asylums brought the issue of language into public notice and debate. It was a debate involving a modernising medical rhetoric in which Welsh doctors wished to participate. Thus the multiple layers of the 'language' question in Wales provide an essential background to an understanding of the institutional politics of this period.

The legitimation of the North Wales Lunatic Asylum as the main provider for pauper lunatics in North Wales is illustrative of a successful coalition between a modernising local elite and agents of central government in achieving and enforcing a radical solution to an age old problem. In this regard there are significant parallels with the Devon experience discussed in the essay by Forsythe, Melling and Adair and some interesting variations when we consider the Scottish and Irish studies also presented in this volume. There were peculiarities in the Welsh situation which should be highlighted and differentiated not only from the broader experience of England but also the concerns revealed in the Oonagh Walsh essay on Ireland. Religion was a significant factor but did not acquire the particular form found in Ireland and in contrast to Scotland (and even to some degree, Ireland), the native Welsh language does emerge as a significant issue in the identification of the problem of managing insanity in Wales. We have seen that the patriarchal concerns expressed on behalf of the Welsh-speaking insane served to 'naturalise' an essentially alien institution. The investigatory practices of the state, at both central and local level, are shown to have been key factors influencing the implementation of a new policy. It is clear how, within a Welsh context, the most extreme cases were used to illustrate the weaknesses of the former system, and to impress on a variety of audiences the necessity for change, thereby enforcing a uniform system, every extension of which 'fortified the state'.[77] What does appear to connect the Welsh experience to the other studies in this volume, including those of the colonial possessions overseas, was the rich and complex politics of state management involved in the recasting of provision for insanity in Wales. If we are to explore these issues further we should at least keep one eye on the changing institutional landscape of state administration during these decades.

Acknowledgements

The research on which this paper is based was funded by the Wellcome Trust. The authors are grateful to Neil Evans and Dai Michael for their comments and suggestions.

NOTES

1 E. Halevy, *A History of the English People in 1815*, vol. 1, London, Penguin, 1937, pp. 60–1.
2 J. Innes, 'What would a Four Nations approach to the history of social policy entail?', Discussion paper, conference on 'Integration and Diversity', University of Ulster, 1996. We thank her for permission to cite this paper.
3 T.G. Davies, 'The Welsh contribution to mental health legislation in the nineteenth century', *Welsh History Review*, 18, 1996, pp. 40–4.
4 Letter from John Jones, Clerk of the Peace in *Chester Chronicle*, 28 December 1810, p. 3.
5 Denbighshire Record Office, (DRO) QSD/AL/3/6 letter from C.W. Williams Wynn to the Clerk of Denbighshire Quarter Sessions, January 1811.
6 W. Parry-Jones, *The Trade in Lunacy*, London, Routledge and Kegan Paul, 1972, p. 16.
7 The Shropshire Asylum was opened in March 1845 and in 1846 received a request from Montgomeryshire magistrates to unite with Shropshire magistrates to provide a joint asylum. This was acceded to and an extension built. Shropshire Records and Research, QA/7/1/4, *Second Annual Report of the Lunatic Asylum for the counties of Salop and Montgomeryshire and the Borough of Much Wenlock, 1846–7.*
8 T.G. Davies, 'An asylum for Glamorgan', *Morgannwg*, 37, 1993, pp. 40–55.
9 Public Record Office (PRO) MH51/1/734 Miscellaneous papers, c. 1701–1966.
10 For the debates in South Wales see T.G. Davies, 'Mental mischief: aspects of nineteenth-century psychiatric practice in parts of Wales', in H. Freeman and G. Berrios, eds, *150 Years of British Psychiatry, Vol. II: The Aftermath*, London, Athlone, 1996.
11 A. Scull, *The Most Solitary of Afflictions*, London, Yale University Press, 1993, pp. 96 and 91.
12 P. Bartlett, 'The Poor Law of Lunacy', unpublished Ph.D. thesis, University College London, 1993.
13 A dialogue explored by I.G. Jones, *Mid-Victorian Wales: The Observers and the Observed*, Cardiff, University of Wales Press, 1992.

14 *Carnarvon and Denbigh Herald*, 4 February 1843. Letter from 'A Poor Welshman', referring to the visit of Samuel Hitch.
15 Sir Andrew Halliday, *A Letter to Lord Robert Seymour with a Report of The Number of Lunatics and Idiots in England and Wales*, London, 1829, p. 67.
16 Ibid., p. 59.
17 Ibid., p.74. An early eugenicist view. Perhaps more extraordinarily a recent historical work has identified 'centuries of inbreeding' as a peculiar problem in rural Wales leading to high rates of insanity. See R. Davies, *Secret Sins: Sex, Violence and Society in Carmarthenshire, 1870–1920*, Cardiff, University of Wales Press, 1996, p. 99.
18 Halliday, *A Letter*, pp. 77–8.
19 DRO QSD/AL/1/1–27.
20 DRO PD3/3/1, Vestry Minutes, Abergele, 4 September 1823.
21 Ibid., 5 August 1824.
22 DRO PD/3/3/3 Overseers Accounts, Abergele, 23 May 1825; 30 January 1826.
23 Ibid., 30 October 1830.
24 National Library of Wales (NLW) William Day Mss, 3149, Correspondence with Unions and Circulars, item 1073.
25 Ibid.
26 PRO MH/12/161131, Poor Law Union Files, St Asaph, Letter from William Day to George Cornewall Lewis, 5 April 1841.
27 A.H. Dodd, *The Industrial Revolution in North Wales*, Cardiff, University of Wales Press, 1971, p. 391.
28 M. Finnane, *Insanity in Post Famine Ireland*, London, Croom Helm, 1981.
29 PP (Lords), 1844, vol. xvi, *Supplemental Report of the Metropolitan Commissioners in Lunacy relative to the General Condition of the Insane in Wales, August 1844*, p. 11.
30 W. Day to E. Chadwick, 21 October 1837, NLW William Day Mss, 3146F; quoted in R.A. Lewis, 'William Day and the Poor Law Commissioners', *University of Birmingham Historical Journal*, 9, 1964, p. 179.
31 Ibid., quoting PRO MH32/14, letter Day to J.G.S. Lefebvre, 7 May 1837.
32 Ibid., quoting PRO MH32/14, letter Day to Lefebvre, 10 September 1837.
33 Ibid., pp.178 and 180.
34 Ibid., p. 181, quoting PRO MH32/14, letter Day to Lefebvre, 23 February 1837.
35 Ibid., p. 180, quoting NLW William Day Mss 3146F, letter Day to Sir John Walsham, 9 August 1840.
36 Bartlett, 'Poor Law of Lunacy'; N.B. Hervey, 'The Lunacy Commission, 1845–60', unpublished Ph.D. thesis, University of Bristol, 1987.
37 Hitch, letter to *The Times*, 1 October 1842. On Hitch see L.B. Smith, ' "A worthy feeling gentleman": Samuel Hitch at Gloucester Asylum, 1828–1847', in Freeman and Berrios, eds, *150 Years of British Psychiatry*.
38 PP 1844, vol. xix, Poor Law Commissioners, *Tenth Annual Report for 1844*, p. 19.
39 Ibid., p. 20.
40 *Supplemental Report*, p. 3.
41 Ibid., p. 4.
42 Ibid., pp. 37–44.
43 Ibid., p. 5.
44 Ibid., pp.10–11.

45 *Carnarvon and Denbigh Herald*, 20 July 1844, 'Pauper lunacy in Wales', letter from W.Ll. Caldecot.
46 F.P. Jones, 'The Blue Books of 1847', in J.L. Williams and G.R. Hughes, eds, *The History of Education in Wales*, Swansea, Christopher Davies, 1978, pp. 127–44; I.G. Jones. '1848 and 1868: "Brad y Llyfrau Gleision" and Welsh politics', *Mid-Victorian Wales*, ch. 5, pp. 103–65; P. Morgan, 'From long knives to Blue Books', in R.R. Davies, ed., *Welsh Society and Nationhood*, Cardiff, University of Wales Press, 1984, pp. 199–215.
47 For a discussion of the official representation of the Welsh language see G. Tyson Roberts,' "Under the hatches" – English Parliamentary Commissioners' views of the people and language of mid-nineteenth century Wales', in W. Schwarz, ed., *The Expansion of England – Race, Ethnicity and Cultural History*, London, Routledge, 1996, pp. 171–97.
48 *Hansard*, 23 July 1844, address by Lord Ashley, col. 1,269; *Carnarvon and Denbigh Herald*, 7 September 1844, 19 October 1844; DRO HD/1/502 Minute Book of the Founders, 31 August 1844.
49 *Hansard*, 23 July 1844, col. 1,268.
50 *The Times*, 1 October 1842, letter from Samuel Hitch, dated 15 September 1842.
51 Gloucestershire Record Office (GRO), (Shire Hall Branch) HO22/1/1 First County Asylum, general minutes, 1813–51, p. 486, minute dated 27 December 1841.
52 Ibid.
53 *Supplemental Report*, p. 16.
54 *Carnarvon and Denbigh Herald*, 4 February 1843.
55 DRO HD/1/172, Visitors Book for 1849–53, entry signed by W.H. Owen, 7 February 1849.
56 A. Fletcher, 'Plas Heaton and the Heatons in the nineteenth century', *Transactions of the Denbighshire Historical Society*, 45, 1996, pp. 21–40.
57 *Supplemental Report*, p. 4.
58 C. Philo, ' "Fit localities for an asylum": the historical geography of the nineteenth-century "mad-business" in England as viewed through the pages of the *Asylum Journal*', *Journal of Historical Geography*, 13, 1987, pp. 398–415. C. Philo, 'Journey to asylum: a medical-geographical idea in historical context', *Journal of Historical Geography*, 21, 1995, pp. 148–68.
59 J.W. Pritchard, ' "Fit and Proper Persons" – Councillors of Denbigh, their status and position, 1835–94', *Welsh History Review*, 17, 1994–95, pp. 186–203.
60 J.W. Pritchard, 'Corfforaeth Dinbych a Datblygiadau Bwrdeistrefol 1835–94', unpublished M.Phil. thesis, University of Wales, 1992, p. 9.
61 See published lists of subscribers in *Carnarvon and Denbigh Herald*, 18 February and 14 March 1843.
62 For a detailed discussion of the founding, see R. Olsen. 'Founding of Hospital for Insane Poor, Denbigh', *Transactions of the Denbighshire Historical Society*, 23, 1974, pp. 193–217.
63 GRO (Main Branch), D3848/1/1/58, letter from Charles Bathurst, Chairman of the Visitors, to Hitch, 4 April 1839; (Shire Hall Branch) HO22/3/2 House Committee Minutes, 7 December 1840. We thank Len Smith for this reference.
64 DRO HD/1/502 Minute Book of the Founders, 18 March and 23 April 1843.

65 Morgan, 'From long knives', p. 208.
66 A. Scull, 'A brilliant career? John Conolly and Victorian psychiatry', *Victorian Studies*, 27, 1983–4, pp. 203–35.
67 A. Suzuki, 'The politics and ideology of non-restraint: the case of the Hanwell Asylum', *Medical History*, 39, 1995, pp. 1–17.
68 DRO HD/1/502 Book of the Founders, minute for 17 August 1846.
69 Ibid., minutes for 2 June 1847 and 18 January 1848.
70 North Wales Lunatic Asylum, (NWLA), *First Annual Report*, Report of the Medical Superintendent, G.O. Jones.
71 DRO HD/1/151 House Committee, Minutes, 27 February, 1852; PRO MH/50/6 Commissioners in Lunacy, Vol. 6, p. 250, 21 July 1853.
72 PRO MH50/6 Commissioners in Lunacy, Vol. 6, p.130, 9 March 1853; p. 151, 30 March 1853.
73 PRO MH/50/6 Commissioners in Lunacy, Vol. 6, p. 130, 9 March 1853; p.151, 30 March 1853; p.187, 11 May 1853; p.195, 25 May 1853; p.202, 1 June 1853; p.219, 23 June 1853; p.228, 30 June 1853; NWLA, *Fifth Annual Report for 1853*.
74 NWLA, *Fifth Report.*
75 DRO HD/1/151 Minute Book of the NWLA, 20 April 1855, p. 318.
76 PP 1865, vol. xxi, Commissioners in Lunacy, *Nineteenth Annual Report*, Appendix F, pp. 93–4.
77 G.M. Young, *Portrait of an Age – Victorian England*, Oxford, Oxford University Press, 1977, p. 22.

9

'THE PROPERTY OF THE WHOLE COMMUNITY'

Charity and insanity in urban Scotland: the Dundee Royal Lunatic Asylum, 1805–1850

Lorraine Walsh

The foundation stone of the Dundee Royal Lunatic Asylum was laid in 1812 accompanied by the pomp and circumstance of a major civic occasion,[1] and by the mid-1820s the institution was described as 'the pride and ornament of the town which gave it birth'.[2] While public subscription asylums were not limited to Scotland, as examples such as St Luke's Hospital (1751), the Newcastle upon Tyne Asylum (1764) and the York Asylum (1777) demonstrate, the pattern of development followed by the English asylums differed considerably from that of the Scottish institutions. While the English public subscription asylums subsequently gave way to the county asylum system provided for under the legislation of 1808, and particularly after that of 1845, the charitable institution remained predominant in Scotland. These 'royal' asylums provided the mainstay of Scottish provision for the insane in the first half of the nineteenth century, and were to remain resolutely, and often defiantly, as independent and essentially charitable institutions.

This chapter aims to demonstrate how the distinctiveness of the asylum system which developed in Scotland – part of what Roy Porter has described as the 'oddities' of the development of the institutionalisation of the insane[3] – was the result of three main factors: the distinctive operation of the Scottish Poor Law, the overriding social and economic imperatives of the Scottish towns which founded institutions for the insane, and the importance of lay involvement in the establishment of the Scottish asylums. In these respects this chapter offers parallels with the chapters on Wales and Ireland, emphasising as it does the distinctive characteristics of the Poor Law provision as well as the strength of voluntary organisations. One of the main concerns of my study is to locate the movement to found the Royal Asylum at Dundee within a larger picture of urban voluntary endeavour and to provide some counterpoint to the county asylums in England and Wales, which were often located near to traditional county towns though in pastoral landscapes, by emphasising the connections between an early Scottish asylum and the social networks of an expanding industrial city of the nineteenth century.

The development of the Scottish charitable asylum

Although there was no statutory requirement in Scotland to provide institutional care for the insane until 1857, eight Scottish lunatic asylums of philanthropic origins were founded between 1782 and 1839.[4] By 1827, seven years after the Dundee Asylum had opened, it was noted in the institution's annual report that lunatics were no longer tolerated at large, 'far less to disturb the peace of private families'.[5] The early-nineteenth-century community in Dundee had been directed by philanthropic endeavour towards the acceptance of the asylum as the answer to the problem of how best to deal with the mad. But why an institutional solution? Asylum provision was not the only response to lunatic individuals within the community, and on the whole, Scotland was relatively slow to accept institutional solutions to 'problem' sections of society. While in England local parishes had long been obliged to provide institutional accommodation for society's destitute, sick and unemployed in the form of workhouses, the Scottish parishes provided assistance for their needy only in relation to the available voluntary funds.[6] Poor relief was raised through church door collections and fees for services such as the use of the mortcloth, and was administered through the kirk (local body of the Church of Scotland).[7] Funds were largely dispensed to recipients in their own homes, or were made available for the maintenance of individuals such as orphans or lunatics in the homes of others.

Although urban-industrial growth and development had begun to place strains on this form of kirk-centred voluntary provision by the early decades of the nineteenth century, the Scots were reluctant to abandon their system of poor relief which they believed to be far superior to that which was in place in England. If the situation arose where voluntary contributions were insufficient to provide for poor relief an assessment could be imposed upon the local heritors (landowners) which required them to contribute towards the support of the poor.

However, this course of action was heartily unpopular with both the heritors, who had to raise the supplementary funds, and the kirk, which viewed the system of assessment as inimical to the charitable impulse and therefore the traditional Scottish system of poor relief. The added financial burden which would therefore fall on the heritors if voluntary poor relief was not forthcoming encouraged charitable provision for society's needy groups, including the insane. Charitable institutions could be more economically run by local people who were familiar with local conditions, while an assessment could prove costly. One way to encourage voluntary giving was through the establishment of specific charitable organisations or institutions and thus the creation of new arenas for the raising of funds for the needy.

The faltering Scottish tradition of voluntary poor relief was given a brief respite and found new support in the growth of organised charity in the late eighteenth and early nineteenth centuries, and from this was born the institutional framework of Scottish charitable institutions which included infirmaries,[8] orphanages and lunatic asylums. This pattern of charitable development was an integral part of the social and economic change of the early nineteenth century which witnessed the expansion of industrial towns, the growth of Evangelicalism and the consolidation of the position of the urban middle classes; all of which provided essential support for the fostering of urban charities such as lunatic asylums. Whereas Andrew Scull has argued that the majority of the early English asylums were situated in rural locations, and that a connection between urban-industrial development and the rise of the asylum is a somewhat simplistic interpretation which cannot be substantiated,[9] the reverse is true for Scotland. The establishment of the Scottish asylums in urban areas reflected specific, local considerations. Inextricably bound up with the development of the Scottish asylum as an essentially charitable institutional facility was the promotion of the town with which it was identified, in terms of both civic pride and the demonstration of the humanitarian nature of its citizens. While the town connection did not necessarily mean that asylums were welcomed as part of the urban infrastructure, and they were often sited some distance from the town and moved to new premises as the town expanded in size, nevertheless, the desire to establish an association with the institutions was clearly demonstrated through the maintenance of the name of the town in the title of the asylum.[10] There was a need for individual towns, such as Dundee, to establish themselves as important urban centres and to avoid becoming a satellite to one of the other major Scottish towns.[11] The foundation of large charitable institutions established those towns as focal points in terms of the provision of care.

While Scull may have overstated the case for the rural isolation of the early English asylums, it is clear that the involvement of the Scottish urban middle class was crucial to the development of the Scottish asylums as distinctly charitable institutions in a way which was not so evident for the English asylums. The urban focus of the Scottish asylums was the result of their financial dependence on the larger community and a direct consequence of the central involvement of the urban middle classes in both the financial and practical aspects of their support and development. Only the Crichton Royal Asylum at Dumfries (1839) and the James Murray Royal Asylum at Perth (1827) were generously endowed by individual philanthropists. The asylums at Montrose (1782), Aberdeen (1800), Edinburgh (1813), Glasgow (1814) and Dundee (1820) were all reliant on the support of the public in both a financial and organisational role. The *nature* of the early nineteenth-century town, the social and economic activities of the constituent middle class and their commitment to the traditional Scottish system of poor relief provided the essential requirements for the urban foundation of the Scottish charitable asylums.[12]

Lunatics found their way into the Dundee Asylum by a variety of means, including the kirk session[13] and the commissioners of police, but others were undoubtedly admitted under the authority of relatives or friends. While the middle and upper classes often considered an asylum to be the very last option[14] it is more difficult to ascertain the reasons behind working-class admissions. Andrew Scull has argued that periodic economic depression created an intolerable strain on wage-dependent working-class families, and that the increased burden created by family dependants in these periods resulted in a greater resort to the institutionalisation of the impotent, aged or troublesome.[15] While some of the issues raised by Scull have been challenged in the English context,[16] there are also issues specific to the Scottish situation which suggest that admitting an individual to a charitable asylum was very much the assumption, rather than the abnegation, of a responsibility. Admitting a relative or friend to the Dundee Asylum was no light matter, not only in psychological but also in economic terms. Each patient was to be provided with a mattress and bed linen, and with a not insubstantial wardrobe. Male patients were to be provided with two shirts, two coloured neckcloths, two flannel under-jackets (if worn), two night-caps, two pocket-handkerchiefs, three pairs of stockings, one coat or jacket, one vest, one pair of breeches or trousers, one hat and one pair of shoes. Female patients were expected to be similarly well provided for. All linen was to be 'kept up' or renewed as necessary. Patients in the 'higher classes' were to be provided for 'according to circumstances'.[17] Aside from these requirements, a very real obligation had to be undertaken by a 'person resident in Dundee or neighbourhood' which required that person to take responsibility for the payment of the patient's board while in the Asylum and for that individual's welfare once they left the institution. This situation does not reflect an abandonment of responsibility towards the lunatic family member, as suggested by Scull, but rather the assumption of added responsibility. Insane family members could be concealed at home or within the community for a fraction of the expense of the outlay required by the Asylum, and although families could fall on the mercies of the kirk session the decision to become acknowledged as 'paupers', and the stigma which that carried, was not one which was lightly undertaken. The decision to admit a relative or friend to one of the Scottish charitable asylums was therefore an action which implied the acceptance of not only psychological but also economic and social responsibilities.

As primarily charitable institutions the Scottish asylums were dominated by lay rather than medical influence and control. Only three of the more than forty ordinary directors appointed in the early years following the opening of the Dundee Asylum were medical men. The remainder of the directors were drawn from influential quarters of the town's hierarchy, including the town council, the guildry and the church.[18] As a result of this predominantly lay influence, the anticipated direction of the Asylum may have lain more with the practice of moral treatment rather than with medicine.[19] A conviction of the benefits of moral reform fitted well with the belief systems of the early-nineteenth-century philanthropists, and at Dundee the directors were eager to model their asylum on that 'mild and excellent Institution', the York Retreat, where Tuke had implemented his ideas on moral treatment. Patients were to be treated with 'as much gentleness and indulgence' as their state of mind allowed and if restraint were to become necessary it was to be 'as moderate as is convenient with safety'. 'No harsh treatment' was to be tolerated.[20] W.A.F. Browne, perhaps one of the most well-known figures in connection with the Scottish institutions, was the first to introduce moral treatment into a Scottish asylum during his period at Montrose,[21] but the directors of the Dundee Asylum were also quick to extol its benefits. In 1834 several individuals were noted as having been improved by employment, described as the 'united influence' of 'moral and physical means', while in 1842 the medical report appended to the institution's annual report of that year stressed the conviction that many of those cured were also improved in moral character. Alexander MackIntosh, who was employed at both Dundee and Glasgow 'royals' in the course of his career, favoured a regimen based largely on 'moral and intellectual treatment', whilst considering the value of medical treatment to be somewhat restricted.[22] The important role played by laymen in the establishment, organisation, financing, and also in many ways the ideological structuring, of the charitable asylums meant that their ideas and their opinions were central to the pattern of asylum development in Scotland.

The absence of an early, strong motivational impetus from the medical fraternity establishes a clear divergence in the pattern of development of the Scottish and English asylums. Whereas Andrew Scull has identified the advancement of the medical 'expert' as an important factor in the development of the nineteenth-century asylum in England,[23] this motivational factor is largely absent in Scotland before the 1830s and 1840s, when the residential medical superintendents were appointed on a full-time basis in the royal asylums and paved the way for men such as David Skae at Edinburgh.[24] Although new research, such as Peter Bartlett's work on the concept of the county asylum as a Poor Law institution, has identified the importance of influences other than those of the medical profession in the development of the English asylum system, the involvement of medical men in the establishment of the English institutions remains more pronounced than in the Scottish asylums. While the Scottish institutions were founded predominantly as the result of the interest and support of laymen, who were often largely unconnected with any other medical or poor relief institutions, the English public subscription asylums were often instigated by, or witnessed the involvement of, medical men, such as William Battie at St Luke's. Much of this early development was accompanied by an entrepreneurial spirit which saw public subscription asylums in England become dominated by medical ambition, or used as a platform from which the medical profession could open private establishments.[25] The establishment of famous names in the field of Scottish psychiatric medicine, such as Thomas Clouston and David Skae, however, was very much a feature of the second half of the nineteenth century, following the introduction of lunacy legislation in Scotland and the establishment of the 'royal' asylums as institutions of some renown.[26] In the period before mid-century, and the changes to the Scottish Poor Law (1845) and the introduction of statutory legislation dealing with lunatics (1857), the Scottish charitable asylum was very much the domain of local laymen.

The Dundee Asylum attempted to delay the introduction of a resident medical superintendent for as long as possible,[27] believing that this obligation was only applicable in the case of madhouses rather than asylums.[28] The financial cost of employing a resident medical superintendent may have contributed to the reluctance of the Dundee Asylum to appoint such a person. The charity was consistently underfunded and financial concerns were never far from the minds of the directors in their attempts to establish 'a most rigid attention to economy'. The continued reliance of the Asylum on public funding meant that constant vigilance was required in an effort not to upset public sensibilities, which could result in a corresponding drop in voluntary contributions. In the annual report of 1830 the directors lamented that 'calumnious stories' concerning the institution were more widely circulated and more widely believed than they had considered possible, including 'the most absurd and erroneous notions' that the physician to the Asylum was profiting from huge fees, whereas all such monies went into the general funds.[29] From the early years of the Asylum financial considerations were uppermost.

The development of institutional care for the insane as part of an organisational system which was first and foremost a charitable one raises several questions concerning the motivation behind the founding, and the practice, of the charitable asylums. A charity had to be seen to be accountable and successful in 'value for money' terms, therefore the charitable asylum followed a rather broader agenda than that of a purely medical or custodial facility. What that agenda reveals is that these early examples of Scottish asylum provision were not simply the result of impressively humanitarian communities, but the consequence of more complicated motives, involving cultural, economic and political factors, which resulted in the charitable institution being placed at the forefront of provision for the insane in the first half of the nineteenth century. Having identified the three main general factors which led to the establishment of a decidedly independent course of action in the provision for the insane in early-nineteenth-century Scotland, I will now consider the operation of one of those Scottish charitable institutions, the Dundee Royal Lunatic Asylum, in more detail.

The nature and practice of the charitable asylum

The establishment of a lunatic asylum at Dundee had followed on from the establishment of a charitable infirmary in the town. A report from the committee appointed to carry into effect the plan for a lunatic asylum commented that the 'managing committees' of the Dundee Infirmary had 'had to witness several cases of mental derangement, and to regret that the institution did not enable them to afford any relief to the unhappy persons'; a subject which was 'often pressed upon their attention, and that of the contributors, at their quarterly meetings'.[30] In 1805 the directors of the Dundee Infirmary had felt compelled to take 'immediate steps' regarding the erection of an asylum for 'persons labouring under Mental Derangement',[31] and the town council 'set on foot a subscription'[32] to which they contributed 100 guineas.[33] The increasing discussion of the insane amongst such middle-class committee members undoubtedly increased interest amongst urban philanthropists in the problem of insanity and provided an important impetus to the foundation of new institutions in Scotland.

It would be unwise, however, to attribute this development simply to growing humanitarian concern for the number of lunatics who found themselves in the public eye.[34] For the directors of the Dundee Infirmary lunatic patients were an expensive liability. With a limited number of beds, and no special provision available for lunatic individuals, the institution could ill afford to shelter the insane. In 1800 one William Patton was admitted to the Dundee Infirmary, but only under the proviso that he was to be immediately dismissed upon his becoming 'outrageous'. This implied that while Patton may have been physically ill, he was also suspected to be suffering from a mental instability. Within a week Patton was found to be insane and was 'ordered to be dismissed', although it was later decided that he was to be given eight days grace in which to allow his friends the opportunity to remove him from the Infirmary. Patton's friends did not immediately avail themselves of the opportunity, however, and he was again ordered to be dismissed, indicating that the Infirmary directors felt little compunction in discharging the insane back into the community.[35] Patton had been a patient in the Infirmary for several weeks, and it was likely that his case raised concerns that the institution might increasingly be used as a dumping ground for lunatic individuals. Although Patton had been considered potentially 'outrageous' in his manner it was not until after his admission that he had been found to be 'insane', thus highlighting the prospect of similar difficulties for the charity in terms of diagnosis and the exclusion of undesirable lunatic patients.

The idea that the charitable infirmary was an unsuitable place for the reception of lunatic patients was therefore accepted,[36] but it was not until the early years of the nineteenth century that the majority of the Scottish 'royal' asylums were opened, while examples of charitable asylums had been established in England since the early eighteenth century.[37] There is little evidence that lunatics were posing a problem or were a source of concern to the Dundee community of the late eighteenth and early nineteenth century, although they were a visible minority.[38] The view of a late-nineteenth-century commentator that, prior to the opening of the institution, 'the want of an asylum was very much felt in Dundee',[39] might have been more the reflection of later years when there was a general concern over apparently ever-increasing numbers of new cases of insanity,[40] rather than an accurate reflection of the late-eighteenth and early-nineteenth-century situation in Dundee. There was no mention of lunatics in the first statistical account of the town (1793), and there were apparently no specific orders made in respect of lunatics, although this could have been the result of the grouping of all wandering poor together indiscriminately, who were then dealt with under general legislation such as the 'Act against Beggars coming to Town, and Landlords Harbouring them, 1773'.[41] In many ways the insane only became a 'problem' when a solution – a cure – became a possibility. From its early years the explicit aim of the Dundee Asylum was to provide a cure rather than simply to act as a repository for the insane. Those 'verging' on 'idiocy, epileptic(s)…others whose cure appears to be hopeless' were to be 'dismissed…after a trial of one year.'[42] Moreover, the object of the institution was to 'promote…the public advantage'[43] and to provide treatment through which patients could be 'restored to society'.[44] The role of the new charitable institutions of the early nineteenth century was essentially remedial, as opposed to the palliative function of the older institutions such as the Town Hospitals, and the idea that infirmaries could heal, orphanages could reform and lunatic asylums could cure formed an essential part of the charitable appeal of these institutions.

Raising adequate funds to establish the Scottish asylums was, nevertheless, not always an easy task. The planning committee for the asylum at Dundee discovered at the time of the founding of the institution in 1812 that the funds at their disposal were short of the sum required, which resulted in their having to pledge 'their own security to the contractors; trusting to public support'.[45] While the original contributions to the asylum had raised almost £8,000[46] by the opening of the institution in 1820, hopes for continuing support through subscriptions proved to be short lived. After this point funds raised through subscriptions never reached more than £30 annually and by 1835 annual subscriptions to the asylum had dried up completely. Voluntary contributions did continue but in the more sporadic form of occasional donations and legacies, which also suffered from an overall decrease in value after 1830. What this meant was that the Asylum, although established and recognised as a charity, was largely funded by board received from patients and, after 1835, monies raised from patients' labour.

Why was there a decline in the charitable support of the Asylum? The possibility that lunatics were not regarded by the larger community as suitable objects for a charity has to be considered. Few fund-raising events appear to have been organised by the institution or by individuals for its benefit. The hope advanced in the annual report of 1832, that the 'excellent ladies' who had previously organised a sale of fancy work in support of the Dundee Infirmary and Infant Schools would do the same for the Asylum, came to nothing.[47] The only organised fund-raising events appear to have been sermons and special collections. There had been some early difficulties when the subscribers were disabused of the notion that the Asylum was to be an integral part of the Infirmary – the most consistently well-supported charity in this period – and that their subscription was not in effect contributing to both institutions. There had also been a recurrent doubt that the Asylum could actually be classified as a charity. There were several reasons for this including the fact that the patients paid for their board and, perhaps most importantly, that the lunatic asylum did not fit the typical image of a charity which provided for the poor, as the Scottish asylums including Dundee, accepted wealthy patients as well as the indigent.

Amongst all the institutional developments of the period the lunatic asylum was the only one which provided a facility for the reception of all social classes. At Dundee, in line with many of the other Scottish asylums, the wealthier sections of the community were positively encouraged to send their relatives and friends to the royal asylum. The Dundee Asylum confidently advertised its accommodation for the wealthier classes, noting that it was 'perhaps unequalled, certainly not surpassed, in any similar institution in the Kingdom', with apartments which were 'elegant and commodious'. Advertisements were placed not only in the Scottish press but also in the London *Times* and the *Lancet*.[48] The asylums positively encouraged the admission of wealthier patients in order to elevate their image from that of a poorhouse for insane paupers but also crucially to help finance their institutions. The Dundee Asylum was never intended to be a repository for the poor, but rather an institution where the insane from all ranks of society could find care and hopefully cure, and while all patients were to pay for their maintenance the directors envisaged that it would be 'from their [the patients of superior rank] board that the expense of the institution will be chiefly defrayed'.[49] This financial support did not materialise to the amount that had been anticipated, however, and the number of poorer patients always outnumbered the wealthy at Dundee, as well as at several of the other Scottish institutions. The two most well-endowed

Scottish asylums at Dumfries and Perth were the most successful in attracting wealthier patients. The Crichton Royal was particularly effective in securing wealthy patients from England, for they could find both comfort and seclusion there.[50] Part of the success of these institutions in attracting wealthier patients where the other asylums had failed was undoubtedly their more generous funding and thus their ability to provide more splendid accommodation, but this attractiveness was also supplemented by the correspondingly lesser need to accommodate pauper lunatics.[51]

The greatest part of the funding of the Dundee Asylum was derived from paupers, highlighting the difference between the Scottish public asylum system and the English private system. Charlotte MacKenzie notes that by 1844 a majority of licensed madhouses in England no longer accepted paupers,[52] while an individual private establishment, such as Ticehurst in Sussex, was able to admit its last pauper patient as early as 1825.[53] The 'mixed economy of care', which has been detailed by Len Smith, meant that there were a number of possible alternatives for the reception of pauper lunatics in England made available through the existence of private and public asylum provision and also workhouse accommodation. Scotland, meanwhile, had relatively few poorhouses or private madhouses and as a result the majority of pauper lunatics were directed to the royal asylums. An English private asylum such as Ticehurst could afford to charge a relatively high, and therefore discouraging, fee for paupers, reasonably confident in its ability to attract the better sort of patient. However, the Scottish asylums needed the income from pauper patients to maintain their economic viability and they aimed to attract pauper patients by providing a low rate of board. The outcome of this situation for many of the Scottish asylums was a downward spiral which saw the institutions become clogged with pauper patients, while the English private asylums were able to offer a more exclusive and refined accommodation for their wealthier clients.

At Dundee, 'a pauper' had to be confirmed by four respectable householders as an individual unable to pay the lowest rate of board and with no relation able to assume the financial responsibility on his behalf.[54] The economic necessities of the charitable system made for a brisk trade in the movement of pauper lunatics among the Scottish asylums by the local kirk sessions in search of the cheapest rates of board. In 1827 a number of pauper patients were removed from the Dundee Asylum, with the prospect of further removals, as the new asylum at Perth offered a lower rate of board. This was seen as a 'difficulty' at Dundee, as it would have resulted in a loss of income, and it was decided that the subject of lowering the rate of board at Dundee should be considered. This was duly carried out within a few months.[55] By the 1840s, however, the Dundee Asylum found itself in the position of being the most financially attractive proposition for the disposal of pauper lunatics. In 1842 the directors noted that the Asylum had the lowest pauper rate in Scotland. The following year applications were made from an 'Edinburgh Charity' seeking admission for between ten and forty pauper lunatics and from the Barony Parish of Glasgow which also aimed to board pauper patients at Dundee. The latter request, at least, was refused as the Dundee Asylum was said to be too crowded.[56]

Although the Dundee Asylum was in many ways dependent on the board obtained from pauper lunatics, securing the payment of this board often proved problematic. In 1831 the directors complained of the 'considerable inconvenience' they had encountered in trying to obtain payment due from the Dundee kirk session. The reason given for this was the fact that individual members of the kirk session were themselves security for the payment of the said board.[57] In 1836 it was noted that over £400 was due to the Dundee Asylum from the kirk session in board for pauper patients but despite 'repeated applications for payment' only £100 had been realised.[58] The Asylum was therefore eager to continue attracting voluntary contributions. The charitable aspect of the Dundee Asylum had initially been envisaged solely as being the means by which the original plan of the building, and any extension to the accommodation as and when it became necessary, could be carried out. It was originally stated that the public would be asked to help with the debt and in completing the architectural plan, 'and that only at distant intervals, as the increasing prosperity of the asylum may require',[59] but the constant financial pressures on the institution meant that subsequent annual reports continued to contain regular appeals for contributions.

Resisting legislation

Dundee was not the only one of the Scottish asylums to experience continuing financial problems,[60] and the obvious difficulties in the funding, and therefore the running, of the charitable asylum are at odds with the objections raised by the institutions regarding the implementation of 'reforming' legislation.[61] Although the idea of the lunatic asylum had obviously been accepted by the Scots by the early nineteenth century the concept of a compulsory, as opposed to voluntary, provision for the mentally ill in Scotland was strenuously opposed. There appear to have been three main facets to this protest: fear of assessment, fear of the loss of the traditional Scottish system of poor relief, and fear of loss of local and national control. A bill to provide district or county asylums in Scotland was introduced in 1818, two years prior to the opening of the asylum at Dundee, but it was defeated due to repeated obstruction by petitions from the Scottish heritors and town councils,[62] two groups comprised of those individuals who were most often involved in the management of the local charities. The heritors of the County of Ayr petitioned against the bill stating that:

> the proposed Bill recognises a systematic assessment, which it has been the wise policy of our forefathers to avoid in practice, and that, too, to an amount *at the discretion of Commissioners ignorant of local circumstances*, and perhaps the dupes of misinformation; entertaining, as the petitioners do, deep and well-grounded *repugnance to the means proposed* for carrying this measure into execution, partly injudicious and *partly degrading to the landholders* of Scotland, for it does appear to be a humiliating and, the petitioners may venture to say, an *unconstitutional Act*, which *would place the whole landholders in Scotland in the situation of being taxed for any object and to any amount at the discretion of any set of Commissioners whatever.*[63]

The introduction of the Scottish Poor Law Amendment Act in 1845, and its recommendation that separate asylums should be established for pauper lunatics, raised fresh concern in Dundee. The Reverend Thomson, a local clergyman who was involved with the Asylum, was of the opinion that this was uncalled for in Scotland, and plans were made to contact the Member of Parliament for Dundee and the Lord Advocate if required, as well as the other asylums in Scotland in order to discuss the matter further.[64] It is clear that the separation of the wealthier and poorer classes of lunatic into different institutions would have further increased the difficulties of the Dundee Asylum in its attempts to remain solvent, while the need to establish a completely separate institution for pauper lunatics would have required the implementation of an assessment in order to fund the building and running costs. Furthermore, under the new Poor Law Act, once an assessment had been imposed it henceforth became an annual levy, rather than a temporary expedient as had previously been the case.[65]

The directors of the Scottish asylums were well aware that their institutions, limited in size and funds, could not cater for the apparently ever-growing numbers of insane who needed admission. Provision for the insane within the charitable institution was undoubtedly superior to that offered by the private sector, whether in the form of madhouses or as private homes which accepted boarded-out individuals. However, by concentrating all their efforts on the institution itself, the philanthropists were unwittingly narrowing the scale of provision for the insane in Scotland. Lack of funds contributed to this through a corresponding lack of opportunity for expansion and provision of asylum accommodation. While the first asylums built in England under the County Asylums Act (1808) were of a 'moderate' size, with an average of 115 inmates per institution, that figure had reached approximately 300 inmates for the average English county asylum of the mid-1840s.[66] Meanwhile, by 1855 the Dundee Royal had only reached just over 200 patients. Similarly, the asylums at Aberdeen, Montrose and Perth all had less than 300 inmates, while Dumfries had only just over that figure.[67]

It is debatable whether the restricted size of the Scottish charitable asylums made for a better environment than the larger English county asylums. Moral therapy remained a more enduring force in the Scottish public asylums than in the English county asylum system, where Scull has noted that the decline of the image of the asylum as a curative institution was allied with a similar decline in the exercise of moral treatment, and subsequently the asylum began to assume the appearance of a custodial, rather than remedial, institution.[68] The overriding philosophy of the charitable enterprise and the continuing preoccupation with moral treatment meant that continuing pretensions towards cure in the Dundee Asylum, whether these activities were little more than simply distractions and diversions for the patients, saw the Asylum resist a purely custodial format. The image of the model family continued to be nurtured. Although the pauper and wealthier patients were separated within the institution, events such as the marriage of a female keeper, Isabella Somerville, which was held at the Asylum and celebrated with a grand fête must have impinged upon the whole community and thus reinforced the image of the asylum community as a family.[69] What can be established, however, was that as a result of the continued Scottish resistance to legislation which aimed to physically isolate pauper lunatics from their wealthier compatriots, the retention of wealthy and pauper patients together meant that vital space in the Asylum was sacrificed. In the, often vain, hope of attracting a few wealthy patients, large and commodious apartments were set aside for one or two individuals while the accommodation for paupers was subsequently restricted. Due to the limitations on the number of paupers who could be accommodated by the asylums a significant number of prospective patients also remained outside the asylum system in Scotland. Alternatively they were pushed into private madhouse accommodation, which although always comprising a very small part of the available provision for the insane in Scotland, began to increase by mid-century as a result of the restricted available accommodation and the continued resistance to legislation and expansion of that accommodation.[70]

In many ways the charitable lunatic asylums in Scotland were carrying out a holding operation in the face of economic inevitability. After 1857 a General Board of Commissioners in Lunacy was formed 'to provide for the building of district asylums for the reception of pauper lunatics, and to insure the proper care and treatment of lunatics generally, whether placed in asylums or left in private houses under the care of relatives or strangers'.[71] The separation of the classes of patient and the removal of the pauper patients from the charitable asylums to the new district asylums saw these pauper institutions become little more than dumping grounds for the impoverished and chronically mentally ill, and the chances for the recovery of pauper lunatics became almost negligible.[72] Although this may have appeared as a justification for the former obstinacy of the royals such as the Dundee Asylum, as early as 1826 it had been apparent that the anticipated level of cures within the Asylum was not materialising and that the institution was developing into a holding facility. In 1830 it was noted how 'the complicated and the hopeless' had been received into the institution and 'retained, from motives of the purest humanity, for an indefinite length of time'. At that point, 91 of the 101 individuals in the Asylum were considered chronic cases.[73] By 1832 it was lamented that the Dundee Asylum was encumbered by a 'load of incurable madness'.[74] The charitable asylums had not been providing a more curative or satisfactory facility under their independent management than the district asylums were able to afford.

Conclusion

The picture which emerges from this study is that of an institution which was shaped as much, if not more, by the needs of the heritors, who sought to maintain their control, than the needs of the insane in early-nineteenth-century Scotland. By the 1840s the traditional Scottish system of voluntary poor relief had largely collapsed. The strain put on the system by urban growth, the Disruption within the Church of Scotland in 1843 which rent apart its organisational and financial base, and finally the Poor Law Amendment Act in 1845 meant that the old system was irrevocably changed. However, the continuation of the Dundee Asylum as a charitable organisation despite its financial difficulties, and the sustained opposition from the Scottish asylums to the proposed legislation, indicates that something other than the basic needs of the insane was at stake. Although lunatic individuals had been identified as a distinct category, requiring the establishment of specific forms of provision, the main impetus behind the relatively early establishment of a lunatic asylum at Dundee was rooted in economic and political, rather than wholly humanitarian, decisions. The Dundee Royal Lunatic Asylum began with the aim of being more than simply a repository for the insane; it sought to facilitate the return of mentally – and morally – sound and productive members of society back into the community, to provide an economical form of care for the insane, and to retain local control over that provision.

The development of the institution was central to this process. However, the charitable basis of the Scottish asylum meant that economic viability was a central concern, and while efforts to attract upper-class patients absorbed both vital asylum resources in terms of money and space, poorer patients were relentlessly moved around the Scottish asylums in the local kirk session's attempts to secure the most favourable rates of board. Meanwhile, the refusal of the asylum directors to give way to what was perceived to be reforming legislation, regardless of the fact that many of the asylum's original aims as a curative and charitable institution had largely disappeared, demonstrates a concern which was manifestly rooted in the socio-economic and political requirements of the Scottish heritors rather than those of the insane. Legislation could have eased the financial responsibilities of the asylums and placed the burdens on broader shoulders but the economic concerns of the heritors regarding the implementation of a compulsory assessment for the provision of lunatics in Scotland, further compounded by their concern at the possible loss of Scottish autonomy in local affairs, saw them resist such legislation until it became an inevitability.

Scotland, from the outset, pursued an independent course, with less indication that she was influenced by humanitarian idealism and the eighteenth-century development of asylum provision in England (although many of the Scottish towns, including Dundee, looked to English public asylums for example and advice *after* they had decided to establish an asylum), than by the social and economic concerns of the early nineteenth century and the need to emulate the activities of the other Scottish towns.[75] It is difficult to tell if the sponsors and governors of such institutions stressed the competitive edge of their own institution in a bid to attract subscriptions or if they were saturated with the ideology of market values, though we can see a range of social virtues in play amongst the advocates of these institutions. While the English system of mixed care provided a number of alternatives for the accommodation of lunatics, provision for the insane in Scotland was monopolised by the charitable asylums, and supported in this role by the social and economic importance which was attached to the asylums as civic institutions. Although the essential elements of the provision for the insane in Scotland were rooted in her traditional system of poor relief, this in turn had consequences for more than simply pauper lunatics, and as a result the institution and its ramifications affected the nineteenth-century community as a whole.

NOTES

1 Local Studies, Dundee Central Library (henceforth LS), Lamb Collection (henceforth LColl), 36(2), *An Account of the Dundee Infirmary; and Report of the Committee Appointed to Carry into Effect the Proposal for a Lunatic Asylum at Dundee*, 1815.

2 LS, LColl, 434(13), *Report of the Dundee Lunatic Asylum*, 1826.

3 R. Porter, *Mind-Forg'd Manacles. A History of Madness in England from the Restoration to the Regency*, London, Penguin, 1990, p. 135.

4 Montrose, Aberdeen, Edinburgh, Glasgow, Dundee, Perth, Elgin and Dumfries. Elgin was not a chartered asylum but was an institution for pauper lunatics which had been founded by philanthropic initiative, O. Checkland, *Philanthropy in Victorian Scotland: Social Welfare and the Voluntary Principle*, Edinburgh, John Donald, 1980, pp. 168–9.

5 LS, LColl, 434(14), *Report*, 1827.

6 M.A. Crowther, 'Poverty, health and welfare', in W. Hamish Fraser and R.J. Morris, eds, *People and Society in Scotland, vol. II, 1830–1914*, Edinburgh, John Donald, 1995, p. 268.

7 The town council was also involved to a greater or lesser extent in different areas.

8 Infirmaries had been opened in Edinburgh and Aberdeen in the early eighteenth century but the infirmaries in Glasgow and Dundee were not opened until the closing years of the eighteenth century.

9 A. Scull, *The Most Solitary of Afflictions. Madness and Society in Britain, 1700–1900*, London, Yale University Press, 1993, pp. 28–9.

10 Only the asylums at Dumfries and Perth were known by different names, the Crichton and James Murray's respectively, after the names of their founders. These asylums were endowed by individuals while the other 'royals' had been largely funded by public subscription.

11 Edinburgh, Glasgow and Aberdeen.

12 F. Rice, 'The origins of an organisation of insanity in Scotland', *Scottish Economic and Social History*, 1985, p. 44, also makes the point that there is a definite connection between the building of institutions and urban size in Scotland, but his argument is limited by its narrow focus on population size and density. The important point here, however, is not necessarily the size of the urban area – both Glasgow and Montrose had asylums but their demographic patterns were quite different – but the social and economic character of the towns and their relationship to one another in this period.

13 Local ecclesiastical court body composed of ministers and elders of the parish.
14 C. MacKenzie, 'Social factors in the admission, discharge, and continuing stay of patients at Ticehurst Asylum, 1845–1917', in W.F. Bynum, R. Porter and M. Shepherd, eds, *The Anatomy of Madness. Essays in the History of Psychiatry, vol. II*, London, Tavistock, 1985, p. 153.
15 Scull, *The Most Solitary of Afflictions*, pp. 26–34.
16 J.K. Walton, 'Casting out and bringing back in Victorian England: pauper lunatics, 1840–70', in Bynum *et al.*, eds, *The Anatomy of Madness*, 1985.
17 LS, LColl, 434(13), *Report*, 1826.
18 LS, Pamphlets D4485, *Report*, 1822.
19 This is not to say, however, that medical initiatives such as blistering and bloodletting were not resorted to, although they may have been employed as a means to sedate patients as much as to treat them, F. Rice, 'Care and treatment of the mentally ill', in O. Checkland and M. Lamb, eds, *Health Care as Social History (The Glasgow Case)*, Aberdeen, Aberdeen University Press, 1982, pp. 72–3.
20 LS, LColl, 434(1), *Sketch of a Constitution and Regulations, for the Dundee Lunatic Asylum*, 1817.
21 A. Scull, C. MacKenzie, N. Hervey, *Masters of Bedlam. The Transformation of the Mad-Doctoring Trade*, Princeton, Princeton University Press, 1996, p. 89.
22 J. Andrews, 'A failure to flourish? David Yellowlees and the Glasgow School of Psychiatry: Part 1', *History of Psychiatry*, 8, 1997, p. 182.
23 A. Scull, *Museums of Madness. The Social Organization of Insanity in Nineteenth-Century England*, London, Allen Lane, 1979.
24 Rice, 'Care and treatment', pp. 67–8.
25 Scull, *The Most Solitary of Afflictions*, p. 19.
26 See Andrews, 'A failure to flourish?', pp. 177–212.
27 Nonetheless, by 1833 Alexander MackIntosh had been appointed as resident surgeon and superintendent to the institution.
28 Dundee University Archives (hereafter DUA), THB 7/5/1 (2), sederunt book of the Dundee Royal Lunatic Asylum, 1829–36, February 1830.
29 DUA, THB 7/5/1 (2), August 1830.
30 LS, LColl, 36(2), *An Account of the Dundee Infirmary*, p. 11.
31 Ibid., 279(2), Extract from the *Dundee Advertiser*, 1805.
32 Ibid., 33(1), *Lunatic Asylum, Royal.*
33 Ibid., 279(2), Extract from the *Dundee Advertiser*, 1805.
34 See, for example, Checkland, *Philanthropy*, p. 168.
35 St Andrew's University Archives, M415, minute book of the Dundee Infirmary, 20 January–17 February 1800.
36 The original plan of the Edinburgh Royal Infirmary had included the designation of a large part of the basement or cellar area for insane patients, and while it was found over time that this accommodation was not suitable for the care or treatment of the insane, it was not until the later eighteenth century, with the gradual spread of the acceptance of lunacy as a potentially treatable condition and the idea of the asylum as a potentially curative institution, that the plan to establish a separate asylum received support.
37 Excluding Bethlem Hospital's earlier foundation.
38 E. Gauldie, *The Dundee Textile Industry, 1790–1885: from the papers of Peter Carmichael of Arthurstone*, Edinburgh, Scottish History Society, 1969, p. 25.

39 Dundee Archives and Record Centre, GD/X207/1 *Handbook to the Charitable Institutions of Dundee*, n.d.
40 As late as 1877, an editorial in *The Times* commented that, 'if lunacy continues to increase as at present, the insane will be in the majority, and, freeing themselves, will put the sane in asylums', quoted in Scull, *The Most Solitary of Afflictions*, p. 338. For a discussion of whether cases of insanity were actually increasing in the nineteenth century, see Scull, *Social Order/Mental Disorder. Anglo-American Psychiatry in Historical Perspective*, California, University of California Press, 1989.
41 DUA, Kinnear Local Collection, *Charters, Writs, and Public Documents of the Royal Burgh of Dundee, The Hospital and Johnston's Bequest: 1292–1880*, Dundee, 1880.
42 LS, LColl, 434(7), *Regulations and By-Laws of the Dundee Lunatic Asylum*, 1825.
43 LS, Pamphlets D4485, *Report*, 1822.
44 LS, LColl, 434(11), *Report*, 1824.
45 Ibid., 36(2), *An Account of the Dundee Infirmary*, 1815, p. 15.
46 Ibid., 434(19), *Report*, 1835, treasurer's accounts.
47 Ibid., 434(17), *Report*, 1832.
48 DUA, THB 7/5/1 (2), March 1832.
49 The 'benefits of the institution are not calculated for the poor only', LS, LColl, 36(2) *An Account of the Dundee Infirmary*, 1815, p. 14.
50 Scull, *The Most Solitary of Afflictions*, p. 295.
51 The Dumfries Asylum was in the position to be able to finance the building of a separate institution for paupers, the Southern Counties Asylum, in 1849.
52 C. MacKenzie, *Psychiatry for the Rich. A History of Ticehurst Private Asylum, 1792–1917*, London, Routledge, 1992, p. 90.
53 Ibid., p. 66.
54 DUA, THB 7/5/1 (1) By-Laws 1820–1831, entry for 1822.
55 Ibid. (1), 8 October 1827; 14 January 1828.
56 Ibid. (3), 10 January 1842; February 1843; 18 September 1843.
57 Ibid. (2), August 1831.
58 Ibid. (2), February 1836.
59 LS, Pamphlets D4485 *Report*, 1822.
60 S. Lobban notes that the Aberdeen Royal Asylum was persistently underfunded and yet overcrowded, 'Healing for the body as well as the soul: treatment in the Aberdeen Royal Lunatic Asylum during the nineteenth century', in T. Brotherstone and D.J. Withrington, *The City and its Worlds. Aspects of Aberdeen's History since 1794*, Glasgow, Cruithne Press, 1996, p. 136.
61 Scottish asylums, such as the Crichton Royal at Dumfries, which had a substantial endowment and less funding concerns than others such as Dundee and Glasgow which had been founded on charitable subscriptions, viewed continuing independent control and autonomy as their prime concern.
62 C.C. Easterbrook, *The Chronicle of Crichton Royal (1833–1936)*, Dumfries, Courier Press, 1940, p. 14.
63 D.H. Tuke, *Chapters of the History of the Insane in the British Isles*, London, 1882, pp. 327–8 (my emphasis).
64 DUA, THB 7/5/1 (3).

65 R.A. Cage, *The Scottish Poor Law 1745–1845*, Edinburgh, Scottish Academic Press, 1981, p. 149.
66 Scull, *Social Order/Mental Disorder*, p. 228.
67 *Report of the Royal Commissioners on Lunatic Asylums and the Laws relating to them in Scotland (1857)*, Shannon, Irish University Press, 1969, p. 50.
68 Scull, *The Most Solitary of Afflictions*, p. 277.
69 LS, LColl, 434(25) *Report*, 1843.
70 *Report of the Royal Commissioners (1857)*, p. 100.
71 Checkland, *Philanthropy*, p. 174.
72 Ibid., p. 176.
73 DUA, THB 7/5/1 (2), August 1830.
74 LS, LColl, 434(17), *Report*, 1832.
75 The Dundee Royal Asylum was closely modelled on the York Retreat.

10

RAISING THE TONE OF ASYLUMDOM

Maintaining and expelling pauper lunatics at the Glasgow Royal Asylum in the nineteenth century

Jonathan Andrews

Historians of psychiatry are now broadly appreciative of the complexities of the relationship between institutions, lunacy administration and the socio-cultural construction of insanity in nineteenth-century Britain. However, their discussions have not yet comprehensively explored the distinctive content of these relationships in such diverse societies as those found in Scotland, England, Wales and Ireland. This chapter seeks to delineate some of the peculiar characteristics of the making of the asylum in Scotland, with particular reference to the Glasgow region. It will demonstrate that the divide between the pauper and the private in lunacy provision had to be carefully negotiated at different levels with different parties. It will examine the circumstances under which the Glasgow Royal Asylum reneged on its original commitment to provide for Glasgow's poor insane, and what this says about the broader problem of pauper lunacy in Victorian Britain. Elucidation shall also be sought of the interplay of medical and lay ideologies which led to the designation of pauper lunacy as a profound social and a medical problem. Additionally, attention shall be given to the extent to which lunacy and institutional policies were arbitrated consciously or unconsciously along ethnic and religious lines.

Andrew Scull argued that most of the fundamental changes in terms of the establishment of the asylum as a solution for the problems of lunacy, pauper lunacy in particular, were in place by 1850.[1] He also asserted that the growth of the pauper lunatic populations in the period preceding mid-century signified a new level of acceptance amongst poor families for incarcerating their insane members.[2] Furthermore, contended Scull, the new museums of madness were filled by the aggrandising activities of the psychiatric profession itself, extending the boundaries of what constituted madness, and remodelling the old regime madhouse so as to sharply mitigate the stigma of incarceration. Scull confined this explanatory model to England and Wales, recently arguing explicitly[3] that the pace of change and the type of provision for lunacy in Scotland were in some respects different. There will always be specific geographical and institutional exceptions to more broadly constituted models. Yet arrangements in Scotland and differences with England have received scant attention from modern historians of psychiatry. Furthermore, it may also be the genuine similarities between the two countries which indicate that previous historiography has not got the balance of factors affecting pauper lunacy quite right. In Scotland parochial authorities and families had at least as vital a role as central and medical authorities in negotiating policy towards pauper lunatics. And this may constitute mainly a difference of degree by comparison with England. Numerous regional variations prevailed in Scotland and there was continuing and vigorous resistance to the asylum solution before (and after) 1857. But similar trends may be found in England and Wales too.

Pauper lunacy in Glasgow and in Scotland as a whole

There were fundamental differences between England and Scotland in both the timing and type of provision developed for the pauper insane. Many of the pivotal changes with regard to Scottish lunacy administration were only comprehensively effected after the mid-nineteenth century, especially after the passing of a host of new lunacy legislation from 1857. The apparatus that came with the 1857 Act, in particular the establishment of a Lunacy Commission and the compulsion for district asylums, came twelve years after the English Lunacy Act. Most of the limited institutional provision in Scotland before 1857 was provided by the seven royal or chartered asylums founded during 1781–1839; by the pauper lunatic asylum at Elgin; and by the lunatic wards of poorhouses,[4] with a minority of pauper inmates in private asylums. In Lanarkshire, there were only 663 pauper lunatics registered with the Lunacy Commission by 1859, 84 per cent of whom were in institutions, almost half of the latter being in poorhouses, over one-third in public asylums and nearly one-fifth in private asylums.[5] Poorhouse accommodation for lunatics had existed in Glasgow and the west of Scotland for well over a century. Yet many poorhouse lunatic wards were not established or subjected to exacting licensing and inspection until after 1850.[6]

The story of Scottish resistance up to 1857 to large-scale lunacy provision, or indeed to any reform of its Poor Law along English lines, has been well told by other historians,[7] including Lorraine Walsh in this volume, and shall not be recounted in much detail here. Dislike of English interference and pride in traditions of voluntary charitable relief administered primarily through the Kirk only gradually gave way to a grudging recognition of the inadequacy of existing provision for the poor. The 1845 Poor Law Amendment (Scotland) Act, which *inter alia* furnished local authorities with powers of levying assessments to set up their own asylums, marked a much delayed but major threshold in Scottish adoption of English approaches to poor relief and may represent a more crucial historical juncture than the legislation of 1857. As Scull suggested, centralising lunacy reform had little chance of succeeding before the Poor Law question was settled.[8]

Nevertheless, the shock waves caused by exposure of the conditions of lunatics (paupers especially) in Scotland by the 1855 Lunacy Commission Enquiry – the momentum of which carried through the 1857 Act – should not be underestimated.[9] Furthermore, as a combined result of this new Scottish legislation of 1845 and 1857; of spiralling costs of pauper maintenance in chartered asylums; a growing recognition of a genuine or potential increase in pauper lunacy; and the persistent badgering of the Scottish Lunacy Commission, things were to change quite rapidly after mid-century. A growing body of opinion was emphasising the inappropriateness of provision in poorhouses and private asylums for the pauper insane, on the grounds of inadequate size, facilities and sanitation. The Scottish Lunacy Commission in particular was determined to see such accommodation phased out and supplanted by larger-scale, separate provision in public and district asylums,[10] an ambition largely realised by the end of the century. By 1913, less than a fifteenth of registered pauper patients were in poorhouses or private asylums. At mid-century the proportion had been nearly half. It is debatable whether the pauper insane benefited from this redistribution. Indubitably, however, it represented a major change in lunacy administration, witnessing a massive increase in the numbers of pauper patients being incarcerated, as well as a substantial erosion of resistance on the part of parochial authorities and (more controversially) the family to the asylum solution.

Local authorities had not quickly or uniformly taken up the invitation furnished by the 1845 and 1857 Acts to provide accommodation for all their pauper insane, but rather required cajoling from the Lunacy

Commission. They continued to shunt their pauper insane from one institution to another in search of the cheapest rates.[11] Even in counties supporting very few pauper lunatics, Commissioners of Supply still grumbled about the expense.[12] Despite compulsion provided in the lunacy acts for the setting up of district asylums, many local Scottish authorities remained unwilling to foot the bill well into the late nineteenth century. In the west of Scotland, it was not until after 1870 that most local authorities really began to establish their own asylums, six parochial and district asylums being established in the area during 1873–97.[13] It had not been until 1877–87 that local authorities in Lanarkshire and Scotland formed themselves into proactive lunacy districts and. undertook comprehensive responsibility for separate institutional provision for their own pauper lunatics.[14] There is no doubting the magnitude of this new spate of asylum building, nor that it was directed at coping with a perceived escalation in pauper lunacy and its associated problems.

One of the most significant areas of change after 1857 was in relation to pauper lunatics maintained outside of asylums in private dwellings. Prior to the Scottish Lunacy Commission Report in 1857, identification and supervision of such individuals had been rather inefficient. While pauper lunatics had long been subject to shrieval and parochial inspection, many authorities, keen to avoid the extra expense that their maintenance would entail, actually failed to register such cases. Inspectors of Poor emphasised that they were not required to report them, and sheriffs rarely required them to.[15] A number of authorities, in response to the Commission's initial circular about the numbers of such lunatics in their areas, claimed they had only a handful.[16] Yet considerable numbers were concealed or ignored as neither dangerous nor troublesome. There was neither the machinery nor the inclination to identify and dispose of them otherwise than in existing informal ways. The Lanarkshire Sheriff claimed he did not know of any 'pauper lunatics in the custody of their relatives'. Two years later the Lunacy Commission had already identified over eighty.[17] Many families were keen to do all they could to avoid the stigma and loss of rights involved in pauperism. Asylum officers complained that paupers were often sent in long after becoming insane and in terrible conditions, blaming parochial concerns with economy.[18] Although the Lunacy Commission probably exaggerated the neglect of local supervision of lunacy prior to 1857, it is also evident that there was considerable laxity and avoidance of responsibility.[19]

The 1857 Lunacy (Scotland) Act not only divided Scotland up into lunacy districts, each assigned to a Visiting Commissioner, but involved a fundamental broadening of official cognisance of the insane, and the conditions in which they were kept.[20] The requirement that pauper lunatics in private dwellings obtain the sanction of the Lunacy Board, as well as, in certain circumstances, that of the county Sheriff, and novel powers granted to Lunacy Commissioners to demand the removal of such patients to asylums, resulted plainly in the increased identification and sequestration of pauper lunatics.[21] Even after the Act, many families and parochial authorities strove to ignore or circumvent its requirements, emphasising the continuing unacceptability of the asylum solution. Considerable opposition persisted from various groups, including local authorities, families and guardians to removing pauper lunatics to asylums. The Commissioners' pressure for removal often provoked families to take their lunatic or idiot members off the poor roll, thus depriving the Lunacy Board of any authority over their case, and themselves of parochial relief. Commissioners tended to blame locals' ignorance and their own lack of powers for cases where removal was eschewed. Nevertheless, many local officials and families blamed the excessive application of the Act. In one case, having already had their daughter's name removed from the poor roll after the Wick Inspector had initiated removal proceedings with the board, her parents were forced to adopt the same tactic again when a second removal order was issued.[22] It was to prevent this resort, that the 1866 Amendment to the Lunacy (Scotland) Acts made it unlawful for pauper lunatics whose removal had been ordered by the board to be taken off the poor roll – another important legislative change which encouraged committal.[23]

One needs to address broader questions as to the demographic and economic structure of different regions in order to comprehensively assess changing patterns of admission to asylums. Plainly the growth of asylum accommodation in the Glasgow region was in part an outcome of the demographic explosion of early industrial Britain, which saw the Scottish nation double and the Glasgow populace multiply twelve-fold, during 1775–1841.[24] Links between these developments and expanding cycles of boom and bust, poverty and employment–unemployment, such as those attendant on the decline in the cloth industry in early-nineteenth-century Lanarkshire or the depressions of the 1860s–70s, are difficult to demonstrate statistically. New pressures on family structures accompanying this demographic explosion, including changed patterns of living and work associated with industrialised labour and market capitalism, and increased in-migration to the city, may have made the burdens of disabled family members less sustainable. Increased overcrowding in urban living quarters may also have eroded tolerance for the insane, and contemporary observers certainly felt that more and more pauper lunatics were being drawn from insalubrious hovels, wynds and tenements.[25] Yet contemporary analyses of these issues often appear prejudiced and unhelpful. Victorian moralistic and medical testimony looked only infrequently at poverty, crime, squalor and other attendant socio-economic problems and tended to concentrate more on the bad habits deemed to accompany insanity (such as those recorded in Lanarkshire mining communities), to explain apparent rises in asylum admissions.[26]

Explanations from modern historians, notably Andrew Scull, have stressed enhanced pressures on networks of familial support and kinship ties due to the development of a capitalist market economy. These pressures, Scull argued plausibly, were felt most acutely by families with sick and mentally afflicted members, especially those families 'from the lowest socio-economic classes...with fewest resources'.[27] Recent work, however, has seriously questioned the tendency of previous historiography to characterise pauper lunatics and their families as the poorest of the poor, sensibly focusing on the heterogeneous nature of the poor; the variety of reasons and reversals that persuaded poor families to commit a lunatic; the tremendous reserves of resistance they showed, and the arbitrariness of the administrative category 'pauper lunacy'.[28] Throughout the period, poor families from a wide variety of backgrounds continued to worry about the stigma of pauper lunacy. If resistance was focused around that large population sector on the cusp of poverty, the highly transient nature of numerous contemporaries' economic sufficiency meant that many a poor family could find itself in need of poor relief at one time or another. The pauperising effect of lunacy itself, something that was a growing subject of concern amongst medical experts and officials in lunacy, alongside the evident greater availability of institutional care and the normalisation of committal procedures, may have presented greater enticement and impetus for families to accept poor relief. As local authorities began to set up or extend their own asylums, poor families, under increasing pressure to succumb, still proved resilient. The Provost of Glasgow emphasised the numbers of people able at best to afford asylums' lowest rates, but 'yet unwilling to have resort to the Parochial Asylums, as they wished to avoid the discredit of being placed as Paupers'.[29] The problem of high and rising fees at private and chartered asylums only exacerbated the problem.

English and Scottish Lunacy Commissioners were highly appreciative of the disinclination of many parishes either to take advantage of expensive asylum accommodation, or to properly supervise pauper patients in private dwellings.[30] It was partially to combat this trend and the tendency of pauper lunatics to end up in English workhouses and Scottish poorhouses that they lobbied for a government grant-in-aid for the support of pauper lunatics under their sanction (available respectively from 1874 and 1876). Before this date, local authorities had nothing but the rates and limited contributions from poor families to defray the costs of their provision. This grant constitutes another important change after 1850 which fostered the identification and sequestration of the pauper insane. Nevertheless, it also seems to have provided local authorities and the Lunacy Commission itself with a subsidised and widely approved alternative to institutionalisation. Commissioners had previously felt obliged, sometimes against their own discretion, to remove paupers to asylums who were not adequately maintained in the community. With the Commission's encouragement, local authorities seem to have taken much more advantage of the government grant in Scotland, than in England. At its height the Scottish boarding-out system provided for over a quarter of registered pauper lunatics. In England the proportion was never more than 16 per cent.

While non-institutional solutions to the problems of pauper insanity received less support in England than in Scotland, David Wright and others have emphasised the high levels of discharge from nineteenth-century English asylums. This finding may also be endorsed for Scottish institutions.[31] It suggests that previous historiography may have been overly concerned with asylum care, with chronic insanity and with the 'increase' of pauper lunacy, echoing Victorian commentators' own over-preoccupation with these matters.

Pauper lunacy at Glasgow Royal Asylum, Gartnavel

Examining a specific case like Gartnavel Royal is not a wholly satisfying way to test paradigms applied generally to pauper lunacy in recent historiography. Yet, none of the Scottish chartered asylums, as privately established and subscription sponsored establishments, supporting both pauper and private patients, would accord entirely comfortably with the English historiography on asylumdom. While founded in 1814 largely in reaction to the poor standard of care for pauper lunatics in Glasgow's poorhouse, or Town's Hospital, Glasgow Lunatic Asylum, like the other six chartered asylums, was intended to be a mixed institution. Initial lobbying for the erection of the asylum assumed the unity of 'the private and public good' in this cause: for 'the wealthiest citizen as well as the poorest labourer may require to be secluded'.[32] The 'principle' behind this type of provision was 'that the profits arising from boarders, are to assist in furnishing good accommodation for the poor'.[33] The building's very look was supposed to enshrine a happy consensual medium, the directors were keen to 'avoid' both 'unnecessary expense, and...a mean and sordid appearance'.[34]

In most contemporary asylums, stress was placed on segregating pauper from private patients, a reaction against the lack of classification in old, 'unreformed' asylums. The emphasis on segregation by class (and by diagnosis) was taken even further at Glasgow Asylum, owing to the panoptic elements incorporated into its design by the architect, William Stark. The context and ideology of panopticism has already been admirably discussed by other historians.[35] However, the extremity of the concern in Glasgow's case is noteworthy. As Stark put it, the idea was of a total classificatory quarantine, precluding those in one 'class' from being able 'to meet with, or even see, any individuals belonging to the other classes'.[36] Accommodating the genteel in inferior situations, it was believed, would offend their own and their families' feelings, and retard their recoveries. Association with the pauper ranks would also expose them to the shock and infectious influence of bad habits and manners. Asylum reformers were very concerned that in older establishments 'persons of liberal education, and of respectable rank in society, are unavoidably mixed with those of the lower rank, of the most brutal manners, and of the most profligate habits'.[37]

Nevertheless, the situation at Glasgow Royal was to change considerably as the century progressed. Under increasing pressure of space, the asylum was soon to deviate from its original ideals, the strict classification Stark envisaged proving unfeasible in practice. Furthermore, the apparent consensus between private and public interests was an uneasy alliance. While paupers consistently outnumbered private patients for most of the century, their interests were consistently subordinated to those of private patients. Even with respect to the early asylum's design it was felt that, as it was private patients who would defray the institution's expense, the 'external appearance' should attract their 'attention' and 'correspond' with their 'habits and feelings'.[38] Only during the 1870s and 1880s, long after the rebuilding of the asylum at Gartnavel in 1843, was the somewhat uneasy balance between private and pauper patients resolved. Now the asylum actually transformed its identity from a mixed institution to an establishment catering exclusively for private patients.

The asylum was from the beginning designed first and foremost to service Glasgow citizens. Paupers from the city were received on a privileged rate of board, and tended to make up between 30 and 40 per cent of the population. In addition, between seventeen and twenty-four parishes (mostly those around Glasgow who used the asylum regularly) gained admissions for their lunatic poor at privileged rates, on payment of a subscription scaled in proportion to their population.[39] Yet the institution's catchment area extended much more widely than this, it acting in effect as 'a district asylum for the whole of the West of Scotland',[40] also drawing small contingents from the outlying highlands and islands.

The major changes in Gartnavel's catchment population came during 1850–90. With the exodus of all its paupers, including large contingents of patients from Argyll and Bute, the Inner Hebrides, Paisley and Greenock, and the loss of a further influx from the City, Barony and Govan, to the multiplying parochial and district asylums, Gartnavel became a private institution of national appeal. Private patient numbers rose steadily at the asylum after 1814, but peaked dramatically after 1874, under Yellowlees' superintendence. From this date, Gartnavel Royal became an increasingly exclusionary asylum, with private patients outnumbering paupers for the first time in its history. In 1897 the Directors proudly announced that not a single pauper remained.[41]

Yet, as late as 1880, contemporary authorities were still expressing the belief that the asylum 'would always' cater for a substantial number of paupers.[42] Here, then, is a new chapter in the saga of lunacy, an apparently radical, unanticipated departure from previous practice that needs explaining. It was significantly, of course, the result of a declared and genuine crisis in the accommodation of pauper lunatics at Glasgow Royal (where patient numbers had peaked at almost 600 in the 1870s, two-thirds of whom were paupers), and in the Glasgow region as a whole. Superficially, the end of pauper admissions to Gartnavel was a logical consequence of, and an extra spur to, the establishment of the parochial and district asylums. Gartnavel was also adopting a policy already being practised at the Murray Royal Asylum, in Perth, and at some English asylums. Dundee Royal too was soon to follow suit. In so far as it was conceived of as a means of raising the profile of such asylums and psychiatry within them, off-loading of pauper populations on parochial and district asylums might accord well with Scull's models of professional medical imperialism. However, this policy was not advocated only by the royal asylums and the medical profession. Furthermore, it implies less about the profession's winning over of the families of the pauper insane and the erosion of the stigma of mental illness than it does about the continuing vigour of that stigma.

To some extent, the total exclusion of paupers from Glasgow Royal was a fulfilment of the implications of earlier policy. Long before the 1870s, the asylum had been choosy about pauper admissions. While private cases were rarely turned away, paupers who were destructive, pregnant, chronic, moribund or infectious were quite frequently refused or discharged. Asylum officials had regularly complained about the 'trouble and expense' the institution was put to by such paupers.[43] Although therapeutic concerns clearly informed criticisms of patients being kept too long at home by their penny-pinching families or parishes, there was also concern with the deleterious impact these cases had on the asylum's statistics and reputation. The Physician-Superintendent objected (vainly) to the Lunacy Commission about patients who had perished on arrival being included on the asylum's death roll.[44] By an informal and unreliable arrangement with parochial authorities, the asylum had long attempted to reserve for itself the best cases. The resident surgeon at Barony Poorhouse asserted that Gartnavel sent them 'very bad cases – people worn out by excessive drinking', and 'a great many old people'.[45]

Yet parochial and asylum officials had different balance sheets, and their interests were not infrequently at odds. Of course, there were clearly variations in the relationship of asylums to local authorities over time, and from place to place. Sometimes local authorities were quite active in removing dangerous and curable pauper cases to Gartnavel. Yet often their priorities were economy and security, rather than therapy, in getting 'quit of these patients'.[46] Most contemporary observers would have agreed with the Lanarkshire Sheriff that parochial boards 'almost [n]ever look to anything else' but 'economy'.[47] However, some observers plainly stressed the negligence of parochial boards for their own ends. The minutes of their own proceedings and the contemporary testimony of inspectors of the poor emphasise that such boards were also concerned with patients' recovery and welfare. Some conducted searching visitations of their lunatics in asylums and were even prepared to remove their paupers to more expensive asylums if 'not satisfied with the treatment and accommodation'.[48]

Leading psychiatric opinion was generally 'against sending patients to lunatic wards in poorhouses', and was concerned to get such accommodation replaced by district asylums.[49] While local officials often agreed that the poorhouse was not a fit place at least for curable patients,[50] parochial boards had many other costs to bear. Many members of these boards regarded lunacy provision as a secondary concern, and saw poorhouses as adequate enough for chronic patients. Parochial boards can hardly be expected to have treated lunacy as a priority given 'the great mass of people under their charge'.[51] Even in poorhouses with large lunatic wards, like the Barony, lunatics represented less than a tenth of the population, and medical staff had often felt frustrated by narrow-minded parochial boards when trying to introduce putative (but cost-bearing) improvements.[52]

One should not overemphasise the tensions and differences between lay and medical, and parochial and asylum authorities, or the negligence of local authorities towards pauper lunacy. Pauper lunatics in asylums were rarely visited by Board of Supervision inspectors, and the Sheriff visited only twice a year. Yet they were generally scrutinised weekly by the parochial boards in poorhouses and parochial asylums, and tended to be seen at least quarterly in chartered asylums. Whereas ordinary paupers were 'frequently removed' from asylums like Glasgow Royal by parochial authorities, the asylum rarely seems to have had much reason to object. Mackintosh could only recall one case in which he objected in 1855, namely because the patient was 'dangerous'.[53] By contrast, tensions were probably greater and the asylum more discriminating when it came to the relatives of pauper lunatics, Mackintosh sometimes declining relatives' requests for removal unless the inspector concurred.

While, in the 1850s, Mackintosh could see no 'objection to pauper and private patients being in the same asylum', and authorities appreciated some of the practical advantages for paupers in mixed asylums,[54] their successors were to have rather different ideas. In publications between 1874 and 1901, Gartnavel's Physician-Superintendent, David Yellowlees, explained in detail the rationales behind the exclusion of the pauper insane from the asylum. First, the policy was supported in terms of therapy: of expelling the most chronic cases from the asylum, who, it was adjudged, predominantly belonged to the pauper classes;[55] and of permitting the earlier treatment of the acute insane, who, it was asserted, were being 'kept at home as long as possible…in order to avoid the expense of asylum treatment'.[56] Second, it was advocated in terms of improving the asylum environment: reducing overcrowding and upgrading patient accommodation.[57] Third, justification embraced a renegotiated, class-mediated economics that substantially reneged on earlier commitments to supporting the poor on the bounty of the rich. Proponents now claimed that they were relieving the ratepayers of the inequitable burden of having their payments for asylum care supplement the deficiencies of pauper rates.

In addition, the policy was espoused for social reasons. As Yellowlees put it: 'The removal of the Parish Patients tends to raise the social tone of the Institution, and removes from the minds of patients all ideas of such association.'[58] Not only would patients and their friends no longer be deterred from seeking asylum care by the threat of having to share accommodation with socially repellent paupers, in addition they might benefit psychologically from an environment where 'they are associated with persons of their own rank'.[59]

It was a policy that was predicated also on a long history of perceiving and portraying pauper admissions as of an inferior sort, both in terms of their prognosis and their morals. Paupers were bad for asylum statistics, because as Yellowlees put it, they 'must adversely affect the proportion of recoveries'. Additionally, they were regarded as of a less 'favourable type' because they were drawn mainly from 'the squalor and crime' of the city.[60] Yet for much of the period there was actually little difference between recovery rates of private and pauper cases at Glasgow Royal. In general pauper rates were slightly better.

By the 1870s, the asylum was obliged to lodge pauper East House patients on 'camp-beds and shake-downs', and to commandeer 'vacant space...in the West House...as sleeping accommodation for [them]'.[61] Overcrowding had been a problem since at least mid-century, but a new determination to deal with it by ousting lunatic paupers was encouraged by an enhanced emphasis on their greater infectiousness as a class of patients. Growing awareness through developments in public health and hygiene of the association of disease with overcrowding caused clinicians increasing concern about the threat of infection and 'the appearance of any epidemic malady'.[62] When cholera had afflicted Glasgow in the 1850s, Gartnavel 'refused a great many, principally pauper patients, for fear of infection'.[63] Later, this rationale was prominent amongst the directors' declared reasons for terminating the contract with the Glasgow District Board for the admission of its paupers.

Gartnavel's managers agreed that 'chronic patients...could not fail to have a depressing influence upon the house'.[64] More and more concerned then about the demoralising and damaging accumulation of chronic, if not infectious, pauper patients, Gartnavel's directors and medical officers thus sought to raise the asylum's tone and extend the available space for less wealthy middle-class applicants. Purging the chartered asylum of paupers, it was believed, would make it more acceptable to those middling sort whose income and sensibilities barred them from poor relief, but who were too poor to afford the cheapest private rates at asylums. The lowest rates of board for private patients had been subject to a creeping inflation. In 1876, however, they were reduced to 15s., maintaining this rate with only a slight increase until the cessation of all pauper admissions in the 1890s. Partly as a result, more and more private patients were received into Gartnavel.

Nevertheless, the effects of economic depression in this period and endemic reversals in families' fortunes meant that such patients' status was far from assured. At least 6 per cent (60) of private admissions during 1878–86 were demoted to paupers – a reminder of the pauperising influence of insanity and the ambiguity inherent in contemporary distinctions between private and pauper. Furthermore, while private patient numbers at Gartnavel had more than doubled between 1875–1900, from around 150 to over 400, in real terms the asylum population had actually declined from its former levels. Aside from meeting a newly clamorous social and demographic need from 'the respectable part of the lower middle classes', the ambitions of Gartnavel's promoters had to do with converting it into a smaller, 'acute' hospital of the front rank.[65]

Further bias and selectivity in ridding the royal asylum of paupers

In practice, ridding the royal asylum of the pauper insane was a form of social cleansing of which the psychiatric establishment, which had long stressed the need for strict social segregation in the asylum, also approved in theory. It was a policy broadly, although less emphatically, endorsed by social values in wider society. In addition, gender, religious and racial exclusions were also entailed by the practical consequences of this policy, although largely unacknowledged by asylum officials. Throughout Glasgow Royal's early history, male admissions and male residents had consistently, although far from spectacularly, outnumbered females. This disparity was reversed from the later nineteenth century. By 1878–86, pauper male admissions outnumbered pauper female admissions by more than 2:1, while private admissions generally sustained an equal gender ratio. It was the male paupers who comprised the majority amongst those removed to parochial and district asylums, and it was female private patients who primarily took their places.

The exclusion of paupers (especially male paupers) from Glasgow Royal also entailed the exclusion of Roman Catholic patients, a large number of whom must have been Irish immigrants. Glasgow Royal had always been a highly Presbyterian, Protestant establishment. But Catholics had always comprised a significant minority of the asylum's patients and, even during 1878–86, still made up more than 10 per cent of admissions. Almost 87 per cent of these admissions, however, were paupers, and it was this coterie that represents one of the most conspicuous disappearances from the religious-racial landscape of the asylum. The asylum had from its earliest days prided itself on its multi-denominationalism, and the freedom it allowed for Catholics, as well as other religions, to observe their faith. By the later nineteenth century, discussion of such issues was no longer a feature of asylum records, nor indeed an especially noticeable feature of asylum life. Recent scholarship has identified similar rationales operating at some American asylums that were contemporaneously redefining admissions policies.[66]

At Gartnavel and elsewhere an important agenda behind the policy of excluding paupers was consolidating the hierarchy of Scottish asylums, with royal asylums securely on top of the pile. There is partial linkage here with wider moves towards 'the hospitalisation of the asylum', as touted by Scottish alienists like George M. Robertson.[67] Some colleagues, including Yellowlees, who were convinced as to the superior benefits of moral over medical means, remained dubious as to the virtues of the hospitalisation movement and defensive towards the critique of their own records it carried.[68] Yet Yellowlees and most contemporary alienists were certainly concerned to free their asylums from the 'incubus' of the chronic lunatic. Indeed, they were very keen to promote their asylums, in Yellowlees' evocative phrase, as 'brain infirmaries', conditioned so as to perform 'the highest function of the Asylum, which is cure and not merely the care of the insane'.[69]

Royal asylums also succeeded in restricting their provision for another type of pauper lunatic at this time: the criminal. In 1871, for example, Gartnavel and four other royal asylums had objected to the Lunatics (Scotland) Bill, which sought to compel them to receive over-spillage in 'criminal lunatics' from Perth Criminal Lunatic Department and other institutions.[70] Emphasising the sensibilities of their private patients, and claiming that the proper place for undesirable, insane 'criminals and convicts' was 'the District Asylums', they had succeeded in obtaining an amending clause requiring that managers at chartered and licensed asylums consent to such admissions. Asserting additionally their origins in 'voluntary subscription' and questionable status as 'private corporations', and able to exploit their stronger links with influential politicians and patrons, this was far from the only time that royal asylums had combined successfully to protect their interests at the evident expense of parochial and district asylums.

Such episodes still remind us that pressure for contemporary changes in accommodating paupers was far from confined to royal asylums. There were additionally the significant compulsions of legislation, central government and its offspring (including the Lunacy Commission). Nor did such pressure emanate solely from the psychiatric community, or from central authorities. The parochial authorities were also prime arbiters. As discussed above, these authorities had long been choosing to remove their paupers in favour of cheaper or more local accommodation, even if their decisions sometimes cut across the more medically oriented interests of asylum clinicians. However, as Peter Bartlett has argued,[71] asylums should in part be seen as adjuncts of the overarching system of magisterial and parochial administration with which they were more often at one than in conflict. Previous historiography may have exaggerated the differences between the concerns of the psychiatric establishment and the local authorities. Mackintosh was highly complimentary, in the 1850s, as to the co-operation he received from the Lanarkshire Sheriff and inspector of poor when it came to disposing of patients.[72] Occasionally, members of parochial boards and asylums served concurrently on the boards of chartered asylums, like A.H. MacLellan, Chairman of Gartnavel's Contributors and one-time member of the Barony Parochial Board, or else, were former members of staff of chartered asylums.[73] Moreover, parochial authorities worked substantially under their own steam in setting up alternative establishments to provide more economically for their pauper insane after mid-century. MacLellan himself emphasised in 1875 how keen parochial boards had been for a long time to provide for their own pauper insane. Gartnavel's managers spoke of having 'relieved the District Boards of Lanarkshire...from the legal obligation to send...Patients to Gartnavel' and claimed that this was 'greatly to their [the Boards'] satisfaction'.[74]

Even if this came to be the case, however, as clearer economic and demographic incentives emerged for pauper lunatics' care to be more exclusively the responsibility of local authorities in their own asylums, it also represents a new gloss being put on past relations. For, previously, parochial authorities with limited alternative options had been keen to retain their access to chartered asylums and their privileged rates, while their own institutions had been much criticised for poor standards of care. The Glasgow District Board fought hard to keep some limited space available in Gartnavel for its paupers, after the cancellation of its contract in 1878.[75] Moreover, despite, or perhaps because of, feeling that they were leading actors within Scottish lunacy administration, parochial boards had complained bitterly (if in vain) during the 1870s and 1880s about their lack of representation on the boards of chartered asylums, and of being marginalised by the Scottish Lunacy Board.[76] Scottish parochial boards, including those within the Glasgow district, had themselves gathered together on a number of occasions to air such complaints, typically seeing and presenting themselves as the defenders of the ratepayers. In 1885, for example, they presented a joint memorandum objecting to existing legislation regarding pauper lunatics and the 'extravagant and unnecessary expense to ratepayers'.[77] And on this and on other occasions their complaints had been far from sympathetically received by royal asylums.

Growing economic disparities between the rates being charged by chartered and parochial asylums must also have favoured shifts in negotiating the balance of provision in the region. Before 1857, there had actually been little difference between privileged and non-privileged rates of board for admissions to Gartnavel. After this time, however, the divide widened sharply, and parochial boards complained about not being consulted on gradual increases. Rates at Glasgow (which were between £31 and £35 per annum in the 1880s) were higher than at any other chartered asylum, comparing especially unfavourably with those achievable in the new district asylums. In the Lanarkshire region, Govan had found this situation especially hard. Indeed, partly as a result the parish had been spurred on to provide its own separate accommodation earlier than some other parishes. Yet despite offering licensed accommodation for its paupers in its poorhouse from 1857, and erecting a new parochial asylum at Merryflats in 1872 at a cost approaching £70,000, Govan was still to be assessed for the erection of a district asylum by the Glasgow District Lunacy Board. And its desire for Merryflats to be recognised as a district asylum (and the parish thus freed from a 'double' assessment) had been frustrated by the Lunacy Board's judgment that the asylum was unsuitable.

Nevertheless, after considerable efforts, the parochial boards eventually got more or less their own way with regard to the reorganisation of lunacy districts in the west of Scotland during the 1880s. A united front of objections by Govan and Barony to the plans for the erection of a new district asylum for Glasgow succeeded in delaying the new asylum's erection at Hartwood.[78] Govan, in particular, had led the protests against the district board's plans, worried about yet another assessment for lunacy, but also criticising the proposed asylum as too far away and inconvenient for relatives; over-large for efficient management; and extravagant and exorbitant for prevailing needs in the district. Govan also questioned the very existence of so extensive a lunacy district as comprised by Glasgow. This and more widespread agitation from the parochial boards in Scotland helped to effect legislation nationally for lunacy districts to be altered by the 1887 Lunacy Districts (Scotland) Act. Locally, it saw a radical reorganisation of Glasgow's lunacy administration. Immediately after the Act, Glasgow district was divided or rationalised into the smaller lunacy districts of Govan, Barony City and Lanarkshire (with a portion of

Govan going to Renfrew) – granting each district board and parish greater authority over lunacy provision in their own area. That, despite divisions in their own ranks, the parochial boards could find sufficient common ground to collaborate and force through changes in lunacy administration helps to explain why it was neither possible, nor strongly in the interests of chartered asylums, to ignore their views. The Scottish parochial boards were far from completely satisfied with the 1887 Act. In 1888, they collectively protested against their restricted but continuing dependency on chartered asylums for accommodating their pauper lunatics and their lack of say over these asylums' policies. And they had blamed the provisions in the acts for favouring 'the interests of these institutions' and for the very failure historically of district asylums to be erected in areas where there was a royal asylum.[79]

It must be said, none the less, that the expulsion of all paupers to parochial and district asylums and their replacement by private admissions was far from wholly advantageous to asylums like Gartnavel. The irony was that chronic patients continued to silt up the institution, paupers being replaced by larger numbers of chronic, elderly and often female cases from the 'lowest social grade of Private Patients'.[80] It was found (at least in the short term) not only that the new 'provision for this class of Patients...greatly lowers the Recovery rate', but that it was 'disastrous' in this respect.[81] This was primarily attributed to the new private patients being mostly 'hopeless cases', who had been insane for long periods of time.[82] It was believed (something that can be partly supported by quantitative analysis) that 'in the case of Parish Patients Asylum care is much sooner resorted to', and that as a result their cure rates were actually often superior to those amongst private cases.[83] Furthermore, expelling paupers had also entailed forfeiting the income from their labour. However, this latter loss, which had been foremost amongst the anxieties of the asylum's administrators when considering the policy, was to more than be made up for by private patients' fees.[84]

It would be a mistake to see the divisions between private and pauper patients at Victorian asylums like Gartnavel and even the subsequent off-loading of pauper patients to other asylums as something imposed entirely from above and wholly against the interests of parishes and paupers. Segregation by class was not only advocated by officials and administrators, but was called for by many patients and their families[85] – although, predictably, by those of private means more than by those on parish rates. When Renfrewshire patients were transferred from Gartnavel to Langdale at mid-century, the Renfrewshire Sheriff could 'not recollect any objection having been made by the friends'.[86] A medical inspector of Glasgow asylums, Harry Rainy, testified in 1855 that Paisley paupers 'felt…lost in Gartnavel', and 'wished to get back to Paisley'.[87] Nevertheless, it seems highly unlikely that all paupers were, or thought themselves, better off in their local asylums than they had been at Gartnavel. Some removed during the 1870s and 1880s must have been less than content – particularly those hailing from nearer Gartnavel, whose poor relations would have been forced to travel greater distances, or been deterred from visiting them. Furthermore, in prioritising private over pauper interests and in the extremity of their conviction in fitting asylum conditions to social and economic background, contemporary authorities were also justifying a neglect of paupers. It was a common belief, as Scottish Lunacy Commissioners expressed it, that, as a result of their ingrained 'previous habits', the poor were actually unable to appreciate the superior comforts of the richer classes and 'generally prefer an inferior description of accommodation'.[88] This argument was ready-made to excuse evident deficiencies in provision for pauper lunatics, while serving to retard the progress of amelioration. It was on the basis of similar ideology, and of contemporary stigmatising of the low morality of the poorer classes, that the apparent increase of pauper lunacy was often attributed to the increased prosperity of the poor, rather than to deprivation and depression.

Conclusion

There are a number of conclusions which are particularly worth noting from this chapter. Much of the apparatus for the identification and sequestration of pauper lunacy was not developed or applied in Scotland until after 1850. Both local authorities and the relations of the pauper insane proved strikingly resilient to the asylum solution to the problems of pauper lunacy before and for some time after the 1857 Lunacy (Scotland) Act. Scottish evidence reinforces evidence in other recent studies that too little attention has been paid to the views and strategies of local authorities when it came to the arbitration of pauper lunacy in this period. Rather than solutions to the perceived problems of lunacy provision being imposed from above, I have traced wide areas of negotiation operating at a local level and informing decision-making as to where to accommodate the pauper insane. The vicissitudes and variety of actors and factors involved in this negotiation, from economic to medical rationales, and from parochial authorities to the family, have further been underlined. The significance of sectarian, social and racial lines according to which the boundaries of lunacy provision were being drawn in this period has also been elucidated.

Considerable vagaries and changes over time have been charted in the pauper lunatic population of Glasgow, and more especially its royal asylum, which emphasise the importance of local variations in lunacy provision for paupers. In analysing the reasons for these patterns, I have stressed that most were predicated on an attitude to pauper lunacy that perceived it as of a more vicious, more morbid, more pathological state than lunacy amongst the middle and upper classes. Contemporaries also emphasised the potential infectiousness of the pauper insane and their inequitable economic drain on the moneyed classes. Such conceptualisations must have chimed in with wider concerns in late Victorian society about the preservation of bourgeois values against the threat of the unruly poor, about hygiene and sanitation in fast growing, particularly urban, poor areas, and about the advancing spectres of hereditary taint and degeneration.

A somewhat transformed or intensified disposition towards providing separately for the pauper insane in late Victorian Glasgow fitted in – if somewhat ambivalently – with contemporary ideologies, particularly those of its medical profession, who sought to revamp and remodel the leading asylums, and to raise their own status. While characterised as a return to 'the benevolent function for which it was founded', the 'privatisation' of Gartnavel meant, in fact, departing from the ethos of 1814 of providing 'Asylum to the wretched' insane, amongst both 'the wealthy and the poor'.[89] Indeed, this chapter has generally emphasised how careful one must be to sift contemporary testimony, whether medical or lay, for its underlying ideologies.

NOTES

1 Andrew T. Scull, *Museums of Madness: The Social Organisation of Insanity in Nineteenth-Century England*, London, Allen Lane, 1979; *Social Order/Mental Disorder: Anglo-American Psychiatry in Historical Perspective*, London, Routledge, 1989; *The Most Solitary of Afflictions. Madness and Society in Britain, 1700–1900*, New Haven, London, Yale University Press, 1993.

2 Ibid. and see also Scull, 'Was insanity increasing? A response to Edward Hare', *British Journal of Psychiatry*, 144, 1984, pp. 432–6. For a contrasting view, see Edward Hare, 'Was insanity on the increase?', *British Journal of Psychiatry*, 142, 1983, pp. 439–55.

3 Andrew Scull, Charlotte MacKenzie and Nicholas Hervey, *Masters of Bedlam. The Transformation of the Mad-doctoring Trade*, Princeton, NJ, Princeton University Press, 1996, pp. 93–4.

4 Scottish poorhouses were loosely equivalents of English workhouses, except that they were not supposed to house the able-bodied poor, and were all parochially managed institutions, rather than farmed-out to private contractors.

5 *First Annual Report* (henceforth AR) *of the General Board of Commissioners in Lunacy for Scotland* (henceforth GBCLS), Edinburgh, HMSO, 1859, p. 112.

6 The lunatic wards in Paisley Poorhouse were rebuilt in 1854. Greenock, Govan, Dumbarton, Bute and a number of other localities adjoining Glasgow had no institutional provision for pauper lunatics until after 1850; e.g. *Scottish Lunacy Commission Report*, Edinburgh, HMSO, 1857, pp. 442, 448.
7 David Gollaher, *Voice for the Mad: The Life of Dorothea Dix*, New York, London, Free Press, 1995; R.A. Cage, *The Scottish Poor Law, 1745–1845*, Edinburgh, Scottish University Press, 1981, pp. 133–42.
8 Scull *et al.*, *Masters of Bedlam*, pp. 93–4 and refs 34 and 35.
9 See Jonathan Andrews, *"They're in the Trade... They 'cannot interfere' – they say": The Scottish Lunacy Commissioners and Lunacy Reform in Nineteenth-century Scotland*, London, *Wellcome Trust Occasional Publication*, 8, 1998, forthcoming.
10 *Scottish Lunacy Commission Report*, 1857, p. 473; 2nd AR of GBCLS, 1860, p. iv.
11 This point is also made about Dundee Kirk Sessions in Walsh's chapter.
12 *Scottish Lunacy Commission Report*, 1857, p. 449.
13 After Argyll and Bute District Asylum's foundation (1864), these were: Govan Parochial (Merryflats) Asylum (1873); Barony (Barnhill) Parochial Asylum, at Lenzie, Woodilee (1875); Glasgow District Asylum, Bothwell (1881); Govan (Hawkhead) District Asylum and Lanarkshire District Asylum (Hartwood) (1895); and Glasgow District Asylum, Gartloch (1897).
14 The power to divide lunacy districts was inadvertently granted through the passing of the Prisons (Scotland) Act of 1877, which saw the revitalisation of the Glasgow District Lunacy Board. This power was not revived until the passing of the Lunacy Districts (Scotland) Act of 1887. See, 30th AR of GBLCS, 1888, p. xliii.
15 *Scottish Lunacy Commission Report*, 1857, p. 473.
16 Even by 1859, for example, Peebles was registering just 3 and Kinross just 8; 1st AR of the GBCLS, 1859, pp. 112–13.
17 1st AR of the GBCLS, 1859, p. 101.
18 Ibid., p. 462.
19 Friedrich Jolly, 'On the family care of the insane in Scotland', *Journal of Mental Science*, 21, 1875, pp. 40–60, pp. 48–9.
20 See, e.g., 8th AR of GBCLS, 1866, p. 253.
21 See Harriet Sturdy, 'Boarding-out the insane, 1857–1913: a study of the Scottish system', Ph.D. thesis, University of Glasgow, 1996.
22 See *WRH MS MC1/4*, Minute Books of the Lunacy Commissioners for Scotland 1873–80, fols 116, 87, 94, 151, 167 and 258; 21 August and 15 September 1874, 6 January, 8 June and 7 September 1875, and 3 January 1877, Scottish Record Office, Edinburgh.
23 29 and 30 Vict., Cap. 51, x, and 9th AR of GBCLS, 1867, p. xxix.
24 T. C. Smout, *A Century of the Scottish People, 1830–1950*, London, Collins, 1986, p. 8
25 *Scottish Lunacy Commission Report*, 1857, p. 462.
26 E.g. *63rd Annual Report* (henceforth AR) *of Glasgow Royal Asylum* (henceforth GRA) *for the year 1876*, Glasgow, James Hedderwick, 1877, p. 11; 65th AR, 1879, p. 11; 66th AR, 1880, pp. 3–4, 11–12.
27 Andrew Scull, 'A convenient place to get rid of inconvenient people: the Victorian lunatic asylum', in A. D. King, ed., *Buildings and Society*, London, Routledge and Kegan Paul, 1980, pp. 37–60.

28 Bill Forsythe, Joseph Melling and Richard Adair, 'The New Poor Law and the county pauper lunatic asylum – the Devon experience, 1834–84', *Social History of Medicine*, 9, 3, 1996, pp. 335–56.
29 66th AR of GRA, 1880, p. 3.
30 E.g. 8th AR of the GBCLS, 1866, pp. iii, 239.
31 E.g. Gillian A. Doody, Allan Beveridge and E. C. Johnstone, 'Poor and mad: a study of patients admitted to the Fife and Kinross District Asylum between 1874 and 1899', *Psychological Medicine*, 26, 1996, pp. 887–97; Allan Beveridge, 'Madness in Victorian Edinburgh: a study of patients admitted to the Royal Edinburgh Asylum under Thomas Clouston, 1873–1908', *History of Psychiatry*, 6, 1995, pp. 21–54 and 133–56, esp. pp. 43–4.
32 Robert Renwick, ed., *Extracts from the Records of the Burgh of Glasgow*, Glasgow, Corporation of Glasgow, 1914, vol. ii, entry dated 1804, p. 442.
33 *Report of the General Committee Appointed to Carry Into Effect the Proposal for a Lunatic Asylum in Glasgow*..., Glasgow, James Hedderwick, 1814, p. 5.
34 Ibid., p. 8.
35 Stark's building was not a Benthamite panopticon, but rather had panoptic features. See Anne Snedden, 'Environment and architecture', in Jonathan Andrews and Iain Smith, eds, *'Let There Be Light Again'. A History of Gartnavel Royal Hospital*, Glasgow, Gartnavel, 1993, pp. 31–50; Thomas A. Markus, ed., *Order in Space and Society. Architectural Form and its Context in the Scottish Enlightenment*, Edinburgh, Mainstream, 1982, esp. pp. 25–114 and 'Buildings and the ordering of minds and bodies', in Peter Jones, ed., *Philosophy and Science in the Scottish Enlightenment*, Edinburgh, John Donald, 1988, pp. 169–224 and 'Class and classification in the buildings of the late Scottish Enlightenment', in T. M. Devine, ed., *Improvement and Enlightenment. Proceedings of the Scottish Historical Studies Seminar, University of Strathclyde, 1987–88*, Edinburgh, John Donald, 1989, pp. 78–107.
36 William Stark, *Remarks on the Construction of Public Hospitals for the Cure of Mental Derangement*, Edinburgh, James Ballantyne, 1807, pp. 15, 17.
37 Ibid., p. 10.
38 Ibid., p. 9.
39 *Report of the General Committee*, 1814, p. 19.
40 *Scottish Lunacy Commission Report*, 1857, p. 379. In actuality, Gartnavel became the district asylum for Lanarkshire from 1865, when it contracted to take all pauper lunatics from the area.
41 84th AR of GRA, 1897, p. 7.
42 66th AR of GRA, 1879, pp. 3, 8.
43 *Scottish Lunacy Commission Report*, 1857, pp. 374, 461.
44 *WRH MS MC1/4*, fols 142, 146, 150, 4 and 18 May, and 8 June 1875, case of Mary Adams or Anderson; 62nd AR of GRA, 1875, p. 23.
45 *Scottish Lunacy Commission Report*, 1857, pp. 489, 494.
46 Ibid., pp. 372, 376. Economy e.g. had been behind the removal of Barony and Govan patients from Gartnavel in the 1850s; see, ibid., pp. 377, 474, 490.
47 Ibid., p. 377.
48 Ibid., p. 475.
49 Ibid., p. 470.
50 Ibid., p. 479.
51 Barony poorhouse in the 1850s held around 1,400 paupers, only 100–130 of whom were in the lunatic wards. See ibid., p. 378.

52 Ibid., 1857, pp. 491–2. For a fuller discussion of lunacy provision at Barony Poorhouse, see Jonathan Andrews, 'A failure to flourish? David Yellowlees and the Glasgow School of Psychiatry. Part 1 and Part 2', *History of Psychiatry*, 8, 1997, pp. 177–22, 333–60
53 *Scottish Lunacy Commission Report*, p. 466.
54 Ibid., pp. 381, 470.
55 E.g. 67th AR of GRA, 1880, pp. 7–8, 10–11; 69th AR, 1884, p. 9.
56 69th AR of GRA, 1882, p.10. See, also, 65th AR of GRA, 1878, p. 9; 74th AR, 1888, p. 9; 76th AR, 1889, p. 11.
57 E.g. 81st AR of GRA, 1894, p. 13.
58 84th AR of GRA, 1897, p. 11.
59 Report of John Fraser, Scottish Lunacy Commissioner, quoted in 84th AR of GRA, 1897, p. 9.
60 63rd AR of GRA, 1876, p. 11.
61 64th AR of GRA, 1877, p. 11
62 Ibid.
63 *Scottish Lunacy Commission Report*, 1857, p. 460.
64 81st AR of GRA, 1894, p.4.
65 66th AR of GRA, 1879, p. 9.
66 E.g. Ian Dowbiggin, ' "A life free from unpleasant associations": policy, charity, and social class at the Butler Hospital, 1847–1921', unpublished paper given at EAHP meeting, Friends House, London, August 1993. Dowbiggin found that policy at the Butler, justified in terms of achieving a 'better class of patient', entailed the removal of significant numbers of male and Catholic paupers, many of whom were Irish (and other foreign) immigrants.
67 George M. Robertson, 'The hospitalisation of the Scottish asylum system...', *Journal of Mental Science*, 68, 1922, pp. 321–33.
68 E.g. 88th AR of GRA, 1901, p. 17.
69 Yellowlees, quoted in BMA discussion, *Journal of Mental Science*, October, 189, p. 590; 67th AR of GRA, 1880, p. 7.
70 GGHB13/10/37, Lunatics (Scotland) Bill, 1871 and Memorandum on Behalf of the Royal Edinburgh Asylum for the Insane on the subject, 1871; GGHB13/10/38 miscellaneous correspondence on the matter; and the Criminal and Dangerous Lunatics (Scotland) Amendment Act, 1871, 30 and 31 Vict., Cap. 55, clause 4, p. 3.
71 See Peter Bartlett's chapter in this volume. See, also, Bartlett, 'The Poor Law of Lunacy: the administration of pauper lunatics in mid-nineteenth century England with special emphasis on Leicestershire and Rutland', Ph.D. diss., University of London, 1993; Forsythe, Melling and Adair, 'The New Poor Law'.
72 *Scottish Lunacy Commission Report*, 1857, pp. 463, 466.
73 62nd AR of GRA, 1875, p. 3; 63rd AR of GRA, 1876, p. 17.
74 82nd AR of GRA, 1895, pp. 7–8.
75 E.g. GGHB13/10/37, Minutes of the Directors at Glasgow Royal dated 23 July 1878 and of the Glasgow District Lunacy Board dated 20 June 1876; and Notes regarding Asylum Accommodation for Pauper Lunatics, 1878.
76 E.g. GGHB13/10/37, Lunacy Law in Scotland. Memorandum on Behalf of the Parochial Boards..., 2 July 1885, and Memorial to...the Marquis of Lothian by Parochial Boards...as to Constitution of Royal Asylums, 29 March 1888.

77 GGHB13/10/37, Lunacy Law in Scotland. Memorandum...1885.
78 GGHB13/13/34, typescript notes on Govan District Lunacy Board, Govan Parochial Asylum and Govan Poorhouse, by Dr Andrew Bell, c.1972.
79 GGHB13/10/37, Memorial to...the Marquis of Lothian...1888.
80 E.g. 75th AR of GRA, 1888, p. 10; 85th AR, 1898, p. 9; 87th AR, 1900, p. 10; 88th AR, 1901, p. 13.
81 78th AR of GRA, 1891, pp. 11–12; 79th AR, 1892, p. 11.
82 78th AR of GRA, 1891, pp. 11–12.
83 Ibid., p. 12.
84 See e.g. 81st AR of GRA, 1894, p. 14; 82nd AR, 1895, pp. 3–4, 8; 84th AR, 1897, pp. 7, 11.
85 See e.g. case of George Reid, *GHB13/5/47*, fols 117, 207 and 151–2, who protested about the placing of John Tudehope in the same ward, feeling 'much wronged' in being 'classed with this poor creature'.
86 *Scottish Lunacy Commission Report*, 1857, p. 479.
87 Ibid., p. 443.
88 See ibid., pp. 61, 66 and 73–4.
89 81st AR of GRA, 1894, p. 5; op. cit., ref. 29, pp. 3, 5.

11

'THE DESIGNS OF PROVIDENCE'

Race, religion and Irish insanity

Oonagh Walsh

In this chapter I wish to explore several aspects of the cultural and historical significance of the Connaught District Lunatic Asylum in Ballinasloe, Co. Galway,[1] and draw some, necessarily tentative, conclusions regarding its position in Irish society. The concern of the chapter is to determine the historical context for the establishment of the asylum, and its relationship to the introduction of the Irish Poor Law. In this context, I wish to highlight the various ways in which religious tension was displayed and controlled within the asylum, through, for example, the struggle between the Protestant management and the Catholic priest who tended to the patients over the construction of a Catholic church in the asylum grounds; the debate over differing rates of admission for Catholic and Protestant patients, and the machinations behind the admission of professed religious. The chapter also discusses the increasingly racial, certainly pseudo-scientific, discourse employed by certain members of the hospital medical administration to describe patients, and examine whether the presumptions implicit in these representations made any difference to power relations between physician and patient.[2]

The Ballinasloe Asylum, despite its formidable physical presence, with high walls and barred windows, was not isolated from contemporary political and social developments. The patients reflected the various bodies of opinion outside the asylum on Home Rule, land reform, agrarian outrages, and the Gaelic Revival. The present chapter therefore attempts to locate the asylum within the flux of historical and social considerations from which it often appeared remote. In this and other respects my contribution can be compared with the chapters on Wales and on the colonies, where the relationship between the politics of lunacy administration and the wider concerns of the British state became apparent in the deliberations of the local institutions as well as the more obvious policy debates within the political system.

The development of the asylum

The development of the Irish asylum system was contemporaneous with the creation of the Irish Poor Law in 1838, which was itself a consequence of broader political developments. From the Act of Union in 1800, Irish administration became increasingly centralised: 'In the fields of education, economic development, police, prisons and public health – to take but leading examples – the state intervened to a degree and in a fashion scarcely conceivable in contemporary Britain.'[3] This rush to direct the country's affairs as far as possible from London, via the Lord Lieutenant's Office in Dublin, reflected insecurity regarding the state of the country, and a determination to prevent the establishment of local nationalist power bases. The Irish Poor Law System was formed by the Poor Relief Act of 1838, and under its auspices the poor of the country were to have recourse to medical care through dispensaries and hospitals, and to workhouses as a final resort. There has been a good deal of debate over the efficacy of the Irish Poor Law and its appropriateness for Ireland's particular circumstances, but what is of interest here is the position of asylums within the system. In 1836 The Commissioners' Report on Irish poverty had recommended that asylums be brought under the direct control of the Poor Law Commissioners.[4] However, this advice was rejected, on the grounds that the insane needed specialist attention, and a separate administration developed. This strategy allowed for a rather more enlightened attitude towards pauper lunatics, as they were defined and treated on the basis of their mental state, and not on their poverty.[5] Irish asylums were under the direct control of the Lord Lieutenant, and any changes in asylum administration, funding or construction had to be approved by Dublin Castle. The asylums were inspected at least once a year, by the Inspector of Prisons, but the day-to-day administration was undertaken by Boards of Governors. At Ballinasloe, these men[6] were all members of the Protestant middle and upper classes, mainly local landowners and businessmen, and they worked closely with the asylum manager and physician in the running of the asylum. They approved staff appointments, decided upon punishments for unruly nurses, set asylum wages, and signed release forms on the advice of the physician. They were however limited in their powers – decrees issued by the Lord Lieutenant's office over general asylum regulations, or admission and release procedures, had to be obeyed.

The asylums did have a certain degree of autonomy, however, which set them apart from the more repressive regimes implemented in the workhouses. Joseph Robins has argued that Irish asylums were fortunate to escape being linked with the construction and administration of workhouses after 1842, describing the latter as 'harsh and forbidding in character, planned deliberately to facilitate the creation of an "irksome" and unsympathetic environment where paupers would have no inclination to dally at the expense of the ratepayer.'[7] The formation of Irish lunatic policy did not take place in a vacuum, however, despite its distance from the Poor Law. On the contrary, legislation governing lunacy was shaped within a highly politicised environment, in which issues of security, and the necessity to establish and maintain order, were paramount. This concern was signalled at an early stage by the passage of the so-called 'Dangerous Lunatics' Act of 1838[8] which, in the early years of asylum construction in Ireland, established an intimate link between insanity and criminality. The provisions of the Act, which did 'not extend to England or Scotland', were to haunt asylum administrators and inspectors for the remainder of the century. The Act placed an extraordinary degree of power in the hands of medical, judicial and security figures, but also of ordinary citizens. Under its terms, an uncorroborated sworn statement, made before two justices of the peace, was enough to secure arrest and admission to gaol of an alleged lunatic, and then onward to a district asylum. However, many alleged lunatics actually spent up to a year in prison before being transferred to the asylum and, in the case of Ballinasloe, they frequently arrived with little or no information as to relatives, home life, or basic details regarding age and marital status. These patients formed a core of life-long asylum inmates, and were a permanent drain on institutional resources. Moreover, the intervening period in gaol frequently served to weaken family ties, associate the lunatic with 'the degradation of prison', and make eventual reintegration into society more difficult.[9]

After decades of objection on the part of inspectors and asylum personnel, the 1838 Act was amended, although the new act of 1867 simply compounded many of these difficulties. After 1867 any alleged lunatic could be committed direct to the asylum and indeed it was now illegal to send a 'dangerous lunatic or dangerous idiot' to gaol. The asylum inspectors welcomed this rather more humane attitude towards the insane – they had long protested about the distressing effect prison had upon lunatics awaiting transfer – but they were cautiously pessimistic:

> but what is to be feared is that they [justices of the peace] will consider nearly every case of lunacy brought before them as a fit one for committal; and we know of our own experience....that parties bringing lunatics before justices have found no difficulty in deposing to facts sufficient to give a colour to the case, even though the individuals might be perfectly harmless, and thus secure their committal as 'dangerous'.[10]

Within just one year, the inspector's fears were confirmed: 'The operation of the Act...has also contributed materially to crowd the District Lunatic Asylums with patients – magistrates, we regret to say, giving the widest possible interpretation to the term "dangerous lunatic".' The coercive nature of the Act, under whose provisions no asylum could refuse a patient, led to an immediate and dramatic rise in the number of patients committed as dangerous. For example, at Ballinasloe, in 1867, a startling majority of admissions were linked to the Act:

> The increase of room [through new buildings] will not, however, be available a moment too soon looking to the wholesale committal of lunatics by justices under the recent enactment, for out of 88 admissions 79 were in the category of 'dangerous lunatics' so that the Governors and Medical Officers had a voice in the admission of only nine cases.[11]

The principal concern amongst officials, reiterated in successive asylum reports, was abuse of the act to secure the admission of unsuitable cases who were a burden on the workhouses. This following example, from Co. Cork District Asylum, indicated the absurd extent to which some justices could be persuaded to apply the term 'dangerous':

> P.S., an idiotic child of apparently about ten years old, diminutive even for that age, and still in petticoats, was received on 6th July, 1869, under warrant. He was seen shortly after by one of our Inspectors, to whom he appeared to be an inoffensive quiet little creature, and the R.M.S. [Resident Medical Superintendent] reported that he had not shown the slightest tendency to violence from the time he was placed in the asylum; yet this mere infant was sent from Berehaven to Cork, a distance of more than 120 miles, under a constabulary escort at the public expense, as a 'dangerous lunatic'.[12]

As late as 1912, a majority of admissions nationally were still being made under the Act.

Throughout the nineteenth century several attempts to reform lunacy and create a system linked to the Poor Law, as in England, met with failure. In addition to crowding Irish asylums with cases which, as the inspectors regularly pointed out, would be more appropriately and cheaply cared for in workhouses, the Act created a significant body of long-stay patients, whose cases had no automatic right of review and who, once admitted, could be detained indefinitely. However, the Dangerous Lunatics Act was a symptom rather than a cause of the huge increase in asylum inmates throughout the nineteenth century. This period witnessed an unprecedented expansion of the asylum system in Ireland. The Act of Union in 1800 had brought 'a host of institutional innovations to Ireland',[13] one of which was the creation of a comprehensive system of district asylums throughout the country. At the beginning of the century, the principal establishment for the care of pauper lunatics was the Richmond Asylum in Dublin. By 1835, nine such institutions were in existence, and by 1869 there were twenty-two district asylums, offering accommodation for 7,593 individuals.[14] This growth[15] is all the more remarkable when one considers that the total population in Ireland fell drastically from 8,175,124 in 1841 to 4,458,775 in 1901.[16] In attempting to explain the increase the asylum inspectors came up with the intriguing suggestion that 'a cause of the large existing number of lunatics in Ireland can be traced to a greater longevity from an improved treatment of mental diseases generally, and the quietude of life enjoyed in district asylums'.[17] The asylum at Ballinasloe demonstrated one of the most dramatic increases in patient numbers. Originally built in 1833 to accommodate 150 people, it housed over 300 in 1853, and just over one thousand in 1896.[18] Given that the catchment area for the asylum had shrunk from the five counties of Galway, Roscommon, Mayo, Sligo and Leitrim in 1833 to just two, Galway and Roscommon in 1866, the increase was significant.[19]

The wider society

Outside the asylum walls in the late nineteenth century there was a politically active culture in which continuing high rates of emigration, the beginnings of large-scale transfer of property from landlord to tenant under various land acts, and the growing strength of nationalist opinion, created a sense of political restlessness which occasionally percolated through to the inmates and hospital staff. Indeed, there was one issue that bound staff and inmates, the asylum and the greater society, firmly together: religion. Tension between Catholicism and Protestantism was a constant factor in Irish politics. Although Catholic Emancipation had been achieved in 1829, Protestant dominance in trade, government and higher employment remained steady throughout the nineteenth century. However, in the 1880s and 1890s, Catholics increasingly encroached upon these fields, and particularly at the level of local government. Institutions such as the Ballinasloe Asylum came under increasing pressure to appoint Catholics to senior positions, demands which were successfully resisted until the first Catholic Manager was elected in 1904. Prior to that date, all of the asylum guardians, the physician, the manager, and most of the senior nursing staff were Protestant, a profile sharply at odds with a Catholic patient population of over 90 per cent. The asylum administration argued that their religious profile was irrelevant, but it remained a source of tension, which manifested itself most obviously in the battle to have a Catholic church built in the asylum grounds.

In Ballinasloe, the board of guardians allowed a Catholic Mass to be celebrated every Sunday in the asylum grounds, but refused permission for the construction of a chapel, and would not permit a daily service. Individual patients were allowed to attend Mass outside the asylum[20] if accompanied by a nurse, but the board had to be satisfied as to their pacific nature. There was a genuine fear that some patients would disrupt the service, or behave in a blasphemous manner, but there was an additional factor in the board's determination to maintain the asylum's secular state. In the post-famine period the number of professed religious in Ireland had risen dramatically, from, in the case of nuns, 1,500 in 1851, to over 8,000 in 1901.[21] Teaching and nursing orders had in particular expanded, and had from 1850 onwards made increasing inroads upon schools and hospitals. The assumption of financial responsibility by the Catholic Church in these areas had been tacitly welcomed by the government, as it represented a significant saving, but some individuals were concerned about the possible religious consequences of such developments. Thus when successive Catholic priests appointed to the institution bitterly protested about the lack of a chapel, the board remained unmoved, refusing to allow the priest a permanent base inside the walls. On one occasion, the priest pointed to an attendance at Mass of 'one hundred and sixty patients and thirty servants', and declared that the service improved their mental health:

> Of the patients several are usually convalescent, others have at intervals often of several weeks duration the full possession of

> their faculties, and [it] profits them of course when allowed to be present at Mass, whilst many others are, although habitually monomaniacs, perfectly susceptible of religious impressions, alive to the loss of religious opportunities, and duly appreciate the ministrations of religion.

Hinting that the board, as Protestants, could not understand the spiritual needs of Catholic patients, the priest declared:

> As to the spiritual advantages of the arrangement, they can be duly appreciated only by Roman Catholics. Very many of the patients are in a state of mind that fully warrants the administration of Sacraments to them, and at the approach of death very many indeed become quite sensible of their religious responsibilities.[22]

The board continued to refuse the plea, on the grounds that it was a considerable expense, and because it was not a standard provision in Irish gaols. This rather disingenuous argument[23] – religious attendance was compulsory at most prisons, and was regarded as an essential part of the disciplinary process – was used to prevent Church advances until the 1880s. It is clear that the board at Ballinasloe feared that the establishment of a permanent Catholic base within the asylum would lead to a Catholic take-over of the institution itself, and their refusal to permit a Catholic church on asylum grounds reflected a broader contemporary political concern.

General professional opinion in this period varied over the usefulness of religious practice in lunatic asylums. While ministers tended to argue that religion was crucial in assisting recovery, asylum authorities feared the effect which religious ritual might have on already distressed imaginations. Patients pondering such issues as salvation and the existence of God, it was argued, might have their recoveries impeded. W.A.F. Browne, in 1837, expressed reservations about the potentially stimulating nature of religious celebrations. He feared that 'the excitement to which the mind is exposed by the imposing aspect and duration of the ceremony and the mingled feelings of awe, and penitence, and hope to which it gives rise', might unsettle certain patients further.[24] Interestingly, however, he claimed that a respectful participation in religious ritual should be taken as grounds for immediate release from an asylum:

> I am, however, inclined to think that when patients have advanced so far towards restoration as to be intrusted with such high and holy privileges, that they should not longer be detained in an asylum, but should be reinstated in society, and in the possession of rights, and the discharge of duties of an important but less exciting character.[25]

Visitors to Ireland frequently debated the wisdom of increasing asylum places, on the grounds of expense as well as efficiency. However, the Reverend James Hall, a Scot who travelled throughout the country in 1813, argued that in placing lunatics in asylums the authorities were negating the purpose for which they were created by God.[26] As far as Hall was concerned, lunatics were put on earth to act as a reminder and a reproof to the sane population of God's just wrath. No effort should therefore be made to rehabilitate the insane, an opinion which ran contrary to the prevailing mood of the nineteenth century, with its increasing emphasis upon institutionalisation:

> Lunatic-hospitals, and places set apart for the convenience of those deprived of reason, have, no doubt, their advantages; but they partly frustrate the designs of Providence in so ordering matters, that here and there individuals are deprived of the reasoning faculty, to be an admonition to all.[27]

In a country where religion had frequently been used as a means of establishing superiority, the question of whether Catholicism or Protestantism inclined followers more towards insanity had broad implications. On the one hand, Protestantism, with its rational basis, its emphasis upon an individual relationship with God, and its logical interpretations of the Bible, seemed to suggest a measured approach conducive to sanity. Catholicism, with its dependence upon the mediating power of the priest, its sumptuous rituals, Latin incantations, and suggestions of the supernatural through an intimate association with spirits and saints, might lend itself to diseased imaginings. However, Protestants seemed plagued to a greater degree with issues of worthiness and salvation than were Catholics. A Catholic was unquestioningly 'saved' from the cradle, or at least from baptism, and provided the rituals and a godly life were followed, was assured of entry to heaven on death. This is not to say that Catholics were without doubts regarding religious worthiness, but the process of confession – the most widespread 'talking cure' – and communion provided a continual assurance of sanctity. Protestants, on the other hand, were encouraged to question their personal spiritual states, and to explore the validity of their religious existences. On the evidence from Ballinasloe, it would seem that Protestants, rather than Catholics, had a propensity towards what was diagnosed as 'religious excitement'. The total Protestant population[28] of Co. Galway stood in 1891 at 2.5 per cent, and in Co. Roscommon the figure was slightly higher at 3.5 per cent.[29] In the 1890s, Protestant admissions to the asylum ranged from 5 to 8 per cent of the total, but Protestants were 30 per cent more likely to be diagnosed as suffering from religious excitement than Catholics.[30]

Despite these figures, there remained a fixed belief amongst certain Protestant ministers that Catholicism lent itself more readily to inflamed imaginings. A case from 1893 neatly encapsulated this belief, despite solid evidence to the contrary. A Protestant man was admitted to the asylum, suffering from religious mania. The case notes record that the patient had Christ-like delusions. He patrolled the asylum armed with an iron bar, which he said he needed to fight off those who were preventing 'the little children from speaking to him'. The physician was plagued by a series of petitions from the man's minister,[31] who demanded the patient's release. The minister argued that the man was self-evidently sane because he was a prosperous farmer and a regular church-goer, but more importantly, because he was a Protestant. Protestants in Ireland, it seemed, could not be insane, since God had appointed them over Catholics to organise and administer the country. The physician commented:

> [The] clergyman seems to have thoroughly assimilated to himself all the patient's persecutory delusions and to have allowed them to take irradicable root. He is a ready apologist for all his 'eccentricities' of behaviour as he terms them and says [the patient's] frequent vigils armed with iron bars and hurling denunciations are mere 'peculiarities' which none of us are free from: To a professional opinion that [the patient] was insane he opposed an emphatic denial with rude haste and clerical dogmatism.[32]

The diagnosis of religious excitement was applied to between 10 and 15 per cent of the admissions to Ballinasloe throughout the 1890s, although there were particular periods in which such admissions would sharply rise. The curious thing about religious excitement is that it was a diagnosis which was rarely applied to any of the professed religious who entered the asylum. They were admitted suffering from mania and melancholia, but it was lay patients who were specifically diagnosed as labouring under religious excitement or religious hyper-ecstasy.

However, throughout the nineteenth century, there was a steady rate of admission of priests, but very few nuns. In the 1890s none of these cases was diagnosed as suffering from religious excitement, and the physician made no note of religious delusions or preoccupations. What emerges from the admission records is the unsurprising fact that the Catholic Church appears to have made considerable efforts to cope with mentally ill priests outside of the asylum in the early stages of illness, and only resorted to admission to public asylums as a last resort. In nineteenth-century Ireland, priests occupied not merely positions of importance in the community generally, but acted as advisers to the Catholic population in matters outside of religious affairs. Thus the spectacle of a lunatic priest would implicitly undermine the local authority of the Church. In one case from 1896, a priest based in Dublin had been treated at a private institution for a considerable period of time. He appeared to recover, but on his relapse, and when signs clearly indicated that he would not be able to resume his religious duties, he was transferred as a paying patient to Ballinasloe. He had relatives in Galway who made the necessary arrangements, but there was a clear concern on the part of the Church to remove him from the area in which he was best known.

Despite the very large expansion in the numbers of professed religious in nineteenth-century Ireland, nuns were rarely admitted to the Ballinasloe Asylum. One possible explanation is the large number of enclosed religious orders in Ireland, such as the Poor Clares. These nuns spent the whole of their lives inside the convent walls, offered prayers for the benefit of the population, but never directly engaged with the outside world. In this context, insanity and manifestations of aberrant behaviour may have been more easily dealt with, and mentally ill individuals allowed to remain within the community. On a literal level, however, it was extremely difficult for these women to leave the convents, as they had taken vows of renunciation. A nursing sister attended ill individuals within the convents, although in cases of serious illness doctors could be admitted. Even outside of the enclosed orders, with the teaching and nursing sisters, who had a far greater degree of contact with the non-religious community, there was still scope for the relatively secret treatment of a disturbed woman, since not all of the community was involved with the outside work of the convent. A priest on the other hand was an active, integrated member of the population, with duties to fulfil which brought him into the closest of contact with others. In this environment, aberrant behaviour was much more difficult to conceal, which may explain the greater representation of priests than nuns in the asylum.

Another possibility is that the vocation and training which nuns possessed may have left them better able to cope with mental illness than others. Within many of the women's orders there was a constant emphasis upon the abnegation of self, and on conquering one's will. Mary Aikenhead, the founder of the Sisters of Charity, wrote:

> Our consideration of our interior state will show each the deficiencies in her own self; and by fervent prayer, and devout reception of the Holy Sacraments, we shall conquer self and the enemy who is actively engaged in raising obstacles to our perfection. We must be watchful and active to oppose our enemies (for assuredly self is the worst enemy).[33]

This constant emphasis upon self-control and self-examination could have a negative effect upon a susceptible individual perhaps, but could one argue that it might also keep a potentially unstable person under control?

Religious difference in Ireland led more often than not to a simple division of institutions into those which served and were staffed by either Catholics or Protestants. Even in those regions and institutions where religious tension was low, Catholics and Protestants for the most part attended denominational schools, hospitals and even universities. Voluntary and involuntary segregation in these areas was well established by the time the dispute over the Catholic chapel arose in Ballinasloe, and an underlying presumption that encroachment into such an institution would lead to take-over was difficult to overcome. The board's resistance towards the building of a church may have had a negative impact upon the patients' spiritual well-being, as the priest feared, but the institution, unlike the general hospitals, schools, charitable organisations and political groups in Ireland, remained secular and mixed, in the twentieth as well as the nineteenth century.

Scientific discourse and racial difference

The 1890s was an important decade in terms of Irish political life, but it was also the period of high imperialism, during which intense discussions regarding the fitness or otherwise of subject nations for self-government were taking place. Many of these debates drew heavily upon the discourse of racial difference, which was in turn dependent to a significant degree upon physical characterisation. In Ireland, where issues of nationality and government dominated in the nineteenth century, there were several attempts to establish whether the Irish were racially equal to other 'high' European civilisations, or whether they constituted a mixed-race sub-grouping, which demanded a more traditionally colonial administration. The theories which evolved, and which were based upon supposedly distinctively racial physical characteristics, may be seen in the language employed by senior administrative and medical staff to describe patients. The physician's notes reflect a highly stylised form of representation which resonates elsewhere, and which suggests a significant development in the power differential between physician and patient.

The stereotypical view of the asylum, as a weapon of social control used by authoritarian individuals, did undoubtedly exist in the nineteenth century. For vulnerable individuals the threat of confinement was a potent one, and the asylum records include many instances of admission of patients who were clearly not insane. Social factors including pressure of resources, or quarrels over inheritance, could be resolved through the convenient expedient of committal. A public consciousness of this use of the asylum as a place of incarceration is indicated by a poem, published in the *Western Star and Ballinasloe Advertiser*, in 1846:

> Feel I not wrath with those who sent me here?
> Who have debased me in the minds of men,
> Debarring me the usage of my own;
> Blighting my life in best of its career,
> Branding my thoughts as things to shun and fear?[34]

Clearly the asylum physician played a key role in determining the extent of a patient's illness, and ultimately decreed whether an individual was sane or otherwise, and when they ought to be released. He exercised tremendous power in an obvious sense, and although subject to inspection and advice from others such as the asylum inspector and the keepers and nurses, was at the head of an autocracy as far as patient care was concerned. The increasing professionalisation of medicine, and the extension of an indisputable scientific discourse into Irish lunatic asylums at the end of the century, made the physician's position sacrosanct. In the case notes from Ballinasloe one can see an increasing emphasis upon the positivistic – a good deal more attention was being paid to the physical condition of the patients, which was capable of being described within an evolving medical discourse. However, the physician was still heavily dependent upon his own interpretation of patient symptoms, and this, along with his informal knowledge of their family circumstances, determined to a great extent the length of a patient's stay within the asylum.

Diagnosis of sanity and insanity in the late nineteenth century was a highly subjective and speculative affair, even for those who spent their working lives in institutions such as the Ballinasloe Asylum. Broad classifications of disease and behaviour were available, and each patient was categorised as suffering from something, usually mania or monomania. However, beyond these vague categories, there was a distinct lack of a sophisticated vocabulary with which to embrace and delineate degrees of madness. In an increasingly scientific environment, as far as general medicine was concerned, psychiatry was at something of a stand-still. Invasive surgery was not available, and drugs were employed for sedation rather than therapy. Thus as far as the insane were concerned, there was a limit to what science could offer. It is at this point that the physician at Ballinasloe began to place an increasing emphasis upon apparently physical manifestations of mental disease, which might be amenable to treatment. Indeed, it becomes clear from the case notes at the end of the nineteenth century that the Ballinasloe physician believed that insanity literally inscribed itself upon the body of the sufferer, and that the face and head, in particular, could be read as a text of abnormality, or excess, or mania.

This development needs to be viewed in a broader political context. Since the 1860s, a body of literature had been published regarding the characteristics of differing races, which drew heavily upon established theories in science and anthropology. By the 1890s, with the culmination of high imperialism, several texts had been published which suggested that superior and inferior races could be distinguished by physical appearance – colour of skin and hair, stature, physiognomy – and judgments concerning intelligence and fitness for self-rule were made on that basis. In the 1860s it had been proposed that a team of physicians and anthropologists be sent around the country to categorise, and ultimately, comprehend Irish society. Initiated by Francis Galton and others,[35] and based upon studies conducted at Eton and Cambridge, these anthropomorphic laboratories would, it was believed, reveal the truth about the Irish. Following on from these forays, there were a significant number of texts published from the 1880s onwards which sought to prove that the Irish were in fact racially linked to the Negro, and on that basis, were unfit for self-government. The anonymously published 'What Science is saying about Ireland' of 1882, H.S. Constable's racial musings on the Irish,[36] and the anthropological theories of figures such as John Beddoe and others,[37] did much to establish Ireland as a racially and, more importantly, politically backward realm. Thus, the argument ran, although the Irish were white, their inherent incapacities could be distinguished by other physical signs.

Using the same sorts of categories and descriptions, what the physician at Ballinasloe was undertaking was an attempt to characterise lunatics physically, who might otherwise be unrecognisable, and pass for sane. Drawing upon mid-nineteenth century phrenological beliefs that 'the face was an outward sign of the inner soul…[and]…the bony head an outward reflection of the structure of the different organs of the brain'[38], the physician described some patients thus:[39]

> His skull is peculiarly formed; very narrow and low in front and capacious in depth and breadth at the back. His eyes are set wide apart. There is very little expression in his face except that of strong animal passion.[40]
>
> Has a stooping gait and very large feet.[41]
>
> Patient has a heavy sullen expression but talks in a quick suspicious way.[42]
>
> Has coarse heavy features; quiet dull voice.[43]
>
> Has a stolid stupid expression evidently indifferent to all his surroundings.[44]
>
> Has a heavy sensual face.[45]
>
> Has a heavy sullen expression and talks in a quick suspicious way; hair grows very low on forehead which is narrow and receding.[46]
>
> Has a quiet downcast sullen face and restless staring eyes.[47]
>
> He has a receding forehead, an apathetic stare and very ill shapen ears.[48]
>
> Has a typical epileptic gait and dull heavy immobile face.[49]

Clearly, in the absence of scientific classifications the physician was suggesting that mental illness could be read in the face of the sufferer, just as a visible physical illness could. However, it should be noted that none of the above patients were recorded as suffering from mental handicap, such as idiocy, imbecility or mental defectiveness, which, it was believed, might produce a particular physical type, but rather psychiatric disturbances only. The language employed simply linked patients with a series of racially specific terms which had a currency, and a level of popular scientific respectability, in this period. Moreover, the terms used hold particularly negative connotations. The body was coarse and ungainly; its features seemed either enlarged, or disproportionate to the rest of the torso. Dull, stupid and heavy, the Irish patient appeared to represent all that was intransigent or threatening about mental illness, but also about Irish social and political life. The language used echoes that employed by physiognomists such as Wentworth Webster, who described the Irish as having 'a lower facial angle, and a tendency to prognathism', in contrast to the Saxon.[50] Similarly John Beddoe made a connection between facial expression and character, such as that indicated by the physician, when he described the Irish as being of low intelligence, cunning and suspicious, and Ireland as the centre of the 'prognathous type'.[51]

The late Victorian belief in the expression of mental disturbance through the physical body had many literary parallels. Texts such as R.L. Stevenson's *Dr Jekyll and Mr. Hyde*, and even Oscar Wilde's *The Picture of Dorian Grey*, associated the corruption of the body with increasing mental instability. These literary texts were obviously concerned with a good deal more than medical and psychiatric opinion – such as the duality of man and the sexual hypocrisy of the late Victorian era – but the implications of such texts would have had a resonance for educated British society more generally. All this is not to say however that the Ballinasloe physician was consciously stereotyping patients in a wilfully negative manner. Rather his use of an established scientific, anthropological and racial discourse indicates his anxiety to emphasise the professional classification of the insane within the asylum. The concern to categorise and identify strengthens the psychiatric claim that insanity could be recognised by the trained eye, but it was also employed as a reassurance that the apparently hidden nature of lunacy was not sustainable.

The physician at Ballinasloe also devoted some considerable time to the treatment of physical illness, and not merely the routine care of those patients who fell ill after admission. He conducted operations to remove growths and rectify hare-lips, and treated surgically patients who had years-old injuries. In this way, the patients at the Ballinasloe Asylum allowed him to exercise his medical skills and authority, for the body, if not for the mind. More importantly, however, the physician made a direct link between a 'normal' physical appearance, and a restoration to mental normality. It was not merely the case that a calm visage and placid expression denoted a return to sanity, for the reverse very often accompanied insanity. Rather, a successful operation to rectify a physical abnormality was linked to a belief that the patient had been similarly transformed mentally. In March 1893 a patient was admitted for assaulting his wife. Three months later he was operated upon to remove a growth on his lip, which required extensive surgery and a lengthy period of nursing. He was discharged as soon as he had healed, and the case notes make little reference to his mental state, other than to indicate 'improved'. It would appear that the success of the operation overshadowed other considerations, however, as he was subsequently readmitted for again assaulting his wife.

Relatives and others

All power within the asylum, such as it was, did not necessarily lie with the physician alone. The classificatory impulse, and the association between physical and mental states, was not necessarily internalised or adopted unquestioningly by the patient population. They could temper the administration of the hospital, not merely in regulating its process through non-co-operation or obstruction, but through an active use of its provisions for their own benefit. If patients were not physically dangerous, they could enjoy a certain freedom of behaviour and privileges. One man, for instance, was permitted to remain in women's clothes for a period of years, and was commented upon in bemused tones by the asylum inspectors in their annual reports. Ironically, this patient was allowed the freedom to indulge his desire to dress as a woman inside the asylum, in a way which was far less likely outside it.

Relatives, however, were clearly in the strongest position, as far as gaining some advantage from the asylum system was concerned.[52] In the first instance, they had recourse to law to have their relatives admitted, and the institutional authorities had no power to refuse cases, under the Dangerous Lunatics Act, if violent behaviour was alleged. However, it was not always for economic gain that relatives abused the asylum system. In some cases people admitted family members in exasperation at their conduct, knowing they were not insane. In January 1893, a patient was admitted with no discernible symptoms of insanity, but whose relatives had clearly reached the end of their collective tether. The principal source of conflict, according to the case notes, was the patient's refusal to work. He had been evicted from his holding because of non-payment of rent, in accordance with Land League protests against unfair rents, and was in receipt of an allowance from the organisation up until his admission. Because of this allowance, he refused to do any work for his family. They alleged he 'spends all the day moping through the woods and comes home at night fall when he goes to bed'. The physician found him to be 'an affable little man without much originality and an easily provoked complacent smile'. After some months observation, it was concluded that there were no symptoms of insanity. In fact, the 'treatment' – admission to the asylum – appeared to have worked to the family's satisfaction. It was noted some five months after his admission that 'He is slightly weak-minded and rather sorry not to have worked when at home and anxious to get back to the chance again.' He was discharged cured in March 1894.

However, when the physician's advice to family and friends was disregarded, and he was proved right, he found it difficult to resist the temptation to record his 'victories' in the case notes. A man who had been admitted as suicidal, and who remained depressed when in the asylum, was removed by friends who felt he would recover more quickly at home. The physician strongly advised them to leave him at Ballinasloe, but they insisted on taking him out. However, the professional slight was more than compensated for by the instant display of instability on the patient's behalf:

> Friends had him at the gate on bail about one month since when he expressed his delight at the opportunity his freedom would give him of burning himself, hanging himself, drowning himself, cutting his throat and doing various other felonial acts some of which included his wife and relations as participating victims. They immediately brought him back. He remains in much the same condition.

The Ballinasloe Asylum might seem at a glance an institution on the periphery of Irish life. Located in the economically disadvantaged west, catering for the pauper population, and geographically remote from the seat of power at Dublin: all this would seem to suggest that the institution was distanced from contemporary social and political developments. However this was far from being the case. Asylum administration responded swiftly to alterations in power structures outside the institution, and, in the case for example of Catholic advances within the walls, rapidly closed ranks. The decision to forbid the establishment of a church was taken more as a result of contemporary sectarian developments in Irish society than on the religious rights of the majority of the patients. Similarly, the adoption of a particular descriptive terminology by the Ballinasloe physician to categorise patients emphasises both the existence of an intellectual community, and the anxiety to present the custody and treatment of lunatics as a scientific undertaking. Finally, the responses of both patients and relatives, and indeed of the officials of other institutions such as workhouses and gaols, indicate that the asylum was not necessarily viewed as a simple vehicle for the incarceration of the insane, but as a resource, to be used for reasons other than the strictly medical. In these ways, the Ballinasloe Asylum was characterised not by a distance from personal and political influences, but on the contrary a responsiveness, which shaped and moderated life within the walls.

NOTES

1 Known from the 1850s simply as the Ballinasloe Asylum.
2 This section of the chapter will concentrate on the male experience of admission and classification. For a comparative discussion of male and female experience during the famine years, see Oonagh Walsh, ' "A lightness of mind": gender and insanity in nineteenth-century Ireland', in M. Kelleher and J. Murphy, eds, *Gender Perspective in Nineteenth-Century Ireland: Public and Private Spheres*, Dublin, Irish Academic Press, 1997.
3 Oliver MacDonagh, 'Ideas and institutions, 1830–45', in W.E. Vaughan, ed., *A New History of Ireland V: Ireland Under the Union I, 1801–70*, Oxford, Clarendon Press, 1989, p. 206.
4 Report of commissioners for enquiry into the conditions of the poor classes in Ireland PP 1836, vol. xliii, xxx.
5 The association of pauperism with lunacy, and the attendant focus on the first part of the equation, could have a detrimental effect on lunatic care, as both Jonathan Andrews and Lorraine Walsh point out in this volume in relation to Scotland.
6 At Ballinasloe the Board was all-male until well into the twentieth century.
7 J. Robins, *Fools and Mad: A History of the Insane in Ireland*, Dublin, Institute of Public Administration, 1986, p. 88.
8 I Vic., Cap. xxvii, 1838.
9 M. Finnane, *Insanity and the Insane in Post-Famine Ireland*, London, Croom Helm, 1981, p. 94.
10 *Seventeenth Report on the District, Criminal, and Private Lunatic Asylums in Ireland*, PP Vol. XXV, 1868, p. 11.
11 Ibid.
12 *Nineteenth Report on the District, Criminal, and Private Lunatic Asylums in Ireland*, PP Vol. XXXIV, 1870, p. 17.
13 Finnane, *Insanity and the Insane*, p. 18.
14 Census of Ireland, 1871, *Vital Statistics*, pp. 84–5 HC (1873) lxxii, pt. 2.
15 The asylum system continued to expand into the twentieth century. By 1904, there were beds for 16,537 patients in Ireland. Finnane, *Insanity and the Insane*, p. 227.
16 R.F. Foster, *Modern Ireland 1600–1972*, Allen Lane, 1988, pp. 606 and 611.

17 *Twenty-second Report on the District, Criminal, and Private Lunatic Asylums in Ireland*, PP Vol. XXX, 1873, p. 6. It was also felt that 'with the process of enlarged accommodation, cases which were before unrecognised come to the surface from year to year, and obtain admission', p. 5.
18 Additional mid-century building accommodated this increase in numbers, after years of overcrowding.
19 Sligo Asylum was built in 1855, and took responsibility for patients from the counties of Sligo and Leitrim. Castlebar Asylum took Co. Mayo patients from 1866. Both of these institutions admitted existing patients from Ballinasloe on their opening, as well as new county admissions.
20 There was a Catholic church opposite the asylum, and another ten minutes' walk away in town.
21 Maria Luddy, *Women and Philanthropy in Nineteenth-Century Ireland*, Cambridge, Cambridge University Press, 1995, p. 23.
22 Board of Guardians Minute Book, Connaught District Lunatic Asylum, 21 September 1851.
23 The Catholic Church was in fact prepared to fund the church construction themselves, but the freedom of action which this might imply with regard to work within the asylum merely strengthened the board's opposition.
24 W.A.F. Browne, *What Asylums Were, Are and Ought to Be* (first published 1837), in A. Scull, ed., *The Asylum as Utopia: W.A.F. Browne and the Mid-Nineteenth Century Consolidation of Psychiatry*, London, Routledge, 1991, p. 213.
25 Ibid.
26 Rev. James Hall, A.M., *Tour Through Ireland*, 2 vols, London, R.P. Moore, 1813.
27 Ibid, p. 178.
28 Episcopalians, Presbyterians and Methodists combined.
29 *General Report of the 1891 Census*, p. 447.
30 Register of Admissions to the Ballinasloe District Asylum, 1890–1899.
31 Not the asylum minister.
32 Physician's Case Book: Male Case Book, no. 2, case no. 3282.
33 Quoted in Luddy, *Women and Philanthropy*, pp. 28–9.
34 'The reputed lunatic', in *The Western Star and Ballinasloe Advertiser*, 10 January 1846.
35 Francis Galton, F.R.S., *Memories of My Life*, London, Methuen and Co., 1908, p. 244.
36 H.S. Constable, *Ireland: From One or Two Neglected Points of View*, London, Liberty, n.d.
37 John Beddoe, *The Races of Britain*, London, 1885; James Bonwick, *Who Are The Irish?*, London, 1880 and John Mackinnon Robertson, *The Saxon and the Celt: A Study in Sociology*, London, 1897.
38 Nancy Stepan, *The Idea of Race in Science: Great Britain 1800–1960*, London, Macmillan, 1982, p. 21.
39 All of these admissions took place in just one year, indicating how important physical characterisation had become. The physician was, in other words, not merely noting especially unusual physical types.
40 Physician's Case Book: Male Case Book, no. 2, case no. 3,528, p. 35.
41 Ibid., case no. 3,376, p. 67.
42 Ibid., case no. 3,281, p. 9.
43 Ibid., case no. 3,307, p. 25.
44 Ibid., case no. 3,321, p. 31.

45 Ibid., case no. 3,327, p. 34.
46 Ibid., case no. 3,328, p. 35.
47 Ibid., case no. 3,333, p. 38.
48 Ibid., case no. 3,338, p. 42.
49 Ibid., case no. 3,343, p. 47.
50 Quoted in L. Perry Curtis, *Apes and Angels: the Irishman in Victorian Caricature*, Bristol, David and Charles, 1971, p. 19.
51 Beddoe, *The Races of Britain*, pp. 10–11.
52 For a fuller discussion of this issue, see Oonagh Walsh, 'Asylums, gaols and workhouses: lunatic and criminal alliances in nineteenth century Ireland', in P. Bartlett and D. Wright, eds, *Outside the Walls of the Asylum: Historical Perspectives on 'Care in the Community' in Modern Britain and Ireland*, London, Athlone Press, forthcoming.

Part IV

THE COLONIAL VISION

12

OUT OF SIGHT AND OUT OF MIND

Insanity in early-nineteenth-century British India

Waltraud Ernst

As the chapters by Len Smith, Peter Bartlett and others in this volume indicate, asylum provision in Britain during the early decades of the nineteenth century was still restricted in terms of the size and number of institutions for the confinement of the mentally ill. Scholars such as Andrew Scull and Roy Porter have shown that the total number of asylum inmates was low and the consolidation of psychiatry as a specialised medical discipline had not yet occurred. Yet insanity and attempts to control and cure it by means of management techniques and science-based medicine appeared to capture the interest and imagination of medical professionals and the wider public alike. Insanity was widely characterised, in the contemporary mode of expression, as the 'most grievous malady to which the human family is subject'. It was even seen to stride 'like a Colossus in the country',[1] so that 'the asylum took on for a time a status as panacea equivalent to the steam engine, the rights of man, or the spread of universal knowledge'.[2]

A similar process was at work in India, where the East India Company had established itself not only as a dominating trading concern but also as the representative of British colonial power. The Anglo-Indian[3] community in the various provinces under British rule did not escape the allure of the asylum as a marker of Western progress and civilisation. In British India, too, the institution-based management of insanity had a significant public profile. Moreover, the British in India were keen to prove that their organisation of social and political life in the East compared favourably with the way in which things were done 'at home'. Surgeon J. MacPherson was one who pressed for this when he pushed for an expansion of asylum provision in the 1850s: 'we have our jails, our schools, and our dispensaries in almost every Zillah [district], and why should we not have our asylums too?'[4]

Lunatic asylums were designed on a practical level to protect the Anglo-Indian public – the mad were securely locked up, and 'violent maniacs' as well as irritating 'idiots' were thus kept at bay. More importantly, however, within a colonial context where the 'rights of man' were British and where the spread of specifically British (rather than merely Western, let alone universal) knowledge and civilisation were believed to be at stake, asylums assumed a more complex role. The main concern was not so much with the merely practical and instrumental aspects of psychiatric institutions. Like other public institutions established by the East India Company they became symbolic markers of British superiority.[5]

Lunatic asylums, alongside manufactories, schools, dispensaries, hospitals, court rooms, and gaols were not only necessary parts of the administrative fabric of the colonial state, but they were also showpieces and justifications of British colonialism at work in India – bricks-and-mortar manifestations of patriotic pride and self-satisfaction: symbols of the assumed benefits of an allegedly superior and rational, enlightened civilisation. This idea of the civilising mission had been expressed succinctly by such influential Company officials as Charles Grant, who had aimed at opening India not only for commercial enterprise but also for the spread of 'our light and knowledge'.[6] His argument appealed to many members of the Anglo-Indian community for generations to come.[7]

The progressively emerging consensus among the British on the assumed superiority of Western civilisation did, of course, not go completely unchallenged. The prolonged debates following the resolution of 1835 that 'the great objects of the British government ought to be the promotion of European literature and science' are but one indication of the multiplicity of prevailing colonial discourses. In the area of lunacy provision, too, variety existed in the different areas under Company rule both in terms of the policy and practical arrangements, and in regard to the therapeutic and institutional approaches taken.[8] However, notwithstanding diverse administrative set-ups and therapeutic diversity, there still prevailed consensus on some central issues.

The governors of the various provinces under British rule – both those who were utilitarian-inclined and those favouring a liberal, laissez-faire or autocratic approach to administration – were in principle united by a trust in the practical, therapeutic and symbolic value of psychiatric institutions for both the European and the Indian insane.[9] What is more, the first half of the nineteenth century in particular saw the extension of the administrative apparatus and of civil institutions concomitant on the rapid expansion of Indian territory under British rule. As indicated below, there was a steady increase in the number of lunatic asylums and of asylum inmates during this period and this was fuelled as much by the expansionist tendencies of the British 'garrison state'[10] as by any tendency in Britain itself to consolidate and regulate the public asylum system. The sort of changes that occurred are best illustrated by the contrasts between the early days of Company rule and the middle of the nineteenth century.

Institutional provisions in colonial India

Haphazard provision for European as well as Indian lunatics was made by the British in Bombay (today Mumbai), Madras (today Chennai) and Calcutta as early as 1670, 1787 and 1793 respectively. These facilities were small scale, and they were run, as was then common in Britain, as private enterprises, typically attached to doctors' private practices. The number of inmates consequently amounted to as few as five to fifteen. By the 1850s, however, each of the three asylums in the major provincial capitals confined as many as 100 to 150 patients – mainly of European and Indo-British extraction. In addition asylums in major district towns were reserved for the exclusive reception of 'Native Lunatics' – mainly of Indian and lower-class Indo-British background.[11] In Bengal and the North-Western Provinces alone in the mid-1850s between 52 and 189 patients were admitted to each of the seven 'Native Lunatic Asylums', bringing the total of Indian patients in that area to a little over one thousand.[12] Further institutions for the mentally ill had been established in more recently annexed areas, such as Burma, the Punjab and Sindh, as well as in the coastal centre of Sri Lanka, and in Penang and Singapur. In addition to these specialised receptacles, lunatics in inaccessible and desolate areas 'up-country' would be locked up for shorter periods in the more ubiquitous local gaols and in cells adjoining dispensaries and regimental hospitals.

The Company's provision for European lunatics in fact extended back into the colonial motherland itself. In England, Pembroke House, a privately managed madhouse, specialised in the treatment of insane Europeans sent home from India by the East India Company.[13] Distinguished places such as Ticehurst Asylum[14] also received officers and gentlemen or ladies said to be insane whose fortunes allowed for confinement in style. Haslar and Great Yarmouth Hospitals as well as Chatham Asylum[15] made provision for former Royal Army servants who were not eligible for maintenance in Pembroke House at the East India Company's expense. At the bottom of the social scale guardians of the poor in sea ports where East Indiamen put ashore reluctantly made provision in public asylums or workhouses for pauper lunatics found wandering at large subsequent to their arrival from India, or following an eventual relapse after temporary spontaneous recovery on board ship.

Such a network of lunatic asylums expanding from Britain all over British India and back again thus seems to have realised early-nineteenth-century asylum reformers' dreams and the ambitions of utilitarianism and Britain's civilising mission. It also neatly conforms with Foucauldian assumptions about the gradual, all-pervasive spread of Western reason. Both in terms of the number and scope of institutions for Europeans and Indians, as well as in terms of the absolute number of patients admitted during the period from about 1800 to 1858, the impression of increased consolidation and of a progressively expanding, well-coordinated 'system' of asylum provision appears to emerge. When the British Crown took over the political administration of British India in 1858, it was to inherit the Company's impressive legacy of gaols, penitentiaries, hospitals, lunatic asylums and dispensaries, as well as some orphanages, workhouses and schools. The network of mid-Victorian institutionalism, it would appear, closed in on mad Europeans and colonial subjects in the East alike – from Lahore to Colombo and from Madras to the Straits and back to London.

However, what appears like a tight network on the map of British colonialism, does not bear too close scrutiny for a variety of reasons. If the huge geographical area and the overall number of both Europeans and Indians resident in the 'pink' areas under British rule are considered, this new network was by no means as pervasive as its counterparts in Britain or in France in particular. The European lunatic asylum in Calcutta, for example, contained, even in the late 1850s, only around 100 Europeans, while the asylums in Bombay and Madras provided on average for not more than ten to fifteen Europeans each.[16] This is out of an estimated Anglo-Indian military population of some 40,000 before the 'Mutiny' of 1857–8, and a combined European civil and military population in 1861 of 125,945 (of whom 84,083 belonged to the military service).[17]

The small number of European patients is of course partly a result of the Company's policy of repatriating the European insane at least once a year. However, Pembroke House, the major institution for the confinement of 'Indian Insanes' – as one medical records keeper in London evocatively named returned mental patients of European parentage – did not see an extraordinary number of patients pass through its premises either.[18] From its opening in 1818 until 1858 about 500 lunatics with previous Indian experience had been on this institution's books. Even if one allowed for roughly as many patients again ending up (rightly or wrongly) in one of Britain's military, pauper or private asylums, and for deaths during the then arduous and lengthy sea journey round the Cape of Good Hope, the total number of Europeans certified 'mad' and confined in a mental institution of one kind or another on arrival from India was probably not much more than a thousand. It has of course to be conceded that the number of *European* lunatics would play only a minor part in any account located within a colonial setting. However, in regard to *Indian* asylum inmates, too, a similar tendency is evident. Although the absolute numbers of Indians involved sound more substantial, they were by no means high in proportion to overall population figures.[19] Even if it is taken into account that further provision for lunatics was made in gaols of smaller stations, it is still only a 'small proportion' of Indians said to be insane who were institutionalised by the British .[20]

How can we explain the apparent gap between the rhetoric of the asylum as a panacea on the one hand and the actual developments on the ground on the other? To a certain extent the development of British institutional psychiatry in India mirrors the way in which a fledgling psychiatry struggled to come of age in Britain itself. Very much in contrast to the situation in post-revolution France, lunacy provision on the British Isles was in the early nineteenth century characterised by diversity rather than uniformity, by a variety of practices rather than one orthodox psychiatric approach, by various different institutions rather than a coherent 'system' of psychiatric provision, and by relatively small numbers despite proclamations to the contrary. Furthermore, these characteristics were not confined to lunacy provision. Other measures in the area of health and social welfare provision (most well-researched in regard to Poor Law provision) were not characterised by large numbers of institutionalised people, uniformity and centralisation of services either.[21] Last, but not least, in Britain the gap between reformers' rhetorical proclamations and actual practice indicates, in Foucauldian terms, the point that discourses of power do not always reflect actual social practice, but create and define a society's perception of reality.

Verbal overstatement was then characteristic of colonial and British social policies in general. For example, James Mill, an influential member of the Company's executive government in England, did not hesitate, in the words of Stokes, to point proudly 'to the kingdom that had been delivered into his hands', when he asserted that he was 'the only man whose business it is' to deal with 'the internal government of 60 millions of people'.[22] Similarly, Wilberforce, drawing on Grant, pointed not only to the 'vast superiority even of European laws and institutions, and far more of British institutions, over those of Asia', but appealed to the British government to 'endeavour to strike our roots into the soil by the gradual introduction and establishment of our own principles and opinions; of our laws, institutions, and manners'.[23]

Such statements could of course be brushed aside as overblown rhetoric, were it not for the fact that they had a vital impact on the way in which policy matters were, and continue to be, judged. In regard to British psychiatry, for example, the contemporary rhetoric of the lunatic asylum as a showpiece of colonial humanitarianism and scientific progress in India may well sound overblown set against the relatively small number and scale of the institutions actually established. Yet it is exactly this overstatement, and the disproportionate claims made for psychiatry that helped to foster the self-image of the British as a race of humanitarian and rational rulers, whose scientific achievements endorsed claims for the benevolence and legitimacy of colonial rule. The rhetorical and ideological pillars of colonialism were essential to the preservation of its image and authority and are vital for an understanding of its character. It is in this context that the discourses of an emergent psychiatry possess an importance that goes far beyond their more limited practical role in treating or controlling a few deranged individuals.

Psychiatric practice and Indian experience

Within the wider context of colonial rule Mill's and Wilberforce's evocation of the assumed spiritual consensus underlying colonial power has been as enduring as statements about the experimental nature of colonial administration.[24] India still keeps being characterised as having been 'a kind of laboratory for experiments in administration' if not medicine.[25] There is of course some truth in such statements. A variety of different approaches towards administration flourished in the presidencies and districts of the fledgling colony. But this was also true for Britain's various counties, districts and Unions. However, it would be equally wrong to assume that colonial policies and administrative experiments merely mirrored ideas and institutions in the British Isles. This would imply that the colonial discourse was enforced in diverse, yet pre-determined ways, bound to succeed in subjugating local conditions and indigenous responses. More recent historical writing has challenged such premises as constituting part of the enduring myth of empire,[26] and more attention has been given to Foucault's hitherto less emphasised, yet very crucial, contention that where there is power, there is resistance.

In the case of psychiatry the British vanguard ideologies and practices of moral management and asylum science were indeed transplanted to the East. Yet they were trimmed to fit better the very different conditions in diverse colonial locations. It is important to be aware of the prevailing limits which confronted an, allegedly superior, British institution-based psychiatry within the context of Company rule in India. In regard to lunatic asylums for Europeans, some of these limitations were intricately bound up with the idiosyncrasies of Anglo-Indian social life and the politics of colonial rule: first, the prevailing ideology of the assumed prestige of the ruling elite, and second, dominant public and medical perceptions of the Indian environment as hostile and pathological.

The preservation of the rulers' prestige had by 1800 become a local government concern and a crucial factor in the way in which affairs of daily life had to be seen to be conducted.[27] The behaviour of the steadily increasing number of lower-class Europeans such as soldiers, sailors and minor clerks, and, in particular, the presence of down-and-outs, deserters, vagabonds, prostitutes and drunkards worried the British colonial elite. Such worries were of course common in Britain, too. There they were responded to by the emerging ideology surrounding the discussion of the New Poor Law which was designed 'not so much...to help the unfortunate as to stigmatise the self-confessed failures of society'.[28] Within the colonial context European vagrancy, destitution and lunacy were seen to bring 'the ruling race into contempt in Indian eyes' and 'the reaction was to make them invisible' by means of institutionalisation or deportation.[29]

For example, when sailors jumped ship or soldiers deserted from military stations and started roaming the country, they invariably drew the uneasy attention of civil authorities and political agents. Although it was asserted that 'pecuniary aid is easily given in these cases', the main problem was rather that of 'lowering the European Character in the eyes of the Natives'.[30] The measures resorted to were punishment and incarceration in India, followed by deportation back to England. Whilst all Europeans were equally subjected to English constitutional principles, special legal provision was made to restrict the influx to India of poor Europeans, and to punish and deport undesirable down-and-outs who were, in Grant's words, thought to 'vex, harass and perplex the weak natives' thereby harming the prestige in which the British liked to believe they were held by Indians.[31] Presidential governments agreed that it was imperative to prevent destitute sailors, vagrants, deserters, lunatics, and such like from becoming a 'threat and nuisance' on every street corner of the trim European parts of their towns.[32]

Time-expired soldiers as well as civilians such as European women of 'bad character', vagabonds and lunatics, were provided with passages back to Europe, where they would be left to their own fate or, in the case of those said to be insane, received into 'Pembroke House'. Deportation was costly, but less so than prolonged confinement in India. Furthermore, it also guaranteed that unwanted and unproductive elements of colonial society, including those 'out of mind', would be permanently 'out of sight'. The early-nineteenth-century practice of repatriating the mentally ill certainly owed much to the Company's protectionist immigration policy and to a general distaste among the ruling elite for lower-class people.[33] It was however also the velvet glove of measures for the control and relief of Europeans in India. Unlike European mendicants and vagrants, the mentally ill were not punished for their state. On the contrary, lunatics had to be treated with 'great care and attention', whilst institutions for the poor aimed at providing undesirable conditions for their inmates.[34]

The less censorious attitude towards insanity was to a large extent the result of the fact that madness, unlike destitution, crossed barriers of social class. It was true that great (and little) fortunes could be as easily lost as gained in the East. But rarely would a gentleman fall victim to destitution and end up in the city's gutters. Madness in contrast could reduce any bright officer's or government servant's intelligent conversation to incoherent babble. Ever since the opening of lunatic asylums in India they had been occupied by inmates of all social classes. As a consequence, the authorities did not measure lunacy against the same yardstick of culpability as destitution and mendicancy. The presence of higher-class patients in the provincial asylums therefore ensured to a great extent that the European asylum sector (despite its auxiliary role within colonial society of ensuring peace and prestige) would not yet be intrinsically linked with the policy towards European pauperism.

Medical considerations as to the healing power of repatriation were at work, too. That these were part of a wider debate about the nature of colonial power is signalled, for example, by the title of an article of 1843 by assistant surgeon A.S. Thomson: 'Could the Natives of a temperate climate colonise and increase in a tropical country and vice versa?'.[35] The question of whether European settlers should be allowed to set up home in British India had of course been controversial also during earlier decades.[36] However, by the 1840s the central concern was whether European settlers could 'live and produce pure offspring in India'. It was feared that they were 'likely to become degenerate' within a few generations – 'from the climate and connexion with low ignorant women'.[37]

The evidence close at hand was open to diverse interpretation though. People of Dutch and Portuguese descent, for example, were considered 'both mentally and physically degenerate'. Their case was taken as a good illustration of 'the injurious effect of climate on the descendants of Europeans in India', although it was conceded that 'their constitutions are rendered more adapted to the climate by a union with the aboriginal inhabitants'.[38] Such inconclusive evidence was however easily reinterpreted in the light of Anglo-Indian experience. Company servants suffered frequent bouts of debilitating illnesses and their children did not seem to thrive easily in India. 'There is little doubt', concluded assistant surgeon Thomson, 'the tropical parts of the world are not suited by nature for the settlement of the natives of the temperate zone', and if the children of the British were not sent back to Europe, they would become 'stunted in growth and debilitated in mind'.[39]

The alternative theory of 'acclimatisation', which suggested that even the British could eventually habituate themselves to the alien Indian climate, was then prominent in Britain among doctors and those in favour of colonial expansion. Many Anglo-Indians, however, tended to agree with Thomson. The Indian climate was believed to be inhospitable and dangerous. It was seen to get on the nerves and skins of those reared under a less fiercely burning sun, in the gentle tepid drizzle of maritime conditions. The enduring 'solar myth' emerged, of the power of 'heat and dust' to set off a whole range of nagging and unhealthy ailments and impediments, from prickly heat to insubordination, from heat-stroke to adultery and manslaughter, depression and paralysis, nervous exhaustion and irritability.

It was not the Indian climate in any narrowly meteorological sense that upset Europeans. It was the whole range of social and cultural trappings peculiar to their life in the East. The Indian environment was seen to be host to uncivilised and barbaric (yet intriguing and fascinating) practices, and to have a dire, destabilising, if not pathological, effect on the unwary European. Perhaps one of the more poignant expressions of this is the insistence by most medical officers on European lunatics' early removal from India. 'The hills' of India were agreeably cool, relatively isolated from the madding Indian crowd and the hostile climate of the plains. Indeed, they reminded expatriates of the Isle of Wight and parts of Surrey. But they were no match for the green and pleasant lands of home. Medicos held that although 'it affords good ground...for a recommendation that [a patient] should not return to duty', it 'must be admitted, that in no instance, after an attack of insanity should a man be permitted to remain in circumstances and relations which are obviously so likely to lead to a relapse'.[40]

Early-nineteenth-century medical practitioners assigned a crucial role to the Indian environment. Yet the way in which India's 'alien sky' was conceived to impact on Westerners differed fundamentally from later conceptions. Where later generations would talk of an alien environment almost exclusively in terms of 'culture', 'customs' and 'beliefs', contemporaries would elaborate on the 'climate' (in particular on heat and cold, atmospheric pressure, marsh effluvia), on the quality of the water and on geographic features, alongside native customs and beliefs. Early-nineteenth-century medical thought had yet to transcend the Hippocratic corpus of airs, waters and places. The prevalence in far-away countries of environmental conditions so different from those of the British Isles did much to revive this classical body of thought. Further, the process of colonial penetration itself widened the scope for environmental theories by enabling Westerners to come into contact with peoples of hitherto scarcely known lands, and to speculate on how the various living habitats had formed their 'character', and might influence the well-being of European traders, soldiers and civil servants raised under more temperate conditions. Lockean ideas about society's ability to promote moral and social improvement by regulating material and environmental conditions reverberate here.

Apart from medical reasoning, the deportation policy fitted in well also with one of the contemporary images of the nature of British colonialism in India. The British control of its 'Indian possessions' was, despite some early warning remarks, considered to be a lasting engagement. This culminated during the heyday of the British Raj in an 'illusion of permanence'. At the same time there existed strong doubts as to the extent to which a place like India could ever become a permanent home to the British. The majority of Anglo-Indians considered themselves basically as transients who were in search of fortune or took up the highly lauded burden of the white man, but who would eventually, in health or sickness, sanity or madness, be shipped back to Britain. There was no better cure for an ailing and alien Company servant than 'home'. This view was cherished by Anglo-Indians, and shared by most medical practitioners in India. It became the hallmark and centre-piece of the treatment of those afflicted with insanity. British colonialism in India was conceptualised as a stable, long-lasting, if not permanent, structure, whilst its agents were to be engaged only on a temporary basis.

The colonial regime and life in the 'tropics'

The idea of the pathological effect of the Indian environment on Europeans' physical constitution and psychological well-being was characteristic of public as well as medical perceptions during the early nineteenth century. The factors which were frequently referred to in asylum reports as implicated in Europeans' mental derangement ranged from more specific ones such as 'fear to be caught by a tiger', 'drunkenness', 'hereditary' and 'fall' or 'sudden fright' to vaguer terms such as 'vice' or 'exposure to the sun, hard living and other irregularities'.[41] Some medical officers did however also signal empathy and understanding of their patients' problems and psychological pain. For example, W. Campbell, Superintendent of the Bombay Lunatic Asylum, and an ardent campaigner for improved institutional amenities, wrote in his report of 1853:

> The records of an asylum, if rightly read, are fitted to teach us many touching, and instructive lessons. They tell us of disappointed love, blighted hope, and crushed ambition, of exhausting labour, distracting care, and corroding sorrow, of time mis-spent, and precious opportunities lost, or mis-applied, of unbridled passion, unresisted temptation; weakness, folly, dissipation, and crime.[42]

Skimming through the usually very detailed case reports on individual lunatics it becomes clear what Campbell was hinting at, yet refused to explore and highlight further because, as he pointed out, 'it is not our province to deal' with the 'lessons they inculcate' or 'the moral they point'.[43]

Contemporary medical theories implicated the Indian environment in Europeans' physical and psychological ill-health. However, this presumed aetiology of madness in Europeans was not always reflected in a straightforward way in patients' reported experiences and circumstances prior to the onset of their mental affliction. In fact the case reports which were drawn up by regimental doctors and asylum superintendents in India often suggested that the main problem was not so much the Indian environment but rather British colonial society and individuals' attempts to succeed within it. The life circumstances of the majority of British people on duty in India were determined by the army and navy, and manifestations of insane behaviour were consequently conditioned by people's life within these military institutions. The events giving rise to mad behaviour were in the main strongly related to the demands of the hierarchical and strictly regimented structure of the 'garrison state' itself. Insane Europeans were thus frequently entangled in acts of insubordination and breaches of duty.

It may well be imagined that the Company's soldiers would have been well used to being hard done by and bullied, even prior to enlistment. The idea that the constraints of British military life could have affected the mental state of such people could then be questioned. Undoubtedly, differential recruitment patterns prevailed. Just like other immigrant groups, volunteers for overseas colonial duty, too, were not representative of Britain's overall population. Recruits for military duty in the East were, indeed, largely drawn from the impoverished strata of society. During the first half of the nineteenth century two-thirds of soldiers were Irish. It could be argued that people who volunteered for the Queen's or the Company's shilling, might have experienced life in the army more as a life-saving crutch, than as a cause for despair and breakdown. After all, asylums in Ireland during those decades of acute economic deprivation were important means of 'famine relief' for desperate families.[44] However, even if recruits' prime motivation was economic, and military service was a survival strategy, this did not necessarily preclude them from a sense of dissatisfaction or despair once they arrived in the East. Nor did it exempt them from going mad – for whatever reason.

Company servants, particularly those in subordinate positions, were confined to barracks or ships, excluded as far as possible from too close contact with Indians and their living environment. Civilians' life, too, was characterised by social hierarchy and aloofness from the Indian communities. As pointed out by Ballhatchet,[45] 'the British ensured a physical separation between the life of the official elite and that of the Indian people by planning civil stations adjoining but apart from Indian towns.…A similar seclusion was provided for the soldiers in cantonments, or permanent military camps.'

The enclaves of British military institutions and civil stations, isolated as far as practicable from the Indian environment surrounding them, arguably led to an intensification of those very structures of British military and social life which already put a high degree of pressure on people in the British environment at home. The construction of the Indian environment as 'pathological' had an inverse, catalytic effect on Europeans' mental health. Exclusion from those territories and cultural realms where danger, if not madness, was seen to loom paradoxically then meant that the oppressive aspects of British mores in general and British military life in particular were reinforced and exacerbated. If selected characteristics of British society were indeed reproduced in a more pronounced form in the hot-house atmosphere of colonial society, the famous myth emerging during the course of the nineteenth century of the 'white man's burden' would indeed encapsulate a crucial characteristic of Anglo-Indian life. Paradoxically, what the 'white man' had to bear was the burden of his own social culture which he carried along with him.

Both the myth of the 'white man's burden' and the conceptualisation of (some) non-Western environments as dangerous and pathological have been long enduring.[46] We may of course legitimately ask whether there was not some truth in them. After all, it was not only common lore but an established fact that mortality rates in British India were extraordinary high. For example, the Royal Commission which was set up to investigate the state of health of the army in India reported that the 'healthy army' in Great Britain in the 1850s had an annual mortality rate of 1.7 per cent, whilst the 'sickly army' in India lost 4.1 per cent of its soldiers and non-commissioned officers.[47] And these numbers already constituted an improvement compared to the death rate in 1817, which was 7 per cent (of which only 1 per cent was related to warfare). During the first half of the century, the annual rate of mortality amounted to 6.9 per cent, with most deaths being attributed to 'fevers', dysentery and diarrhoea, diseases of the liver and cholera.[48] The danger of an environment such as that of India then appears substantiated by these figures.

However, even at the time of the Royal Commission it was well understood that death was sensitive not only to the Indian environment. While soldiers and non-commissioned officers died at the rate of 6.9 per cent,[49] officers passed away at the rate of 3.8 and civil servants at 2 per cent.[50] These rates still compare unfavourably with those characteristic of the population at soldier's age in Britain (which fluctuated between 0.8 and 1.2 per cent). Yet, even the Royal Commission concluded that the higher death rates for the lower ranks of society must have been 'due to other causes than the climate of India; to which officers as well as men are everywhere exposed'.[51] While service and life in the colony could well be blamed for the raised mortality rates, it was, as pointed out by the Royal Commission, 'by the diseases not only of India, but of all unhealthy places'.[52] Yet the crucial issue was that 'unhealthy places' tended to be lived in by people of the lower classes, so that the factors which had such a selectively deadly impact on

Europeans were not simply due to the miasma, atmospheric conditions and cultural idiosyncrasies of the Indian environment.

India was pathologised as a disease and cultural environment that allegedly had adverse effects on Europeans' body and mind. At the same time evidence from the Royal Commission and from patients' records pointed at social inequities and the 'pathology' inherent in British social and colonial culture itself. The point here is not so much to highlight this paradox, but rather to show that seemingly mutually exclusive positions and perceptions could indeed complement each other, and even help to facilitate social and political stability within the fabric of Anglo-Indian colonial society. By refocusing attention on the 'enemy without' – on the alien Indian environment – rather than the injustices, inequities and tensions within, potentially politically controversial and socially divisive features seem to disappear from the Anglo-Indian and, in the last instance, British context whence they sprang. The pathologisation of India and the self-imposed mission of British colonialism to come to the rescue by improving the material and spiritual environment in the colony had an important role not only in legitimating alien rule, but also in preserving the power of the colonial elite over the 'other ranks' and the lower classes of its own kind. If the discourse of colonial power builds upon and articulates metropolitan social and political structures, an investigation of psychiatry in colonialism cannot but lead to an inquiry into British society itself and the disciplines which confirmed the structures of power within it.

Provisions for Indians

The Company established institutions also for its 'native subjects'. Some of the main features of European asylums were echoed in the 'Native Lunatic Asylum' sector, such as the tendency towards gradual institutional expansion during the course of the early nineteenth century and the prevailing gap between official rhetoric and actual practice within institutions. In 1802 the Court of Directors had decreed that asylums for insane Indians were to be established.[53] By 1820 lunatic asylums for the exclusive reception of Indians (and of the lowest stratum of the Indo-British community) existed in about a dozen of locations, containing from a few up to 170 people each.

It was on account of this expansion of Indian Lunatic Asylums in Bengal and Madras, that evaluations of India's asylum system such as those by England-based reformer Sir A. Halliday emerged. He considered it, in 1828, very much the equal of the more salubrious institutions in the British Isles, if 'not much further advanced'.[54]

However, his judgement neither reflected circumstances within the existing institutions during that period nor survived the test of time. By the 1850s the idea of large-scale asylums for the Indian insane was no longer judged practicable. It had in previous years been assumed that a few 'Native Lunatic Asylums' here and there would be sufficient. Soon it had come to be acknowledged that there existed geographical as well as financial restrictions to the extension and expansion of asylums for the Indian insane.

When, therefore, in 1853 the project of a new large-scale institution for the whole presidency of Bombay was mooted, it was remarked, not without some acid sarcasm, that it was unlikely that a place could possibly be found that would be 'central' enough in an area where transfer from remote districts to Bombay was almost as nonsensical as shifting lunatics all the way from London to St Petersburg.[55] This was quite apart from the immense financial implications anticipated during a period when patients' numbers were calculated to increase steadily on account of legal enactments that recommended the confinement not only of violent people but also of 'idiots' and 'imbeciles'.[56] Halliday's earlier commendation of the Company's ambition to provide refuge or retreat for 'mad' or 'idiotic' subjects, regardless of whether they were violent, fell prey to the necessities of cost-effective institutional management and considerations for the safety of the expatriate community alone or, as the governor of Bombay, Lord Falkland, put it: 'under the present financial embarrassment before we can attend to the dictates of humanity it becomes our duty to provide for the security of the people'.[57]

Despite the cuts imposed on institutional provision for Indian lunatics, the colonial rhetoric of the superiority of British asylum science and of the adequacy of institutional provision did not abate. On the contrary, the more asylum services were restricted or deteriorated, the more exuberant became the proclamations of some medical practitioners and government officials on the presumed adequacy of institutional provision.[58] In a similar vein, asylum reports and statistics, which had a major role in the revelation of the enormity of the social, institutional and financial consequences of Indian lunacy, became increasingly in themselves a major criterion for judging the efficiency and superiority of the British system of asylum provision.

Yet the extent to which these reports and statistics actually revealed existing practices within the institutions was limited. Most importantly, conditions inside the asylums were not at all solely determined by the influence of British asylum science and its superior practitioners. It was, of course, seen as vitally important that every institution ought to be headed by a European medical officer, and that 'Half-castes and other natives...be confined to subordinate offices'.[59] After all, as pointed out by the Superintendent of the Benares Asylum in 1821, the 'Medical charge of such a place is attended with a heavy responsibility...fine and noble Buildings may be erected and the best Regulations may be written in vain unless the Medical Officer fully and faithfully discharge his duty.'[60] Despite such declarations, the European asylum superintendent of establishments for Indians was usually more conspicuous by his absence than his presence. At the Rasapagla Asylum, for example, it was found in 1821 that the European medical officer in charge pursued various other activities, and was rarely present to supervise the management of the institution. The Medical Board 'doubted' whether 'unremitting attention' could be shown 'by the Medical Officer attached to the Native Lunatic Hospital, whose residence is at a great distance from the Asylum, and whose time is in part occupied by various other professional vocations of an equally important nature'.[61] Others were reported to have been corrupt, pursuing profits by curtailing patients' food provisions and forging accounts for hospital supplies.[62]

Yet a failing could also be made into a virtue. One superintendent pointed out that too close contact was, in fact, undesirable: 'while living absolutely in the midst of the patients, and being thus brought almost hourly into contact with them [the European superintendent's] authority and general efficiency become abridged and impaired, his intercourse with them being virtually rather that of a keeper than of a Supervisor'.[63] In fact, the day-to-day management of most 'Native Lunatic Asylums' appears to have been left entirely to the Indian doctor, usually a Sub-Assistant Surgeon. Despite voluminous routine reports, rules and regulations, it was rarely specified how these men related to inmates and what sort of treatment and care they imparted,[64] although complaints about their assumed ignorance and unreliability were legion.[65]

The 'native doctors' were practically in charge of segregation and discipline, provisions and medicines, and patients' daily routine as well as their general health. These subordinate officers segregated patients according to their caste and tribal background; they organised water-carriers of different religious denominations (for example Hindu and Muslim); and they decided on the details of food preparation which constituted matters of importance to the various groups among the inmates[66] (for example what sort of person was allowed to cook for particular groups of patients; what sort of cooking utensils were to be made available; who was permitted to do their own cooking; which fire locations were suitable for different groups etc.). Even mainstays of early-nineteenth-century Western asylum science such as 'mechanical restraint' and 'non-restraint' experienced considerable modification within 'Native Lunatic Asylums' where the subordinate officers were deemed to be the best judges of which group of patients needed to be subdued by staff of a particular social background or ought to be dealt with only by 'mechanical' means.

Indian patients may have lost their minds but they did not necessarily lose their sense of what was culturally and socially proper and appropriate simply on entering a British institution. European superintendents were, of course, aware of and even remarked with some cynicism on the fact that mentally deranged Indians, too, were subject to the 'prejudices of Cast[e], of which many seem perfectly sensible'.[67] Some also supported – yet did not themselves engage in – the application of non-Western modes of healing (such as acupuncture) and non-orthodox methods (such as mesmerism).[68] However, even those who spent at least a reasonable proportion of their time at the 'Native Lunatic Asylum' could not be expected to have shared the depth of cultural and social knowledge that enabled their Indian subordinates to enforce restraint, organise food and cooking provision, washing facilities, segregation, work routines and treatment.

Patients tended not always fully to appreciate rules and regulations laid down by British superintendents keen on promulgating in the colony the sort of psychiatric doctrines developed in Britain. Work and employment routines, in particular, met with eventual resistance by some groups of Indian patients. This became more apparent towards the middle of the century, perhaps not least because European superintendents' awareness of native responses to colonial administration was heightened around the time of the 'Mutiny' of 1857–8. In addition, financial considerations had by then led to the preferred admission of 'dangerous' lunatics rather than 'idiots'. The former were more likely to enjoy lucid intervals and thus were, just like European asylum inmates, potentially aware of their former social position, religious beliefs and customs. An asylum superintendent in Bengal reported that the introduction of 'voluntary manual labour' was 'a task less easy to accomplish at [Dhalanda] than it proved in the Lunatic Asylum at Pinang' where the patients, mainly 'Malays, Chinese, Klings, Burmese, Siamese, Cochin-Chinese and Hindostanees', all 'took kindlier to a variety of light work than has been found the case with the Bengallees'.[69]

Colonial rhetoric and its impressive bricks-and-mortar manifestations notwithstanding, institutional practices were still to a large extent determined by Indian staff, Indian healing practices, Indian customs and values. In some instances European superintendents did succeed in the imposition of unpopular work routines[70] – if only by introducing 'diversified' or considerably reduced dietary regimes for those who were 'idle, unwilling or unable' to work, and by using food as 'an easy and unobjectionable means by which to enforce Discipline amongst the patients...and to encourage exertion, and to discourage idleness or malingering in Hospital'.[71] They would however equally frequently be faced with eventual objection and resistance to work schedules by inmates themselves. As one superintendent put it: 'Employment would be most desirable, but besides their mental unfitness there are the prejudices of Cast[e].'[72]

Predictably, the limits to British enlightened asylum management were only hinted at in official reports. Asylum superintendents and provincial medical boards alike focused instead on statistical data, on the various rules and regulations, and on procedures put in place to disseminate these. Devoid of real, practical control, superintendents concentrated, so it seems, on the paraphernalia and the spectacle of control measures: on detailed regulations for different staff members, on regular roll-calls, on rituals which highlighted the hierarchy among staff members, on inspections, inventories, book-keeping and statistics. The very acts of statistical evaluation, conceptual categorisation and procedural routine became substitutes for the practical control of patients' life and treatment applied by Indian staff.

The actual impact of British-based asylum regimes on Indian patients appears to have been generally restricted to bureaucratic measures and rules of precedence. Yet neither colonial nor medical rhetoric were to suffer from such limitations. It seems that it was not so important what institutionalisation and the work of European medical personnel achieved or failed to achieve in practical terms but rather how effectively the myth of British asylum science as a tool of (and excuse for) colonialism could be nurtured. Only when the medicalisation of asylum management was achieved towards the later decades of the nineteenth century, when asylum inmates become 'patients' and 'medical cases' that could be fitted into and treated on the basis of more complex diagnostic criteria, would European ideas and practices have a more thorough and pervasive practical impact on Indian lunatics' life. However, the story of the rise of British psychiatry during the heyday of British colonialism in late nineteenth and early twentieth-century India has yet to be written.

Conclusions

Recent research has alerted us to the heterogeneity of colonial medical discourse. 'Colonial psychiatry' and 'colonial medicine', in general, were not simply preconceived in the West as homogeneous bodies of knowledge to be transferred to various colonial territories. Rather, they developed in response to and in interaction with different colonial regimes. This is also evident in Shula Marks' essay on the Cape. In the case of colonial India, British psychiatry emerged as much in response to and interaction with locally specific circumstances in the various provinces as to developments in Britain. Despite such heterogeneity, when psychiatry even in Britain itself was not yet firmly consolidated, we can trace some similar features in the various 'colonial psychiatries' which developed in the nineteenth century. They were primarily concerned with the treatment of the European expatriate communities rather than with Indians. On a practical level this preoccupation with 'self' rather than 'other', when undesirable elements within the ruling community that could potentially tarnish the colonial image are purged, is partly accounted for by the early phase of colonial development. European lunatics were made invisible either by institutionalisation or deportation.

Further, British psychiatry and its asylums were seen as elements in the civilising mission and were rhetorically presented as a panacea for both Europeans and Indians. Things Indian, including the environment itself, were frequently pathologised as being implicated in mental breakdown. This was congruent with the necessity to provide a legitimate rationale for British colonial hegemony over indigenous peoples. Such a rationale also served to distract attention from the inequities and inequalities of the colonial regime and from insanitary and psychologically destructive features within the European expatriate community.

Although medicine and psychiatry came to be seen as major features justifying if not completely excusing the hardships of colonialism, British asylum-based psychiatry faced resistance from Indian doctors and patients who were not easily subordinated by the foreign discourse of psychiatry or its institutional management. British psychiatry as an instrument of rational Western discourse remained largely rhetorical and symbolic. Even so, these ideological aspects were central to a Western science which claimed to be not only different from but also intrinsically superior to indigenous knowledge.

Acknowledgements

The author is currently engaged in a project funded by the Wellcome Trust: 'Mental health and British colonialism in India and New Zealand (nineteenth and twentieth centuries): towards a comparative historical sociology of mental health and healing'. The generous support of the Trust in her research and the writing of this paper is gratefully acknowledged.

NOTES

1 J. Reid, 'Report of Diseases', *The Monthly Magazine*, 25, 1808, p. 166, quoted in W.L. Parry-Jones, *The Trade in Lunacy*, London, Routledge and Kegan Paul, 1972, p. 11.
2 'Introduction', in W.F. Bynum, R. Porter, M. Shepherd, eds, *The Anatomy of Madness*, Vol. III, London and New York, Routledge, 1988, p. 3.
3 The term 'Anglo-Indian' here denotes members of the British community in India. The term 'Indo-British' will be used for people of mixed Indian–British parentage.
4 J. MacPherson, *Report on Insanity. Royal Commission on the Sanitary State of the Army in India*, Vol. I, London, Eyre and Spottiswoode for HMSO, 1863, p. 605.
5 This point is developed in more detail in W. Ernst, *Mad Tales from the Raj*, London and New York, Routledge, 1991.
6 Quoted from A.T. Embree, *Charles Grant and British Rule in India*, London, Allen and Unwin, 1962, p. 169.
7 Missionary activity and political and administrative innovation was contested during the early decades of the nineteenth century. For an analysis of the debate about immigration restrictions in general, see D. Arnold, 'White colonization and labour in nineteenth-century India', *Journal of Imperial and Commonwealth History*, 11, 1983, pp. 133–58.
8 For the distinctive sorts of institutions that emerged in Bombay, Madras, and Calcutta, see W. Ernst, 'Asylums in alien places', in Bynum, Porter, Shepherd, *Anatomy of Madness*, pp. 48–70.
9 See W. Ernst, 'The European insane in British India, 1800–1858', in D. Arnold, ed., *Imperial Medicine and Indigenous Societies*, Manchester and New York, Manchester University Press, 1988, pp. 27–44.
10 D.M. Peers, *Between Mars and Mammon. Colonial Armies and the Garrison State in India, 1819–1835*, London, Tauris, 1995.
11 On asylums established by the Company for Indian patients, see W. Ernst, 'The establishment of "Native Lunatic Asylums" in early-nineteenth-century British India', in G.J. Meulenbeld and D. Wujastyk, eds, *Studies on Indian Medical History*, Groningen, Egbert Forsten, 1987.
12 See Ernst, 'The establishment of "Native Lunatic Asylums" ', p. 198.
13 For an account of Pembroke House and Ealing Lunatic Asylum (1818–1892) see W. Ernst, 'Asylum provision and the East India Company in the nineteenth century', *Medical History*, 42, 1998, pp. 476–502.
14 C. MacKenzie, *Psychiatry for the Rich. A History of Ticehurst Asylum*, London, 1992.
15 Parry-Jones, *The Trade in Lunacy*, pp. 55, 68, 200–1.

16 See for data collated from India Office Records W. Ernst, 'Psychiatry and colonialism: the treatment of European lunatics in British India, 1800–1858', University of London, School of Oriental and African Studies, Ph.D. thesis, 1986.
17 *Royal Committee on the Sanitary State of the Army in India*, London, Eyre and Spottiswoode for HMSO, 1863, p. XXIV.
18 See Ernst, *Asylum Provision.*
19 The seven 'Native Lunatic Asylums' in Bengal and the North-Western Provinces for example confined in 1854 between 52 and 189 patients, bringing the total to a little over 1,000. See Ernst, 'The establishment of "Native Lunatic Asylums" '.
20 India Office Records, India Public Despatch, 25.8.1852, 43. India Public Letter, 8.4.1854, 53ff.
21 See for example D. Fraser, ed., *The Making of the New Poor Law*, Basingstoke, Macmillan, 1976.
22 E. Stokes, *The English Utilitarians and India*, Delhi, Oxford University Press, 1982 [1959], p. 48.
23 Stokes, *English Utilitarians*, p. 35.
24 For example, Mountstuart Elphinstone (governor of Bombay, 1819–1827) claimed in 1832 that the colonial government 'should still be considered as in a great measure experimental' and that it was 'an advantage to have three experiments [in Bengal, Madras, and Bombay], and to compare them in their progress with each other'. Stokes, *English Utilitarians*, p. 25.
25 'Introduction', in *Anatomy of Madness*, Vol. III, p. 3.
26 See G. Prakash, 'Writing post-orientalist histories of the Third World', *Comparative Studies in Society and History*, 32, 1990, pp. 383–408. R. O'Hanlon and D. Washbrook, 'After orientalism: culture, criticism, and politics in the Third World', *Comparative Studies in Society and History*, 34, 1992, pp. 141–67. G.C. Spivak, 'Subaltern studies: deconstructing historiography', in R. Guha, ed., *Subaltern Studies IV. Writings on South Asian History and Society*, Delhi, Oxford University Press, 1985.
27 K. Ballhatchet, *Race, Sex and Class under the Raj. Imperial Attitudes and Policies and their Critics, 1793–1905*, London, Weidenfeld and Nicolson, 1980.
28 E. J. Hobsbawm, *Industry and Empire. From 1750 to the Present Day*, Harmondsworth, Penguin, 1981 [1968], p. 88.
29 D. Arnold, 'European orphans and vagrants in India in the nineteenth century', *Journal of Imperial and Commonwealth History*, 7, 1979, pp. 104–27, p. 124.
30 Stokes, *English Utilitarians*, p. 10.
31 Ibid., p. 60.
32 India Office Records, Chief Magistrate Calcutta Police to Government, 30.1.1840.
33 India Office Records, Bengal Public Letter, 28.10.1817, 12ff. Bengal Public Letter, 26.1.1819, 1ff. Committee for reporting on the proposed measure of sending Insane Patients to Europe to Government, 12.1.1819, Bengal Public Proceedings, 22.1.1819, 31.
34 India Public Despatch, 1.12.1852.
35 A.S. Thomson, 'Could the Natives of a temperate climate colonise and increase in a tropical country and vice versa?', *Transactions of the Medical and Physical Society of Bombay*, 6, 1843, pp. 112–37.
36 Ibid., pp. 112–37. See also Arnold, 'White colonization'.

37 Thomson, 'Could the Natives of a temperate climate', p. 113.
38 Ibid., pp. 114–15.
39 Ibid., p. 116.
40 Records of Pembroke House, Medical Certificates, 1852, case of H. Strauch.
41 Records of Pembroke House, Medical Certificates, 1818–92. Bengal Medical Board to Government, 30.11.1818.
42 Bombay Asylum Report, 31.3.1852.
43 India Office Records, Bombay Asylum Report, 31.3.1852.
44 M. Finnane, *Insanity and the Insane in Post-Famine Ireland*, London, Croom Helm, 1981.
45 Ballhatchet, *Race, Sex and Class*, pp. 2–3.
46 Compare to present-day anxieties about dangerous diseases originating in the remote steaming jungles of Africa, South America and South-East Asia.
47 *Royal Committee on the Sanitary State of the Army in India*, London, Eyre and Spottiswoode for HMSO, 1863, p. XXIV, p. X.
48 *Royal Committee*, p. XXIV, p. XIII.
49 Which should in fact be 8.3 per cent as this was the rate for the period 1814–1833 to which the officers' and civil servant data refer; the rate of 6.9 per cent refers to the period 1800–1856.
50 *Royal Committee*, p. XXIV, p. xix.
51 Ibid. A similar tendency prevailed in regard to European women. Those married to officers died at a rate of 1.4 per cent, whilst those married to soldiers and non-commissioned officers died at a rate of 3.5 per cent. p. XXV.
52 Ibid., pp. xxiv and xxv.
53 Bengal Judicial Despatch, 30.6.1802, 49 ff. Deputy Register to the Court of Fazdari Adalat to Government. 5.3.1817; Madras Judicial Proceedings, 17.3.1817, 8. Madras Judicial Letter, 11.3.1820, 17.
54 A. Halliday, *A General View of the Present State of Lunatics, and Lunatic Asylums, in Great Britain and Ireland, and in Some Other Kingdoms*, London, Underwood, 1828.
55 India Public Despatch, 9.11.1853.
56 Circulars published in 1847 and 1849 aimed at a restriction of the number of asylum inmates, by decreeing that 'mild cases' of insanity were no longer eligible for admission. Bombay Public Proceedings, 11.7.1849. Bombay Public Proceedings, 11.7.1849.
57 Minute by Governor Falkland, Bombay, 7.9.1850.
58 Civil Surgeon to Medical Board, 16.4.1853, N.W.P. Public Proceedings, 15.6.1853, 7. Medical Board to Lieutenant Governor, 10.10.1854, N.W.P. Public Proceedings, 12.12.1854, 5.
59 General Order of 1826. Bombay Military Despatch, 1826.
60 Medical Board to Government, 6.6.1821; Bengal Judicial Proceedings, 21.8.1821, no para.
61 Medical Board to Bengal Government, 5.2.1821, Bengal Public Proceedings, 20.2.1821, no para. Medical Board to Government, 22.7.1818, Bengal Judicial Proceedings, 28.8.1818, 40.
62 Medical Board to Bengal Government, 22.7.1818, Bengal Judicial Proceedings, 28.8.1818, 67. Military Despatch to Bengal, 26.8.1818.
63 Bengal Medical Board to Government, 1856.

64 Cantor explained that it was 'impracticable concisely to define the duties of each' subordinate officer. He expected them however to 'readily and cheerfully...render their assistance, whenever required'. Bengal Asylum Report, 14.6.1856.

65 In many instances reference to Indian and Indo-British members of the medical service did not fail to express the 'fear' that 'the want of integrity, so general in the Native character, would, notwithstanding their enlightened education, still cling to them as their birthright; and that, on any trying emergency, or dangerous personal illness, they would distrust their European doctrines, and resort to their national empyricism, or to superstitious invocation of the deities of their fathers'. M'Cosh, *Medical Advice to the Indian Stranger*, London, W.H. Allen and Co, 1841, p. 6.

66 Cooking was considered as 'one of the few resources possessed by those who are in charge of Asylums in India, which are not enjoyed by those who treat insanes [sic] in European ones'. Medical Board to Lieutenant Governor, 10.10.1854, N.W.P. Public Proceedings, 12.12.1854, 9.

67 Medical Board to Government, Bengal Judicial Proceedings, 21.8.1821, no para.

68 Medical Board to Lieutenant Governor, 10.10.1854, N.W.P. Public Proceedings, 12.12.1854, 5.

69 Bengal Asylum Report, 14.6.1856.

70 Indian patients at the Rasapagla Asylum raised 'coffee, cotton, sugar-cane, anuath, mulberry, casaiva, tapioca, sapan-wood, alva plant' and 'their coffee in 1832 was highly approved by the London brokers'. Summary of Correspondence relating to the Calcutta Asylum for Insane Patients, 30.10.1847.

71 Civil Surgeon to Medical Board, 11.2.1853, N.W.P. General Proceedings, 15.6.1853, 9.

72 Medical Board to Government, 6.6.1821, Bengal Judicial Proceedings, 21.8.1821, no para.

13

'EVERY FACILITY THAT MODERN SCIENCE AND ENLIGHTENED HUMANITY HAVE DEVISED'

Race and progress in a colonial hospital, Valkenberg Mental Asylum, Cape Colony, 1894–1910

Shula Marks

Unlike in Europe and the United States, where the last two decades have seen a burgeoning of interest in the social history of madness, until recently the social history of insanity and the asylum has not engaged the attention of many historians of Africa; for the most part, the subject has been left to anthropologists or psychiatrists. Like the history of medicine more generally, in Africa the history of psychiatry, of mental illness and of asylums is still in its infancy. There are important issues raised in the scholarship of Roy Porter, Andrew Scull and others for a deeper understanding of the asylum in Africa, though it is also clear that the rich debates on European and north American institutions need to be carefully contextualised within the specific historical circumstances of different African societies. Perhaps not surprisingly, the starting point for historians interested in the social history of insanity and its institutional treatment in Africa has been an attempt to chart the trajectory of psychiatric thought in and about Africa. Thus Jock McCulloch and Megan Vaughan have shown in their different ways and with somewhat different emphases the ways in which psychiatric thinking has been enmeshed in wider imperial discourses about race and has reflected the anxieties and preoccupations of colonial society.[1] It has proven more difficult for historians of insanity in Africa to explore the nature of madness and its treatment in pre-colonial African society, where African nosologies fit uncomfortably if at all with the universal categories of Western psychiatry. Nor has it been much easier to portray what the African mad themselves thought and felt, even in the colonial period, although some historians have now begun to listen to the 'stories' of the African insane, exploring both their content and context for what they can tell us about what can 'be thought and felt at the margins'.[2]

More recently, Sally Swartz has produced a pioneering analysis of the case records and certificates produced by psychiatrists about individual patients in the Cape asylums between 1891 and 1920. In it, she has charted the ways in which she believes the universalism of 'European psychiatry and the certification process imported from Britain' erased racial and cultural difference while constructing a specific form of racial psychiatry which in turn legitimated differential treatment. Paradoxically, she maintains, in their mimicry of metropolitan institutions, 'their discursive production of homogeneity in the insane population' and their failure to take account of the 'unique features of insanity in colonial contexts', psychiatrists at the Cape 'privileged a particular form of knowledge and stripped the indigenous of their identity'. She maintains, further, that between 1891 and 1920 a racist colonial psychiatry emerged as a way of justifying unequal treatment while maintaining a façade of humane care based on universalist principles. Moreover, she suggests, psychiatry, with its claims to understand the 'native mind', has contributed much to the legitimisation of racism in South Africa.[3]

These are powerful and persuasive arguments from which I would not wish to dissent, though I am more cautious about notions of erased identity, given the virtual silence of African voices in the texts. Nor is a study of Valkenberg Asylum an ideal starting point for contesting these claims: as the Cape Colony's first custom-built asylum, it was also the first of the Cape's mental hospitals intended to serve only the white population. Prior to its foundation, mental institutions, like Cape hospitals more generally, had accepted black (largely coloured) as well as white patients, even if wards were segregated in a fairly unsystematic way.[4] Until 1916 when the first black (largely coloured) patients were transferred there, its all-white patients differentiate the story of Valkenberg from the story of the asylum in Africa, and indeed elsewhere in South Africa.

Nevertheless the early history of Valkenberg does serve as a caution to any exaggerated claim about either the innovativeness of colonial psychiatry in these years or its impact on indigenous peoples. Its records reveal the many ambiguities of a marginal institution dependent on the colonial state and the settler populace, and of marginalised professionals anxious to remove the stigma from madness and prove their own progressive credentials. This point may offer a valuable area of contrast with the strategic importance of the asylum's role in colonial India outlined in the preceding essay by Waltraud Ernst. There was, indeed, a massive irony at the heart of the construction of Valkenberg as the model of a modern asylum at the Cape: its universalism was built quite explicitly on principles of segregation which were increasingly being accepted in the Cape and more broadly in South Africa as the 'progressive' solution to the social strains of industrialisation and urbanisation.

The colonial context

Swartz's study is part of the welcome new attention which the asylum in Africa is now beginning to receive.[5] From these accounts, it is not difficult to show that, for the most part, the asylum in Africa has been a poor reflection of the asylum in the metropole: in Nigeria, for example, as Jonathan Sadowsky has remarked, the first asylums 'were, like many colonial imports, already obsolete by metropolitan standards, replicating virtually all the faults British psychiatry had come to pride itself on overcoming'.[6] In his study of the asylum in Sierra Leone, Leland Bell also suggests that the asylum in Africa was in its early days a 'foreign institution, a politically alien place, a colonial establishment...medically and therapeutically removed from African society'. Jock McCulloch goes further: the 'rudimentary and essentially extractive' nature of the state in Africa at the time the asylums were being built, meant that they were never really designed to deal with the psychiatric problems of the indigenous population. Their first function was deal with the white insane; their second to detain the fierce and the fractious in the interests of law and order.[7]

Small, understaffed, chronically short of funds, it is difficult to see the asylum as a major agent of social control, at least of Africans. And while it has been argued – somewhat controversially – that in the British case the asylum arose specifically to address the need of industrial society to isolate a disruptive category of the unemployable from the feckless poor, the better to impose work discipline, it is even more implausible to make this case for sub-Saharan Africa. In colonial Africa, as Megan Vaughan comments, there was no 'Great Confinement' of the insane 'to match that of nineteenth-century Europe, and colonial psychiatric institutions...have their own, rather separate history'.[8]

In many respects the Cape Colony's asylums, and especially Valkenberg, were different to those in the rest of Africa. It is no coincidence that almost all the Colony's institutions for housing the insane – Grahamstown, Port Alfred, Fort Beaufort, and Valkenberg – arose in the wake of South Africa's industrial revolution; only the thirty or so beds in the Old Somerset hospital and the asylum which formed part of the Robben Island General Infirmary predated the discovery of diamonds and gold in 1868 and 1886.[9] While, however, the mineral revolution in South Africa, and the economic and demographic changes which followed in its wake, made the expansion of health services at the Cape both possible and necessary as we shall see, the explanation remains insufficient.

The incarceration of the black insane bore little relation to the labour and social control demands of an industrialising South Africa: given the far more efficient and direct ways in which capital disciplined its black work force and the small numbers of black insane who were institutionalised it would be rash to seek in these the raison d'être of the asylums. Indeed, by comparison with the metropole and other colonies of settlement, the total numbers of the mentally ill in asylums in the Cape Colony come as something of a surprise. As late as 1890–1 within the boundaries of a Colony with a total population of some 377,000 colonists and more than a million indigenous inhabitants, fewer than 2,000 of the total were estimated to be 'lunatic' or 'idiotic'; of these only about a third (595) were actually in asylums, and fewer than half of these were 'Coloured'.[10]

On the eve of the Cape's absorption into the new Union of South Africa some twenty years later, the numbers had more than trebled, yet there were still only just over 2,000 registered insane in asylums in the Colony, of whom now slightly more than 1,000 (around 53 per cent) were black. There were just under 2 million blacks in the Colony in 1911. No fewer than 44 per cent of the white patients were born outside South Africa, although those born outside the Union only constituted 14 per cent of the Cape's white population of some 600,000. As earlier in the nineteenth century, a disproportionate number of the asylum inmates were immigrants with no local kin or community networks.[11] Through the nineteenth century and well into the twentieth, the vast majority of the mentally ill in the Cape, as in South Africa as a whole, were nursed at home, within their families or, in the case of the homeless destitute, the difficult or the dangerous, in small country gaols.

The links between prison, fortress and asylum were never far away. Apart from Valkenberg, the colonial asylums were housed in disused military barracks and prisons, while Robben Island, where the insane joined other poverty-stricken 'incurables' of colonial society, lepers and the chronically sick, had long served as a prison for both criminal and political offenders.[12] Almost as soon as it was established in the mid-nineteenth century, the Island asylum was condemned by a succession of commissions of enquiry as wholly unsuitable for the detention of the insane. Nevertheless, the transfer of its patients to the mainland had to await the wider transformation of medical services at the Cape in the last quarter of the nineteenth century.

From the 1870s to the century's end newly responsible Cape ministries legislated almost annually on a wide range of medical matters, including lunacy,[13] and in 1889 a Visitor to All Asylums (later the Inspector of Asylums) was appointed to advise the government. John William Dodds, then Deputy Superintendent of the Montrose Royal Asylum in Scotland, was chosen for the position. Trained in Edinburgh where he was a gold-medalist, Dodds – as befitted a scion of the Scottish tradition of medical education – was an energetic and dedicated reformer.[14] No theorist, his interests were nevertheless broad, and he became one of the first advocates of a medical school in Cape Town. As Inspector of Asylums no detail, however mundane, escaped his scrupulous attention, and he left his mark both on the lunacy legislation of the Colony, and its institutions. According to the historian of nineteenth-century South African medicine, Edmund H. Burrows, Dodds 'did much to foster the growth of an attitude of mind which viewed the lunatic as patient and a lunatic asylum as a mental hospital rather than a madhouse'.[15]

Dodds was not alone in his desire to reform public attitudes towards the insane, however. By the time that he arrived at the Cape, there was already considerable public and medical pressure on the government to establish a new hospital in Cape Town 'for the better class of patient' – by which was meant generally but not invariably *white* patients. The 'moral management' of the insane had long been a touchstone of metropolitan progress, and the asylum its main curative technique, so that conditions both on Robben Island and in the Old Somerset Hospital were a matter of acute embarrassment to a colonial medical profession beginning to organise its affairs and establish a sense of its corporate identity. Part of Dodds's remit was to supervise the initiation of a 'modern' asylum on 'European' lines, in the city. In July 1891 a sixty-five bed hospital was opened in a 'ramshackle and tumble-down collection of farm buildings' on the Valkenberg Estate. Dodds, still Inspector of Asylums, was appointed as its first Superintendent.[16]

As Superintendent, Dodds examined all new patients on admission, both physically and mentally, and daily thereafter. Responsible for their medical treatment, he also regulated patients' 'bedding, clothing, occupations, amusements, and exercise' as well as their diet.[17] He hired staff from charge nurses and attendants to laundresses and dairymen, kept the accounts and requisitioned supplies from medicines to uniforms and fresh vegetables. In his spare time, he supervised Valkenberg's farming operations. Moreover, until the appointment of an Assistant in 1897 he carried out all these functions on his own. The paper work alone was formidable as the voluminous records of the Colonial Secretary make clear; if the colonial asylum itself was 'one of the symbolic markers of European superiority', proof of 'moral and social progress', as Waltraud Ernst has suggested,[18] so meticulous record-keeping was one of the ways in which the Cape Colony defined its identity as an outpost of civilisation and progress on the 'dark continent'.[19] Dodds prepared annual reports, corresponded with the Colonial Office and with patients' families, and maintained the Visitors' Book; he also was responsible for the case notes, the post-mortem book, the registers of seclusion and restraints, and of accidents. Whatever the surveillance of the patients, it was at least matched by the colonial government's surveillance over the asylum staff, including over Dodds himself. 'Should not the policy of trusting responsible officials a little more, be tried?', he fumed in 1904.[20]

Although there had been previous proponents of 'moral management' at the Cape – it had after all become part of the conventional wisdom among British and American psychiatrists some half a century earlier – no previous medical superintendent of asylums or individual in charge of the insane had as sweeping authority to implement it.[21] Not only was Dodds now head of what was to be the Colony's show-case hospital, as Inspector of Asylums he also visited and reported on all mental institutions in the Colony twice a year, framed the relevant legislation and advised the government on all matters affecting the insane.

Shortly after his appointment, Dodds urged the erection of an up-to-date hospital for the insane in place of the 'inconveniently arranged buildings' at Valkenberg.[22] As elsewhere, 'moral management' was to be accompanied by 'moral architecture' and Sydney Mitchell, Consulting Architect to the Scottish Board of Lunacy, who had built the Royal Edinburgh Infirmary, was commissioned to design a new hospital.[23] Despite half a century of hardly propitious examples to draw on, he remained optimistic about the curative capacity of the asylum; provided patients were admitted promptly to cheerful wards in pleasant surroundings and were treated sympathetically cure would follow.[24] Intended for 'recent and curable cases of insanity', the new institution was to signal to patients and their families a wholly new approach to the treatment of the insane, far removed from the stigma of madness and the brutalities of its past treatment.

Dodds was fortunate in drawing up his plans at an expansive moment in the economic fortunes of the Cape Colony; Cecil Rhodes was its Prime Minister, and the Colony's coffers were feeling the benefits of revenues resulting from the region's mineral discoveries. Moreover, the flood of new immigrants – many of them single men – which followed in the wake of the mineral discoveries made the need for a mental hospital in Cape Town all the more necessary and in 1894 Dodds was able to secure funds in the colonial estimates for a new 200-bed hospital at Valkenberg.[25] This was a matter of self-congratulation for the public-spirited reformers of Cape Town. For them, as for Dodds, the new hospital symbolised the Colony's progress and civilisation. In July 1894, for example, the *Cape Argus* rejoiced that at last 'the scandalous inadequacy and unsuitability of the old Valkenberg' was about to be replaced by a new hospital, and commended the 'thoroughness and general excellence of the plans which have been prepared'. It was, the paper declared, 'the sacred duty incumbent upon the Colony in general and the government in particular to proceed at once to carry out those plans'. Provided this were done,

> the Western Province will ere long possess an asylum for the insane which will combine at once the utmost economy, the best internal accommodation and every facility that modern science and enlightened humanity have devised not so much for the confinement of the lunatic, but for his restoration to health of mind and to the society from which, for his own good and the good of his kindred, he has been temporarily removed.[26]

In the words of Dr Jane Waterston, South Africa's first woman doctor and its most illustrious Official Visitor, the new Valkenberg was to be 'a hospital for the mind and not the sort of dumping ground that the name Asylum means to the popular imagination'.[27]

New initiatives

Waterston had little doubt that with the appointment of Dodds and the new building, a fresh era in the treatment of the insane had been launched in the Cape Colony.[28] Her detailed quarterly reports provide an invaluable account of daily life in the asylum. In line with progressive asylum doctors in Britain and America, she was as concerned with the view of the mountains from the wards, and with the trees, shrubs and flowered walkways, as she was with drains and ditches.[29] Nothing escaped her eagle eye. The clothing sent out from 'Home' she recorded dryly in January 1907 (and it was neither the first nor last of such comments) had been chosen by someone who 'knows or cares little about the business':

> The men's socks are only fit for the North Pole and the men's hats for Sherwood Forest. The thick woollen socks are utterly unsuited for this climate....As to the hats, it is quite against the present treatment of Insanity to make the Patients look as bizarre as possible; their dress is part of the treatment...[30]

Whatever the shortcomings of the sartorial arrangements, however, Jane Waterston could still enthuse in 1906:

> To any one conversant with the bad old times...Valkenberg is a difficult place to inspect. As a Doctor one is so thankful for the comfort of it, and the care...except for the formula 'all right' it is difficult some times to find more to write about...[31]

Being 'one of the few remaining Practitioners who can recollect the times of old when Robben Island was the only Asylum at the Cape for any unfortunate whose mind gave way',[32] Waterston was inclined to be generous. Nevertheless, by 1906 the new Valkenberg hospital, which had been launched with such optimism but a dozen years before, was already beginning to experience the shortfall in income, shortage of staff and severe overcrowding which were to characterise most of its twentieth-century history. Many of the recent accounts of asylums have shown a not dissimilar descent from the euphoria of the early days of individual asylums to their stagnation and decline. In retrospect what is striking is how short-lived was Valkenberg's moment of glory, how rapid its decline, despite its dedication to white patient care.

Valkenberg had barely been built when South Africa was hit by recession in 1897–8 followed by a bitter and costly colonial war and, after a brief post-war boom, yet another depression. This appears to have drained whatever charitable impulse had existed in the colonial exchequer towards the needs of the insane. Thus in the ten years from 1894 to 1903 a total of £174,000 – an average of £17,500 p.a. – was spent on the five Cape asylums; in the six years from 1904 to 1909, the total spent was under £20,000, an average of £3,323 p.a.[33]

Nor were the initial hopes which the colonial authorities had entertained of attracting a sufficient number of the 'better class' patients ever fulfilled: unlike at the Grahamstown Asylum, which garnered considerable sums from its paying patients, the amount brought in by the small number of paying patients in Valkenberg rarely covered their costs. Dodds's belief that early detection made for cure was illusory: about one-third of the *c.*1,500 patients admitted between 1891 and 1908 were discharged as recovered. This is a comparatively high number, and certainly far higher than the black patients discharged from the other asylums, but still left some 60 per cent to clog up the wards.[34]

As elsewhere, the authorities rapidly found that the mere opening of an asylum to which families could entrust their frailer members dramatically expanded the demand for beds, and to this was added a constantly expanding population. From Valkenberg's inception there was barely a year in which there was sufficient accommodation for either the male or female patients. Indeed by 1902 overcrowding was so severe on the female side that it exacerbated the spread of infectious diseases, while the gaols were still widely utilised for the overflow.[35] In 1905 the editor of the *South African Medical Record* called this overcrowding and the housing of lunatics in the gaols, 'the greatest administrative scandal in this Colony'.[36] By 1913 it had become a national scandal, and led to the appointment of a Select Committee to enquire into the 'treatment of lunatics'. By that time the litany of complaints over poor drains and lack of beds had acquired a certain desperation. In his evidence to the Commission, Dodds confessed:

> For years I have been trying to get quarts into pint bottles, I have had no room to take in cases....From 1905 the years had simply been black years. It is impossible to speak of the difficulties experienced...[37]

By 1910–11 Jane Waterston's reports had also become somewhat acerbic, echoing Dodds's frustration. Thus in October 1910 she called attention to the 'shabby' appearance of the asylum and the serious lack of accommodation: there were already 'about sixty patients too many', and the absence of an isolation ward would be serious matter 'should there be an epidemic', as indeed there had been at the beginning of that year. Not only were the vegetables 'sent in by the gardener' unfit for eating; even the patients' underwear left much to be desired. To add insult to injury,

> The coloured lunatics of Robben Island and the paupers in the Old Somerset Hospital have neater underclothing than the European patients in Valkenberg who do not wear their own clothes…[38]

Given that Waterston had been a missionary at Lovedale in the eastern Cape in her young days, and remained renowned as a philanthropist to the coloured population in Cape Town, the unconscious racism of her remarks, and her blindness to the colour bar embedded in the very constitution of Valkenberg is a reminder of the extent to which even colonial liberals had accepted racial segregation by the early twentieth century. They are also a reminder, however, that scandalously poor conditions were by no means confined to black mental patients in South Africa's asylums.

The institutional environment

The problems of Valkenberg – again like its counterparts in Victorian Britain and America – were not confined to overcrowding and the deterioration of the physical surroundings. As in Britain at least as important as the increasing size and bureaucratisation, the absence of cure and therefore the silting up of hospital space with chronic and congenital cases, was the poor calibre of its staff. So long as Valkenberg was restricted in size, the demands for staff were relatively limited and Dodds was able to recruit the majority from the British asylums and maintain a tight hold over their supervision. With Valkenberg's three-fold expansion by the end of the century, however, and with the outbreak of the South African war, he had increasing difficulties in recruiting competent staff. 'Even at our ordinary strength, an asylum cannot be worked with safety with new hands picked up with difficulty from a poor selection of applicants', he complained.[39]

Many of these 'new hands' were untrained and unqualified men and women with a variety of more or less unskilled and labouring backgrounds – the men had been gardeners, coachmen, grooms, watchmen, labourers, soldiers, house painters, salesmen, tailors, bricklayers, blacksmiths and farmers. Mostly they were poorly educated and many were barely literate. In the 1890s the majority seem to have been English-speaking with a considerable number of Irishmen, many of them fairly recent immigrants. By the 1900s there were some with Afrikaans names, and a sprinkling of German and other immigrants were also engaged as nurses although many had difficulty in speaking English.[40] The female nurses were drawn from much the same sector of society as the men, although from the beginning there appear to be a somewhat larger number of Irish and Afrikaans women, at least judging from their surnames, and their previous occupations were less varied. Apart from those few who had previous hospital experience or were recruited directly from Britain, the majority either had no previous occupation or had been dressmakers, tailor's assistants, shop assistants or waitresses. Like their male counterparts, their literacy was not of a high order. The only one who had previously been a teacher lasted 'only a few days'. Dodds took the precaution of appointing all staff on probation for three months, and many did not stay much longer, whether because they were dismissed – more often in the case of male attendants, not infrequently for drunkenness and violence – or because they left of their own accord, as was the case with female nurses, a number of whom left to get married.

Drawn as they were from such a miscellany of occupations from the white working class, Dodds found many of his male attendants sorely wanting. By 1897 he was writing in characteristic vein of his difficulties in engaging suitable men as attendants:

> notwithstanding continued reminders there has been a want of alertness on the part of the attendants that makes one despair of ever training them. I have given notice to two attendants, but I am desirous of leavening my staff with men of some experience in British asylums, instead of trusting altogether to local supplies.[41]

It was no easier to find good female attendants in South Africa, and Dodds was constantly forced to recruit nurses in the UK.[42] Even kitchen staff and laundresses had sometimes to be sought in Britain.[43] Dodds's problems were not unrelated to the poor salaries offered and the arduous nature of the work. The wages of male attendants were frequently lower than those of labourers and artisans through this period, while female nurses received about two-thirds of the male wage.[44] Not surprisingly, staff were dismissed on occasion for petty pilfering.[45]

In 1897 Dodds pleaded with the Colonial Office to raise male attendants' salaries in order to encourage the men to stay on because the service was being 'injured by constant changes', and 'salaries were hardly adequate for married men to live and educate their children'.[46] In fact married attendants were the exception rather than the rule: marriage was regarded as a privilege to be bestowed only on 'our best attendants', perhaps because of the extra cost involved and the necessarily more lax supervision over men who lived in their own married housing rather than in staff quarters under the direct supervision of the Superintendent.[47]

By 1899 attendants' salaries had improved slightly and they received an additional 2d. a day if they managed to take the Certificate of the Medico-Psychological Association. This hardly compensated for arduous and often dangerous work. In the 1890s, attendants and nurses worked from 6 a.m. to 8 p.m. and were not infrequently disturbed at night as their rooms overlooked or adjoined the wards. They worked three Sundays out of four, and most public holidays. In 1899 their leave was increased to two full weekdays and two half weekdays a month.[48] Yet the job called for the utmost restraint. Not infrequently the subject of attack from the patients, staff were under the strictest injunctions not to strike back: those who did seem to have been summarily dismissed, at least during Dodds's day, even when sorely provoked and even if patients did not show any visible injury.[49] At the same time, in line with contemporary progressive thought, mechanical forms of constraint were frowned upon; even seclusion was used sparingly. There is some evidence that tranquillisers were used rather more generously, however, if the evidence of a former matron turned patient is to be believed.[50]

Some flavour of the frequently explosive tensions in the wards is revealed in a description by Dodds of a scuffle between female patients and nurses at the end of 1901 which seems to have developed into a free for all when Nurse Sutton was struck and held by her hair by a Mrs Maitland, 'a dangerous, passionate patient'. Sutton retaliated and a number of patients promptly joined the fray, when Lizzie Styles, 'a troublesome, violent patient', also hit Mrs Maitland in the face and pulled her down, and Mrs Ecksteen, who was sweeping the room at the time, took the opportunity to strike Mrs Maitland with the broom. Nurse Loots who gave evidence against Nurse Sutton 'said she was too excited to help'.

> Whether the slightly bruised eye was done by a knock on the floor, or by the patient Lizzie Styles, or by the Nurse, I cannot say; but my impression is that Nurse Sutton on being taken hold of by her hair lost control of her temper and gave Mrs M a slap certainly on her shoulder and then took hold of her hair. Even under these circumstances [Dodds concluded sternly] an asylum nurse is expected to exhibit complete control, and I therefore propose to give Nurse Sutton one month's notice…

Nor were the tensions restricted to encounters between staff and patients. Tempers among staff were also often frayed. In March 1902, at a time when Dodds was seriously concerned at the calibre of staff he had been forced to recruit during the war, he found it necessary summarily to dismiss Attendant T. Gill; Gill, already under a month's notice 'for disobedience of orders and general unsatisfactoriness', had allegedly called the housekeeper, 'a two-faced bitch'. Gill protested that the report was not wholly accurate: 'He admitted to me calling her a two-faced old cat', Dodds recorded somewhat primly.[51]

Racial perspectives

If thus far Valkenberg is almost indistinguishable from its counterparts in Britain and America, its colonial context sets it apart. In her fine thesis on the medical institutions on Robben Island Harriet Deacon has remarked that, 'medical knowledge about mental illness was closely linked to discourses of race, class and gender at the Cape'. She maintains however that in the Cape Colony racist theorising about insanity was quite slow to take a medical form, only emerging after 1880 'as a systematic theory that justified separate and different psychiatric treatment'.[52] Sally Swartz has elaborated this argument. It was, she maintains, 'classification, segregation and differential treatment according to race and gender in Cape Colony's asylums, and the many texts which defined, justified and described such divisions [which constituted] a distinctively colonial psychiatry'.[53]

As Swartz shows, for Dodds 'adequate care was predicated upon racial segregation. He saw racial mixing in asylums and gaols as detrimental to the process of recovery', and was determined to maintain Valkenberg as a whites-only hospital.[54] In the same way that patients needed to be classified and segregated by gender and handicap, so they had to be strictly segregated by race. Dodds's whites-only policy posed certain problems for the hospital, however, among them the shortage and cost of manual labour. While initially Dodds may have hoped that the patients themselves would supply some of this, he was soon to be disillusioned. As Jane Waterston noted caustically in 1908, 'Even when reason goes in this country the [white] dislike of Manual Labour remains'.[55] By 1913, the Select Committee on the Treatment of Lunatics maintained that it was 'an advantage' to have 'coloured' patients in the same asylum as white patients, so that they could do the menial labour. It was for this reason that in 1916 when World War I intensified the shortage of white male labour, able-bodied black patients were transferred to a site adjacent to Valkenberg.[56]

At a time of creeping segregation in Cape Town's public facilities in the 1890s, paradoxically much of the drive for segregation also came from Dodds's own progressive vision and his desire to remove the stigma of mental illness from white patients. To this must be added his deeply ingrained notions of class, his scientific training and his belief in 'moral management', in which classification was of the essence.[57] Jonathan Andrews in this volume stresses the 'extremity of the concern' in the Glasgow Royal Asylum with 'isolating one class from the other'; in the colonial context this expressed itself in the 'extremity of concern' over racial segregation. Indeed the total exclusion of black patients from Valkenberg has its parallel in the total exclusion of pauper patients from the Glasgow Royal, 'a form of social cleansing which the psychiatric establishment, which had long stressed the need for strict social segregation in the asylum, also approved of in theory'.[58]

In pressing for new buildings at Valkenberg, for example, Dodds complained bitterly that 'makeshift' buildings rendered classification impossible:

> Instead of having separate wards for the sick, feeble, and dying, for recent cases, for convalescent and quiet cases, for epileptics, for dements and cases of degraded habits, and so on, each of them specially designed for the class of cases that occupy it, we have but two wards in each side.... so that all the different classes are more or less associated with one another...[59]

As late-nineteenth-century 'racial science' became all-pervasive, the classification of patients by severity of illness was coupled with an increasing concern with racial classification, which became a matter for constant anxious comment. Thus in his reports as Inspector of Asylums for 1890, Dodds deplored the fact that at the Old Somerset Hospital,

> the only classification possible is into male and female, white and coloured, respectively; no mental classification is practicable; in working parties white and coloured are mixed, and the coloured patients still have to make use of the Europeans' lavatories.[60]

Although in general Dodds approved of the regime instituted in Grahamstown by its Superintendent, Dr T. Greenlees,[61] he used the opportunity of his Official Visit to the Asylum in 1894 to write disapprovingly:

> The classification of the patients – a difficulty in all our Institutions – leaves very much to be desired here.... White and coloured should not mix in walking parties or working parties, as they do at present; it is difficult to make arrangements for a racial classification, but they can and should be made.[62]

There were more material reasons for Dodds's concern: 'let the authorities manage as they may, satisfaction will never be given to the friends of patients and the public until separate blocks for coloured patients are built', he wrote sternly.[63] How the patients themselves felt is rather more difficult to discern. Despite some hostility recorded by violent white male patients on Robben Island to being mixed with blacks, in 1892 Dodds reflected that on the Island 'At dances the white and coloured [women] mix and are said to prefer it, if that is any argument in its favour'.[64]

The establishment of Valkenberg as a 'modern' and 'progressive' hospital was also premised on the existence of Robben Island as a depository for black patients and the dangerous white insane, and the creation of Fort Beaufort as a segregated institution for black patients in the 1890s. In the black wards, food, shelter and treatment were far less salubrious than at Valkenberg, and in general this was taken as 'given', although Dodds also repeatedly urged the government to make better provision for Robben Island's black and criminal white patients on the mainland.[65]

Psychiatric practices and scientific visions

As we have seen, the burden of Sally Swartz's indictment against Cape psychiatry is that on the one hand it applied universal principles without recognising cultural difference, thus stripping black patients of their identity, and, on the other, that it created a knowledge of 'the other', all the more powerful for its scientific credentials. As she puts it:

> It was in the complex tension between universalism, which erased the indigenous as an object of scientific enquiry, and the practice marking race and gender difference in management practice in Cape asylums, which contributed to the constitution of a uniquely colonial psychiatry.

It was, she avers, psychiatry rather than general medicine which 'made a significant contribution to the scientific racism feeding colonial forms of exploitation. This contribution rested on psychiatric descriptions of the "mind", "mentality", or "personality" of colonial subjects.'[66]

In general, both accusations are warranted. Yet it is important not to exaggerate the 'creative' role of psychiatry in producing a specifically colonial psychiatry in the period before World War I. Of the psychiatrists at work in this period, only T. Duncan Greenlees and the first Union Commissioner for Mental Hygiene, Dr J.T. Dunston, appointed in 1916, were in any sense systematic proponents of the view that 'the native mind' had its own special properties, and it is unclear how original their views were nor how widely they were disseminated. Dodds for example confessed in 1913:

> Personally I do not know much about natives. Only a comparatively small number of natives are insane in relation to population. You cannot expect in a race like the natives that you can have anything like the same amount or proportion of insane as among civilised people.

In response to a questioner who suggested that this might be because blacks had a 'prejudice' against sending members of their family to asylums, Dodds responded – 'I have been told that they were proud of having a friend in the asylum.'[67]

Even within the small colonial medical profession, mental hospital superintendents did not enjoy high prestige. Indeed it may have been the very need to gain respectability for their profession that made Dodds into such an ardent advocate of segregation.[68] According to Elizabeth van Heyningen, for the most part before 1910, doctors 'made a modest impact on the cultural and social life of the city outside the sphere of their expertise'. The wealthier sectors of the middle class – 'the merchants, financiers, legal practitioners, local politicians and higher civil servants' – had far higher status.[69] This would seem especially true in the case of colonial psychiatrists, whose activities were still regarded with considerable suspicion by locally born colonists.

Although Harriet Deacon is probably correct in believing that in a general sense a form of racialised psychiatric knowledge had emerged by the 1880s, any systematic scientific colonial psychiatry came considerably later. As she suggests in the earlier period, increasing segregation in the asylum was driven by the intensification of white racism in the Colony during the latter half of the nineteenth century. In the Cape Colony, the tensions between an older liberal universalism and the newer discourse of scientific racism may in fact have set boundaries on the extent of discrimination in medical institutions into the twentieth century. Here a couple of exchanges between Dodds and Greenlees are illuminating. In November 1894 Dodds was shocked to find twenty-two patients in the Grahamstown Asylum sleeping on the floor without mattresses (somewhat surprisingly two white females were among their number) while fourteen slept on mattresses on the floor (including eight male Europeans and a white female). Grahamstown, he remarked tartly, was the 'only Asylum in the Colony where such miserable provision is made for patients at night, and [this] does not reflect well on the Institution'.[70] Greenlees was stung into reply:

> My answer to his [Dodds's] arguments have been reiterated again and again; and everyone consonant with the habits of the crude native agrees with me. I admit it is not the custom of English asylums, nor Valkenberg to admit raw natives who will not and cannot sleep on bedsteads.[71]

To this Dodds responded:

> crude natives are received into other Asylums but they are not offered a blanket and a bare floor to sleep on. Crude natives are received into general hospitals, but once within the doors of the hospital, civilisation is the standard, not barbaric habit. And so it should be in Asylums; and so it is...in every Asylum except Grahamstown.

'Before long', he added caustically, he expected to see 'wattle and daub huts in the female airing court for "crude natives" who object to the provisions of civilisation'.[72]

In his next report in January 1895, Dodds again criticised the Grahamstown Asylum's discriminatory practices, this time Greenlees's failure to arrange daily walking parties for his black female patients. And again Greenlees's answer is instructive:

> Since the new Laundry has been opened nearly every one of our Native Females are working daily. A daily walk would considerably interfere with the working of the Asylum. They get a long walk twice every Sunday which is sufficient in my opinion.[73]

The role of black patients as menial labour in Greenlees's scheme of things is clear.

Equally clearly, however, the classification of patients and their segregation on racial grounds was still based for Dodds on universalist standards which the more thorough-going advocates of racial difference such as Greenlees, based as he was in the racially charged Eastern Cape with its preponderant African population, were happy to transgress. Dodds undoubtedly believed that white and 'coloured' patients should be separated, but for reasons that smack of pragmatism and prejudice rather than any systematic medical or racial theory. As he remarked in 1892, while he did not think it 'right' that the 'two races should mix as they often have to do at present', 'colour should not be a dividing line in medicine and every effort should be made to render happy coloured as well as white'.[74]

Although he recommended, for example, that black staff be employed to attend black patients in Port Alfred and Fort Beaufort his proposal seems purely practical. Under fire from the Colonial Secretary, now the Afrikaner Bondsman, Dr T.N. Te Water, who opposed the employment of 'natives' for any but 'the menial and dirtier parts of the work', he explained that his 'sole object' was to lessen costs as a 'native' attendant's wage would be half that of his European counterpart, and he would 'know Kaffir'.[75]

It may be, as Swartz comments, that Dodds simply wished 'to create and maintain an appearance of "civilised" standards of care for all the insane throughout the Cape' and that 'Black women on asylum floors was at odds with this.'[76] His attitude was none the less a far cry from the stridency of Greenlees, who by this time was beginning to construct a 'scientific' psychiatric theory on the basis of the difference between the 'childlike' brain of the 'native' and the more developed intellectual powers of the European.[77] It was to be equally out of tune with the increasingly segregationist discourse which followed the unification of South Africa in 1910.

In recent years the universalism of the Enlightenment has come under increasing attack from critics who have no difficulty in pointing to the contradictions between its professions and its practices. Yet it is important to note that universalism also constrained the more blatant attempts at discrimination, and ensured at least some provision for black patients. The limitations of Dodds's universalism sprang not so much out of the limitations of universalism *per se*, but out of its precise application as an instrument of power in a colonial situation. As in the Victorian asylum, classification by social status was almost as important as classification by mental state; in a colonial context status and class were translated into colour. This was hardly unique to the Cape or new in the late nineteenth century. There is in the texts of the time a constant slippage between notions of race and notions of class. As Kenan Malik has argued more widely, in the nineteenth century,

> The tendency to view social difference became rationalised through the discourse of race....Race accounted for social inequalities by attributing them to nature. Through this process the universalism of Enlightenment discourse became degraded into a particularist vision of the world.[78]

It was unfortunately this particularist vision of the world which came to characterise care in South Africa's psychiatric institutions for much of the twentieth century.

NOTES

1 M. Vaughan, *Curing Their Ills. Colonial Power and African Illness*, Cambridge, Polity Press, 1991. For McCulloch, see his *Black Soul White Artefact. Fanon's Clinical Psychology and Social Theory*, Cambridge, Cambridge University Press, 1983 and especially his *Colonial Psychiatry and 'the African mind'*, Cambridge, 1995.

2 Roy Porter, *A Social History of Madness. Stories of the Insane*, London, Weidenfeld and Nicolson, 1987 has clearly been the inspiration. The quotation is on p. 2. See Joseph Melling's introductory chapter to this volume for related literature. For the African explorations, see Jonathan Sadowsky, 'Imperial Bedlam: institutions of madness and colonialism in Southwest Nigeria', Ph.D. Northwestern University, 1997, forthcoming, University of California Press, chapter 4; Hilary Sapire and Bob Edgar, *Divine Madness in the Eastern Cape: The Case of Nonteta, c.1918–1935*, forthcoming; S. Dubow and Jacqueline Rose, 'Introduction' to Wulf Sachs, *Black Hamlet*, Baltimore and London, Johns Hopkins University Press, 1996; and Shula Marks, ed., *'Not Either an Experimental Doll': The Separate Worlds of Three South African Women*, London, The Women's Press, 1987.

3 S. Swartz, 'The black insane in the Cape, 1891–1920', *Journal of Southern African Studies*, 21, 3, 1995 and 'Colonialism and the production of psychiatric knowledge at the Cape 1891–1920', Ph.D., UCT, 1996.

4 The racial terminology, which is regrettable but unavoidable, needs some explanation. Contemporaries in the Cape used the term Coloured to refer to the indigenous Khoisan population of the western Cape, ex-slaves, the largely Xhosa-speaking Africans from the eastern Cape who were already working in Cape Town by the last quarter of the century and the products of intermarriages between all of these and whites, to whom the term came increasingly confined in the twentieth century; in the eastern Cape, where Xhosa-speaking people were in the majority, the term 'native' was increasingly used to refer to all 'people of colour'. I have termed this heterogeneous group 'black' except where an alternative term appears in quotation. The term 'European' was used for the settler population; I have used the term 'white', or, when necessary, English-speaking or Afrikaner for this group, again except in quotation.

5 For Zomba, see M.Vaughan, 'Idioms of madness: Zomba Lunatic Asylum, Nyasaland, in the colonial period', *Journal of Southern African Studies (JSAS)*, 9, 2, April 1983, pp. 218–38; for Kissy, Leland Bell, *Mental and Social Disorder in Sub-Saharan Africa. The Case of Sierra Leone, 1787–1990*, New York, Westport, Conn. and London, Greenwood Press, 1991; Sadowsky, 'Imperial Bedlam' deals with Aro and Yaba, and Lynette Jackson deals with Ingutsheni in her doctoral thesis for Columbia University, 1997, 'Narratives of "madness" and power: a history of Ingutsheric Mental Hospital and social order in colonial Zimbabwe, 1908–59'.

6 Sadowsky: 'Imperial Bedlam', chapter 3, p. 1.

7 McCulloch, *Colonial Psychiatry*, pp. 42–3.

8 Vaughan, *Curing their Ills*, p. 101.

9 Of these, Robben Island, Valkenberg and Grahamstown have each found their recent historian. See Harriet Deacon, 'A history of the medical institutions on Robben Island', Ph.D., Cambridge, 1994; Swartz, 'Colonialism and the production of psychiatric knowledge'; Felicity Swanson, 'Colonial madness: the construction of gender in the Grahamstown Lunatic Asylum, 1875–1905', B.A. Hons. thesis, UCT, 1994; and R.C. Warwick, 'Mental health care at Valkenberg Asylum 1891–1909; aspects of its origins and operation', B.A. Hons. thesis, UCT, 1989. Swanson is currently working on the Fort Beaufort Asylum. So far, there has been little recent research on the institutions in the rest of South Africa in Pietermaritzburg, Pretoria and Bloemfontein.

10 According to GH 37-'91, *Annual Report of Asylums, 1891*, p. 5. The total number was 310 'European' and 285 'Coloured', of whom the majority were male: a consistent feature of colonial asylums. According to the Cape census of 1891 at that time 376,987 inhabitants of the Colony were white out of a total population of 1,527,224.

11 G25–1910. Cape Colony, *Annual Reports, 1909. Part II, Asylums for the Insane*, pp. 9, 11; UG 32 1912 *Census of 7 May 1911*, Pretoria, 1912. For a discussion on this issue in relation to nineteenth-century Robben Island, see Deacon, 'A history of the medical institutions on Robben Island', p. 176.

12 Deacon, 'A history of the medical institutions', p. 37.

13 E.H. Burrows, *A History of Medicine in South Africa up to the End of the Nineteenth Century*, Cape Town and Amsterdam, A.A. Balkema, 1958, p. 332.

14 Scottish doctors were prominent throughout the empire. Dodds's Scottish connections may, however, have had 'a more pernicious influence' in forming his racial consciousness, as Elizabeth van Heyningen suggests, because of the 'enduring influence' in Scotland of Dr Robert Knox's racial anatomy. E. van Heyningen, 'Public health and society in Cape Town, 1880–1910', Ph.D. Cape Town, 1989, p. 41. Dodds chose most of his senior staff from Scottish asylums, so that the Scottish influence was quite pervasive. See essays by Andrews and Lorraine Walsh for the 'mixed economy' of care provision in nineteenth-century Scotland.

15 Burrows, *History of Medicine in South Africa*, p. 345.

16 Warwick, 'Mental health care at Valkenberg Asylum', pp. 12–13; Burrows, *History of Medicine*, pp. 344–5.

17 CO 7175 Dodds set out some of these duties in a hand-written instruction to the new superintendent of Fort Beaufort, 'Duties of the Medical Superintendent of Fort Beaufort', 14 March 1894. That he undertook all these

duties himself plus those that follow is clear from the Colonial Office records.

18 Waltraud Ernst, *Mad Tales from the Raj. The European Insane in British India, 1800–1858*, London and New York, Routledge, 1991, p. 64, and chapter by Ernst in this volume.

19 In addition to the case records, many of which are now deposited in the MSS collection in the University of Cape Town's African Library, the CO [Colonial Office] series in the Cape Archives contains a remarkable body of documentation on Valkenberg between 1891 and 1910. Unfortunately after that date jurisdiction over mental hospitals was transferred from the office of the Cape's Colonial Secretary to the new Union of South Africa's Department of the Interior, and in 1948 a decision was taken to destroy the vast majority of their records. South African Archives, ARH 15 C/11/14A/7 Destruction of records Public Health Dept: Cner for Mental Health 1948. This partly accounts for the dates of this paper.

20 CO 7919 Memo by Dodds to CO 26 November 1904.

21 William Edmunds, who was appointed Surgeon-Superintendent of Robben Island in 1862 and inaugurated changes which were sufficiently visible to enable middle-class families to entrust their female members to its asylum, was probably the most notable of these earlier reformers. See Deacon, 'A history of the medical institutions on Robben Island', pp. 82, 102 ff.

22 G37-'91 *Annual reports, 1890*, Inspector of Asylums, p. 15; CO 1488, Medical Superintendent, Valkenberg, to Under Col. Sec. 8 December 1891.

23 CO 1488 8 December 1891 and CO 1527 1892 *passim*. See also Cape of Good Hope, G.17-'93, *Reports on the Government and Public Hospitals and Asylums, and Report of the Inspector of Asylums, for 1892*, I Valkenberg Asylum, pp. 5–6.

24 Cape of Good Hope, G.17-'93, *Annual Reports, 1892*, p. 7.

25 The Colonial Secretary until 1893 was J.W. Sauer (1850–1913), who was regarded as one of the Cape's foremost liberal parliamentarians. Sir Pieter Faure succeeded Sauer as Colonial Secretary when Sauer resigned from Rhodes's first cabinet; he was apparently as enthusiastic in his promotion of Valkenberg. *Cape Argus*, 24 July 1894.

26 *Cape Argus*, 24 July 1894.

27 CO 7971 Official Visitor's Reports [henceforth OVR], Waterston, 2 September 1904.

28 CO 7177 OVR, Waterston, 19 March 1896.

29 'Asylum grounds…though very wet were not so bad as I expected,' runs a typical entry. 'The main avenue to New Valkenberg was wonderfully clean after such weather for making weeds grow.' CO 7977 OVR, Waterston, 23 June 1905. cf. Tomes, *A Generous Confidence: Thomas Story Kirkbride and the Art of Asylum-Keeping, 1840–1883*, New York, Cambridge University Press, 1983, pp. 129–30, for very similar reflections.

30 CO 7971 OVR, Waterston, 7 January 1907. Inspection carried out on 15 December 1906.

31 CO 7971 OVR, Waterston, 8 January 1906. See also ibid. 22 October 1905.

32 CO 7324 OVR, Waterston, 10 November 1902, of visit on 15–17 September 1902.

33 SC-'13 *Report and Minutes of the SC on Treatment of Lunatics, 1913*, Cape Town, 1913, Appx, p. v.

34 G41 – 1909. *Annual Reports: Part II. Asylums for the Insane. Report of the Inspector of Asylums. 2. Valkenberg Asylum*, p. 25. The figure was based on counting as one discharge 'recovered' patients who were admitted and discharged more than once, and excluding those were discharged and then relapsed and not subsequently released. The average recovery rate of whites in colonial asylums in 1908 was 35.71 per cent and for 'coloureds' 25.39 per cent counted on the same basis. Ibid. 1. *Inspector of Asylums*, p. 14.
35 Warwick, 'Mental health care at Valkenberg Asylum', p. 40.
36 *SAMR*, 4, 7, 25 April 1905, p. 106, cited in Warwick, 'Mental health care at Valkenberg Asylum', p. 40.
37 *Select Committee 1913*, pp. 2–4.
38 CO 7971 Waterston to US for the Interior, Pretoria, 24 October 1910 reporting visits on 24, 28 and 30 September 1910.
39 With the outbreak of the war a number of his male attendants joined the British army, while the pool of unemployed white labour at the Cape also dried up. See for example CO 7331 Dodds to CS 19 January 1901 and 28 February 1901 and the notes by Dodds on this correspondence 3 February 1901 and 5 February 1901.
40 This section is based on the forms filled in by all potential members of staff, which recorded – inter alia – their names, addresses, previous occupations, weights and height, as well as on the forms applying for leave or recording promotion, departure, dismissal etc. Around Union, applicants were asked about their education, and knowledge of English, but relatively few were filled in before the series ends. The various forms are scattered through a considerable number of volumes in the CO series, and I have constructed an incomplete data base from CO 7331, 7332, 7388, CO 7424, CO 7501, CO 7972, CO 7973 and CO 7975, variously headed staff applications, appointments and allowances, nurses, attendants etc. or simply 'Valkenberg, Health branch'.
41 CO 7179 Dodds to UCS, 27 November 1897.
42 CO 7501 Folio 610 Dodds to UCS, 4 June 1903.
43 CO 7331 Dodds to Agent General, 8 July 1897.
44 The first clerk/storekeeper was paid 11s. a day without board, the male attendants started at 2s.9d. a day with board, lodgings and uniforms; when an attendant was transferred to the position of dairyman, he received a rise to 3s.4d., with board but not lodging. Female 'nurses' received a starting wage of 1s.11d., which went up to 2s.2d. once they had served their probationary three months, while the kitchen maid received 1s.4d. Two male labourers were hired at 3s. a day, and the man in charge of the garden and farm was paid £10 a month. CO 1488 Dodds to UCS 10 May 1891; CO 1488 Dodds to UCS, February 1891, 18 March 1891, 21 May 1891.
45 E.g. CO 7177 Dodds to UCS, 7 July 1896 reported the pilfering of a shirt and pillow case by the Assistant Laundress, Marie Williams. For this offence she was given five days hard labour, and dismissed.
46 CO 7424 Dodds to UCS, 2 June 1897.
47 See, for example, CO 1576 Dodds to UCS, 16 July 1893; CO 7388 Dodds to UCS, 10 May 1899; CO 7973, Dodds to UCS, 1 June 1906 and CO 7918 UCS to Dodds, June 1909.
48 CO 1576 Dodds to UCS, 16 July 1893; CO 7388 Dodds to UCS, 10 May 1899. Artisans were now being paid between 3s. and 3s.10d. a day while attendants were paid 3s. in their first two years, 3s.4d. in their third year. By

way of comparison, in 1898 good carpenters in Cape Town commanded 11s. a day. CO 7179 Dodds to UCS, 7 May 1898.

49 As Inspector of Asylums Dodds made the extraction of all accidents from the Accident register and their despatch to the Colonial Office compulsory for all asylums. It is of course difficult to gauge how effective this was in practice.

50 CO 7826 'A.P-L' 23–10–10 No addressee. 'A.P-L.', formerly matron at Grahamstown and Robben Island Asylums, was a patient at Valkenberg intermittently between 1899 and 1921 when she died. Her letters preserved in the CO series and directed to – inter alia – the King, the Governor General and the Medical Council provide a rare insight into asylum practices, although they have to be read with caution. I hope to deal with patients' perceptions more fully in another paper.

51 CO 7179 Dodds to CS, 25 March 1902.

52 Deacon, 'A history of the medical institutions on Robben Island', p. 26.

53 'Colonialism and the production of psychiatric knowledge', p. 153.

54 Ibid.

55 CO 7971 OVR, J. Waterston, 28 August 1908, Waterston. Among the first fourteen women students to study at the London School of Medicine for Women, Jane Waterston had experience as a missionary and mission doctor before taking up practice in Cape Town in 1883; in 1887–8 she qualified further, as a surgeon in Edinburgh, and took her MD in Brussels and the Certificate in Psychological Medicine from the Medico-Psychological Association of Great Britain.

56 See SC 14–'13. *Report and Minutes of the Select Committee on the Treatment of Lunatics*, Government Printer, Cape Town, 1913; Swartz, 'Colonialism and the production of psychiatric knowledge', pp. 143–4.

57 For the centrality of classification to 'moral treatment', see Andrew Scull, *The Most Solitary of Afflictions. Madness and Society in Britain 1700–1900*, New Haven and London, Yale University Press, 1993, p. 170. Cf. discussion in Melling essay above.

58 See J. Andrews, 'Raising the tone of asylumdom', above, p. 200.

59 G.17 – '93 *Annual Reports, 1892*, I Valkenberg Asylum, pp. 5–6.

60 G.37-'91. *Annual Reports 1890*, Inspector's Report on the Old Somerset Hospital, p. 19. See also CO 1524: Report of Inspection of Asylums on RI, 7 June 1892.

61 For Greenlees, see S. Dubow, *Scientific Racism in Modern South Africa*, Cambridge, 1995, p. 201; McCulloch, *Colonial Psychiatry*, p. 46; Vaughan, *Curing their Ills*, pp. 121–2.

62 CO 7175 Dodds to UCS, 27–28 June 1894.

63 G.16 – 1895, *Annual Reports, 1894*, 'Report of Inspector of Asylums', p. 156.

64 CO 1524: Report on Robben Island, 7 June 1892.

65 See e.g. CO 7971 Précis of Official Visitor's Report [Dodds] on Inspection of Asylums on RI on 25 July 1901.

66 Swartz, 'Colonialism and the production of psychiatric knowledge', pp. 9–10.

67 *Select Committee, 1913*, Evidence, Dr Dodds, p. 9. For African antipathy to the asylum, see Sapire and Edgar, *Divine Madness*.

68 K. Figlio, 'Chlorosis and chronic disease in nineteenth-century Britain; the social constitution of somatic illness in a capitalist society', *Social History*, 3, 2, 1978, p. 176.

69 Van Heyningen, 'Public health', pp. 101–2.
70 CO 7175 Report on Visit to Grahamstown Asylum, 19–20 November 1894.
71 CO 7175 10 December 1894, cited in Swartz, 'Colonialism and the production of psychiatric knowledge', p. 126.
72 CO 7176 15 January 1895, also cited in Swartz, 'Colonialism and the production of psychiatric knowledge'.
73 CO 7176 Report of Inspector of Asylums Dodds, 14 January 1895 with comments from Superintendent of the Graham's Town Asylum.
74 Cited in Warwick, 'Mental health care at Valkenberg Asylum', pp. 31–2.
75 CO 7177 Minute, Dodds to UCS, 8 May 1896 and Te Water's minute on this 15 May 1896.
76 'Black insane at the Cape', p. 403.
77 See, for example, his 'Statistics of insanity in Grahamstown Asylum', *South African Medical Record*, 3, 1905, pp. 217–24.
78 Kenan Malik, *The Meaning of Race. Race, History and Culture in Western Society*, Basingstoke, Macmillan, 1996, p. 6.

Part V

REFLECTIONS

14

RETHINKING THE HISTORY OF ASYLUMDOM

Andrew Scull

Listening to the papers presented at Exeter's conference of the Society for the Social History of Medicine and revisiting them again as I prepare a response for the present volume, it is an odd feeling to watch one's passage from the status of the arch-revisionist and 'Marxist' *enfant terrible* of the field to the very different position of orthodox authority and Aunt Sally figure against which a new generation of scholars seeks to prove its mettle. The invitation to offer a reflective essay on the research presented in this collection and a considered reading of the chapters thus gives rise to conflicting emotions. These include amusement at the irony of the situation; bemusement at the apparent misconstruing of some of my views (a reminder, one ruefully realises, that texts, once published, are no longer wholly one's own); a natural distaste at having to swallow what I know is a salutary dose of humility when confronted by stark evidence of sins of both omission and commission; and an amply compensating degree of pleasure at fresh opportunities to engage in intellectual debate. There is also the satisfaction in recording how much richer and more sophisticated the historiography of psychiatry has become over the past quarter century, in which one's own ideas, research and writing have played some part.

It should be said at the outset that only some aspects of the intellectual growth and expansion that have marked the field are on view here. Chronologically and substantively, the research reported in these pages pays only passing attention to some of the central themes of much recent historiography, and entirely ignores others. For example, like most of the first generation of what has loosely been called the revisionist history of psychiatry, the attention of the historians in this volume remains almost exclusively focused on the long nineteenth century – the era that, *pace* Foucault, truly marked the birth of the Great Confinement of the mad. Yet one of the most exciting recent developments in the history of psychiatry has been the remarkably expanded temporal sweep that has characterised its scholarship: back into the seventeenth and eighteenth centuries, and forward into what, for a few more months, we can call our own century. Likewise, the present volume pays little attention to medical therapeutics – what alienists did for and to their patients in the name of treatment. It devotes only a limited amount of space to another issue that has consumed much scholarly energy and ingenuity, recovering the perspectives of patients and their families. As for the issues surrounding the constitution of a profession of psychiatry and the content of that emerging profession's claims to expertise, these are at best addressed tangentially and indirectly, though they have been a vexed subject, the site of much lively and provocative debate. Nor can one avoid noticing that the essays in this book are exclusively the work of social historians. Left to one side are the perspectives and preoccupations of a new and more sophisticated generation of clinician-historians, whose work has greatly enlivened and enriched the scholarly conversation about the history of madness.

One could extend this list further without much difficulty, and yet to do so would be, in important ways, to miss the point. For the decision to ignore these wider horizons was, of course, a self-conscious one, and in my view (perhaps entitled to some weight since I had no role in planning the proceedings and hence have no vested interest in defending the choices others made) an eminently sensible and defensible one. To have aspired to a comprehensive overview of the enormous territory the history of psychiatry has now become would necessarily have courted the danger of superficiality, and would certainly have produced an elephantine volume. Moreover, in restricting attention to the rise of the asylum in England and its empire, Joseph Melling and Bill Forsythe have returned us to a set of concerns that were understandably and rightly placed at front and centre stage when the history of insanity first began to command serious attention from professional historians.

The 'revisionist' history of insanity and asylumdom

As its subtitle announced, my own *Museums of Madness* attempted a comprehensive examination of 'the social organisation of insanity in nineteenth-century England'. Looking back some two decades after I completed the book, it occurs to me that my original training as a sociologist is reflected, not just in the kinds of issues and the intellectual resources I drew upon in the course of my research, but also in the *chutzpah* of attempting a grand synthesis of this sort, given the impoverished state of the then-extant historiography. A historian in the early stages of his or her career would almost certainly have chosen (or been counselled) to focus on a more manageable piece of the larger puzzle. In all probability, it was only my status as a disciplinary outsider that allowed and encouraged me, in my first foray into the field, to attempt to provide a global interpretation of such a vast territory: one that sought to encompass the rise of the asylum; the emergence and consolidation of what became the profession of psychiatry; the changing contours of insanity over the course of a century and more; and the relationship of all these to the nineteenth-century revolution in government, to the 'reformed' Poor Law, and to the Great Transformation of English society.

I hasten to add that in speaking of the field as it existed in the early 1970s as 'impoverished', I do not mean to imply that, before I wrote on the subject, it was bereft of scholarship of lasting value. That would be a claim of quite astonishing solipsism and conceit. Moreover, so far from seeking to denigrate the efforts of all those who went before me, I yield to no one, for example, in my admiration for the pioneering researches of William Parry-Jones into 'the trade in lunacy', or the wide-ranging scholarship of Richard Hunter and Ida Macalpine, whether embodied in their remarkable series of introductions to the facsimile editions of nineteenth-century monographs, in their provocative reinterpretation of the 'madness' of George III, or their extraordinarily useful annotated compilation of texts, *Three Hundred Years of Psychiatry*. Yet for all their virtues, these contributions examined only very limited portions of the terrain I sought to explore.

Whatever the merits of the particular answers it provided, I suspect that few would dispute the claim that the polemical edge of the arguments set forth in *Museums of Madness* has served at the very least as a provocation to other scholars. I think, too, that the range of issues addressed in that book has helped to encourage the sustained examination and interrogation of a much broader array of primary materials, as part of the attempt to understand just what was distinctive and different about nineteenth-century efforts to manage the mad. For, regardless of my disciplinary origins, I have always shared the historian's commitment to original archival research and, from the very outset, I insisted on moving beyond the records of parliamentary inquiries and the minutiae of the statute book. Within a few years, Michael MacDonald and Roy Porter had joined the conversation, making the seventeenth and eighteenth centuries the respective focus of most of their scholarship.[1] Gifted historians both, they drew upon a still broader range of source materials, and brought to the fore still other issues that my own work had ignored or distinctly underplayed. The cultural meanings of madness, the role of religious ideas and of the fear of 'enthusiasm', and the effort to recover the patients' perspectives were all especially notable aspects of their work, themes that one can now see being developed in work being done on the nineteenth century, and issues of great importance that I have tried to respond to in some of my own more recent research and writing.

MacDonald, Porter and I all, I think, exhibit a distinctly ambivalent attitude to the work of Michel Foucault, and yet it is also fair to add that in no small measure it was probably his wide-ranging speculations that attracted us to the field in the first place. Indeed, I suppose that the very ambition and sweep of Foucault's scholarship may have found some Anglo-Saxon echoes in our separate efforts to grapple across the centuries with the transformation of social ideas and practices *vis-à-vis* the insane. Our work, too, was very much influenced by and responsive to trends in what was then quite literally 'the new social history', and its emphasis on 'history from below' and recovering the perspectives of the poor and the powerless made it quite natural that this should be so. If my own writing was more heavily indebted than MacDonald's or Porter's to the work of such *marxisant* scholars as Edward Thompson and Eric Hobsbawm, more than likely this once more reflected my sociological leanings. It is to my sociological training, too, that I would trace my persistent concern with trying to link the history of madness to broader changes in English society's political, economic and social structures, and in the intellectual and cultural horizons of its people.[2]

Others have since expanded those efforts in diverse and extraordinarily fruitful directions, many of which are on display in this volume. It is both understandable and essential that much of this recent work directs its attention away from the more macro-social concerns that are a central part of many of my writings, and indeed that much contemporary scholarship uses its tighter focus to hold up to scrutiny some of my bolder and, it may be, ultimately indefensible hypotheses. At the same time, I hope it will not be taken amiss if I hoist a caution flag. We need to be careful lest in our fascination with the details we find ourselves retreating back into a sort of neo-solipsism, a narrow and constricted vision that flattens and distorts our sense of perspective, and leaves in obscurity aspects of historical reality that acquire meaning only when placed in a larger contextual frame. It is well to uncover the premises of what purport to be synthetic accounts of nineteenth-century developments, and to confront general models with detailed empirical analyses. Only in this way can we hope to develop a more subtle and sophisticated understanding of asylumdom and expose the limitations of previous generalisations. But it is equally vital that we acknowledge that we can only achieve this larger aim if we are willing to make explicit how these micro-researches bear upon larger theoretical issues, if we consciously seek to show the more general significance of a given set of phenomena and to transcend the particularities of person and place.[3] Precisely because constructing general models involves intellectual risk, invites inevitable criticism and ultimately must produce understandings later scholars will show are partial or misguided, there are temptations to shy away, to retreat into an increasingly mindless empiricism. That all-too-human tendency must, in my view, be resisted if the field is to develop as I hope it will continue to do.

The new research in insanity and institutions

Lunacy reform in England and Wales, with its emphasis on asylum-based care for the insane, a central inspectorate and oversight from Whitehall, and a compulsory network of institutions for the pauper insane, was in all respects a drawn-out affair. Not least, it depended upon (and helped to produce) an important set of changes in the relationships between centre and periphery, changes that I have long argued were intimately linked to the transformation of the Old Poor Law into the New.[4] In their several ways, the chapters written by Smith, by Bartlett, and by Forsythe, Melling and Adair, are all concerned to address vital aspects of these interrelated phenomena.

Smith's research emphasises the degree to which the new county asylums were in clear competition with the developing private sector, a situation which, as he has discussed elsewhere, gave rise to some well-elaborated and damaging criticism of public asylums by the proprietors of rival private establishments.[5] He underlines, too, some of the obstacles to combining pauper and paying patients within a single institution, difficulties that beyond the mid-century would lead to the rigorous separation and segregation of the two categories into separate systems of care. In my view, however, he underplays some of the connections that clearly existed between all three elements in his mixed economy of care. These include, most notably, the tendency of the new public asylums to draw upon the private and charitable sectors for models of administrative organisation and even for personnel. Here is surely one important source of the diversity in the approaches and therapeutic regimes adopted in the county asylums, corresponding as it did to the considerable variability in the character of the existing madhouses and those who ran them.[6]

On one central conclusion we do concur: that 'the pursuit of "economy" in financial management became a preoccupation of the justices' and was of over-riding importance in determining the character of the emerging public sector in ways that were manifest even before the 1845 legislation made the provision of tax-supported asylum accommodation compulsory throughout England and Wales.[7] We disagree, though, on a central interpretative issue that flows from this reality. I do not think, *pace* Smith, that '[county asylums] evidently succeeded at least sufficiently to provide the lunacy reformers with the rationale for the creation of the universal county asylum system'. Rather, I would argue (and have argued elsewhere),[8] that the reformers were so committed to an institutional approach, and so determined to attribute the defects of existing provision to the intrusion of the profit motive, that they blinded themselves to the accumulating evidence of the contradictions and defects embedded in their schemes, and the fragility of the assumptions upon which their plans rested.

In important ways, of course, the character of the emerging publicly funded system flowed, as Peter Bartlett reminds us, from the fact that 'the county asylum was...an institution legally based in the Poor Law, administered primarily by Poor Law officials, and directed at paupers'. As he rightly insists, one substantially neglected aspect of this connection to the Poor Law was the continuing reliance upon workhouse provision for a significant portion of the pauper insane even in the aftermath of the 1845 legislation. Previous histories, my own prominent among them, have done little more than allude to this continuing role for the workhouse, to the periodic objections of the Lunacy Commissioners to the practice, and to the parsimony of the Poor Law officials whom they blamed for its persistence.[9] But, particularly when one recalls that throughout the century workhouses continued to absorb as many as a quarter of those officially labelled as lunatic, such cursory remarks scarcely amount to an adequate exploration of their role in the overall structure of care and control. Bartlett's own researches, based on materials from Leicestershire, usefully commence that process of exploration, suggesting, for example, that the official mythologies contrasting the intentionally unpleasant workhouse and the much more attractive asylum may represent a substantial over-simplification and distortion of a more complex reality; and that manageability rather than the nature of an individual's mental defect may have strongly influenced consignment to one type of facility or the other.

Forsythe, Melling and Adair emphasise a different aspect of the intersection of the Poor Law and the county asylum system – the persistent and often flagrant disregard of the lunacy laws on the part of both Poor Law Guardians and the Poor Law and Local Government Boards; and the equally persistent efforts of the Lunacy Commissioners to circumvent the passive–aggressive tactics of these authorities by linking up with local elites who sympathised with the Commission's goals. Forsythe and his colleagues suggest that other historians who have examined these conflicts have tended to portray the Lunacy Commission as weak and conciliatory, shying away from conflict and incapable of imposing their will on recalcitrant local authorities. By contrast, using data drawn from their extensive investigation of developments in Devonshire during the Victorian period, Forsythe *et al.* demonstrate that the Commissioners made an active and forceful series of attempts to overcome local opposition, and to compel decreased reliance upon the private madhouse sector or the workhouse, particularly on the part of the boroughs of Plymouth and Exeter. On these central issues, the Commission eventually prevailed (though its 'victories' often had a Pyrrhic quality, in view of the deterioration of asylum conditions that mark these same years).

My own researches suggest that these findings can in many respects be generalised beyond the confines of a single south-western county. In the decade and a half following the passage of the 1845 Asylums Act, for example, the Lunacy Commission was confronted with an array of reluctant and recalcitrant local authorities, ranging from the City of London to such rural counties as Cambridgeshire, Buckinghamshire and Sussex. Continuous discreet pressure from their Whitehall offices eventually wore down the opposition of all but the most determined adversaries.[10] Likewise, there are obvious parallels between the Commissioners' tactics in their long struggle to compel the boroughs of Plymouth and Exeter to construct their own asylums, instead of relying on contracts with the county asylum or the private sector, and their similar campaign in the late 1870s to force the Northamptonshire magistrates to abandon their long-standing contractual arrangement with the local charity asylum, the Northampton General Lunatic Asylum, and instead build a separate rate-supported pauper asylum.[11]

If these findings, and those reported elsewhere in Nicholas Hervey's remarkable path-breaking work,[12] suggest a less passive picture of the Commission's activities and influence than can be found in the work of such scholars as D.J. Mellett[13] and Peter Bartlett,[14] one must none the less be careful not to exaggerate the amount of revisionism they license. For, as a careful reading of the Forsythe, Melling, and Adair chapter makes clear, though the Commission did provide a substantial measure of central regulation over the asylum, its powers in other respects certainly remained sharply limited and circumscribed. As I have noted elsewhere, particularly on such crucial questions as size and overcrowding, and on the use of workhouses as alternative sites of confinement for the chronic and apparently harmless, the Lunacy Commissioners met with nothing but frustration and rebuffs.[15] What Forsythe *et al.* refer to as 'the unrelenting expansion' of asylumdom in the Victorian years was both accompanied by and in substantial measure provoked by the accumulation of chronic patients and a growing pessimism about the prospects for their cure. But if, as they note, 'many of the seminal revisionist texts published in the 1970s' (including my own work) provided an exaggerated portrait of the self-enclosed and isolated character of Victorian museums of madness, scholars in more recent years have rightly insisted on a more nuanced approach. Beginning with John Walton's seminal essay on 'Casting out and bringing back in Victorian England',[16] we have seen a growing interest in uncovering the complexity of the linkages between family, community and asylum, and an insistence that the boundary between the asylum and the larger society was always somewhat more porous than an earlier generation of studies had allowed or implied. Such themes can be seen to emerge indirectly in Hilary Marland's chapter on puerperal insanity, in part because this condition often proved to be a temporary aberration, one that contributed to higher rates of recovery and discharge (if also being a condition that was often treated in non-asylum settings). Here, beyond cavil, was one form of madness that was unambiguously a 'female malady'[17] (albeit one which frequently had an atypically benign outcome), and Marland's chapter serves to remind us that the relationship between gender and mental disorder has been a much studied aspect of the historiography of psychiatry in recent years.

In *The Most Solitary of Afflictions*, I sought to take on board some of the implications of the recent emphasis on the permeability of institutional walls, and to amplify how family and kinship structures were connected to the development of asylumdom and to the rising tide of asylum admissions between 1845 and 1890.[18] There is ample scope, however, for further work along these lines, and we (I) should expect that the findings of these newer, more detailed studies, will extend and modify, perhaps in some highly significant ways, the suggestions I have previously advanced about these connections. Indeed, some of those necessary correctives have already begun to appear, not least in the work of the scholars who have edited this book.[19]

David Wright's chapter on the institutional discharge of lunatics in nineteenth-century Buckinghamshire thus forms part of a larger body of recent scholarship that has begun to open up these issues to sustained scrutiny. His essay is the more notable because so much of the previous work in this area, whether focused on the rich or the poor, has restricted its attention to the social context of the commitment process. Ironically enough, as with confinement, discharge too was something asylum superintendents generally had little control over, with both admission and release of the pauper insane legally left in the hands of the lay committee of magistrates which oversaw each county asylum. Consistent with the findings of other recent studies,[20] Wright's demographic data indicate that as many as one-third of new admissions were discharged within twelve months. More striking, I think, is his marshalling of considerable if fragmentary qualitative evidence in support of a persuasive argument that social and economic factors, together with prudential concerns over potential violent or suicidal behaviour, were more important influences in determining movement into and out of an asylum than were 'medical' evaluations or medical personnel.

Wright's narrative emphasises the importance of a variety of actors in understanding the complexities of the discharge process, in many ways the least prominent of whom are the alienists themselves. Crucially, in the background and influencing much of what occurred is the structural issue of the availability of beds in the asylum. Setting this contextual factor aside, however, it was the ability and willingness of patients' families to absorb particular individuals back into the household, regardless of continuing mental disturbances and infirmities, and the predilections and preferences of the magistrates and Poor Law officials, that together must be seen as the central determinants of decisions over discharge or retention within the confines of the asylum.

Akihito Suzuki's fascinating chapter has a very different focus, but it too emphasises the importance of examining a particular class of events (in this instance the construction of aetiological accounts of the origins of mental disorder) through the prism of the activities and perspectives of several disparate sets of actors: asylum doctors, patients, and patients' families and friends. The relationships between these intimately intertwined groups were far from static over the course of the century, and from the case books of Bedlam itself, Suzuki teases out the ambiguities that surrounded the heightened attention to patient subjectivity that emerged under the superintendency of William Charles Hood. Not least these include the paradoxical and hitherto obscured links between an alienist's struggle for greater authority over his territory and his apparent willingness to listen more carefully to the hitherto hushed voices of the lunatic. The Victorian '*grand refermement*' of the insane[21] has till now been seen as a decisive step to shut up the mad, silencing as well as physically isolating the forces of Unreason. As Foucault memorably phrased it, in the era ushered in by Pinel and Tuke:

> the dialogue of delirium and insult gave way to a monologue in a language which exhausted itself in the silence of others.... Delivered from his chains, [the madman] is now chained, by silence, to transgression and to shame...silence was absolute and there was no longer any common language between madness and reason...[22]

Perhaps, as we are now urged to see, the reality was less straightforward than that.

At the very least, Suzuki succeeds in showing us some very subtle ways by which asylum case books can be exploited to reveal both lay and professional attempts to decode the aetiology of madness; and in making manifest still another dimension of the shifting balance of power and authority over the understanding of madness that was one of the most notable consequences of the triumph of asylumdom in the Victorian age. The case books, of course, constitute one of the most voluminous arrays of manuscript material thrown up by the age of the asylum, and though exploitation of this mass of material remains in its infancy, the very existence of such extensive archival material is now exercising an almost irresistible fascination for historians.[23] Not least, there is the hope that it will offer us a window into the world of the patients, albeit a view refracted for the most part through the eyes and hands of those who ran the institutions in which they were confined, and who recorded the views and behaviours of the inmates for their own peculiar purposes.

Between them, Smith, Bartlett, Wright, Marland, and Suzuki, and Forsythe, Melling and Adair cover a wide range of issues, and approach them from sometimes quite distinctive points of view. They all share, however, a focus on developments in England, and in this they follow in the footsteps of the first generation of modern scholarship that appeared in the 1970s. The English experience, though, was in a number of ways distinct and sometimes radically different from what occurred elsewhere in the lands ruled directly or indirectly from Whitehall, and the remainder of the chapters appearing in this volume both remind us that England was indeed distinctive, and begin the process of specifying the nature of the differences as well as the commonalties among the Celtic fringe, and in more far-flung imperial territories with respect to the treatment of the mad.

The peculiarities and particularities of the Welsh experience are especially fascinating, since the 1845 legislation which made pauper asylums compulsory and established the Lunacy Commission specifically applied to Wales as well as England. None the less, as Pamela Michael and David Hirst make clear, the history of asylumdom in Wales is by no means identical with its English counterpart, despite the common legal framework. In my own work, I have previously stressed the connections between the persistence of subsistence farming and quasi-feudal social and economic structures, and of older, family-based responses to insanity – speculating that the very economic 'backwardness' of the Welsh countryside, bringing with it a certain insulation from the corrosive effects of capitalism on the strength of family ties, perhaps helps us to understand the inhabitants' lack of enthusiasm for consigning their troublesome relatives to the asylum.[24] Certainly, a special case-by-case investigation by the Lunacy Commissioners in 1875 into the care of lunatics kept in the community in Cardiganshire, Carmarthenshire and Pembrokeshire, and conducted with the aid of a Welsh interpreter, found their relatives vehemently opposed to institutionalisation – and these amounted to some 60 per cent of the lunatics known to the authorities.[25] Looking instead at North Wales, Michael and Hirst observe the same 'clear fracture between the new, modern standards represented by asylum care, but requiring state intervention and control, and the older familistic patterns of domestic solutions'. In the process, they provide us with a more detailed and nuanced analysis of the slow erosion of local customs, and once more of the complex interactions between workhouse, asylum and local communities.

Scotland presents a different picture again, for beginning in the late eighteenth century it evolved its own distinctive approach to the management of the mad, a decentralised system which depended upon a combination of family care, the boarding out of harmless lunatics with strangers, and the limited accommodation provided by a handful of charity asylums, the so-called 'royal asylums'. The first of these was the Montrose Asylum, founded in 1781. Others were subsequently established at Aberdeen (1800), Edinburgh (1813), Glasgow (1814), Dundee (1820), Perth (1826) and, finally, at Dumfries (1839).[26] The Scots were determined to resist anything which breached the foundation principles of their own Poor Law system and might set a precedent for replacing voluntary, religiously motivated charity with state-financed relief and compulsory taxation. Parsimonious Presbyterians, they despised the English Poor Law, and fought fiercely against legislative schemes they (rightly) saw would do much to extend Whitehall's control and influence into Scotland. Only the outside intervention of the famous American moral entrepreneur, Dorothea Dix, in the mid-1850s, eventually forced the Scots into a partial retreat, and prompted the imposition of at least some elements of the dreaded English system north of the border.[27] And even then, the Scottish approach to the management of the mad retained some quite distinctive features of its own.

Yet despite its quite distinctive trajectory, the history of psychiatry in Scotland has till recently attracted remarkably little attention from historians. Led by Allan Beveridge and Jonathan Andrews, however, a group of younger scholars has now begun to explore this largely virgin territory. The chapters in this volume by Lorraine Walsh and Andrews himself both exemplify this growing interest, and usefully expand our still meagre knowledge of the foundation and functioning of the Scottish royal asylums. Walsh's chapter provides a series of fascinating insights into the difficulties of the Dundee Asylum, placing her findings firmly in the larger political and cultural context alluded to above. The over-riding importance of the heritors' resistance to interference from Westminster, and the subsidiary but still vital impact of the constant struggle to remain solvent, issues of class and classification, and the shifting balance between cure and custodial care all figure prominently in her account, which paints a dismal picture of the essential demise of an institution intended as 'the pride and ornament of the town which gave it birth'.

Jonathan Andrews' chapter focuses most of its attention on one of these issues – the tendency over time for royal asylums (in his case the Glasgow Asylum) to renege on their commitment to provide for the poor, opting instead to expel the pauper insane and move smartly up-market. His analysis, however, is framed without a larger context, that of examining Scottish developments alongside what he takes to be 'Scull's historiographic models'. And here, I have to say, there is far less in dispute between the two of us than he appears to realise. Indeed, so far from wanting to dispute most of the points he makes on historiographic issues, I find myself in fundamental agreement with him, and am puzzled to find that he discerns such an intellectual gulf between us.

Let me briefly spell out what the apparent points in dispute are, and then clarify my own views on the underlying issues. Andrews criticises my arguments on a variety of fronts: for claiming that the new museums of madness were filled by the aggrandising activities of the psychiatric profession itself, extending the boundaries of madness, and remodelling the old regime madhouse so as to deprive incarceration of much of its former stigma; for failing to acknowledge that 'there continued to be considerable opposition from various groups, including local authorities, families, and guardians to removing pauper lunatics to asylums'; and for neglecting to note that 'there were fundamental differences between England and Scotland in both the timing and type of provision that was available was to be developed for the pauper insane'. These are, if warranted, serious criticisms. But are these really the positions I have taken on the issues at hand?

A great deal of my work has been taken up with the questions surrounding 'the transformation of the mad-doctoring trade', and from *Museums of Madness* through *The Most Solitary of Afflictions* to *Masters of Bedlam* a recurrent theme of much of my writing on insanity has been concerned with issues surrounding the emergence and consolidation of what became the modern profession of psychiatry, and the growth and development of a collective consciousness and organisation among this sub-set of medical men. It is quite reasonable to assert that in these books and elsewhere I portray alienists as seeking to transform the ancient image of the madhouse in more salubrious directions (as indeed they did). It is also fair to suggest that my portrait of the developing profession places considerable stress upon its active and entrepreneurial efforts to define and extend its jurisdiction, in the process providing medical accounts of a wide range of putatively pathological behaviours and mental states. It is quite another matter, however, to claim that I see professional imperialism as the main source of the expansion of the boundaries of madness; or that I view the psychiatric profession as a nefarious, all-powerful entity that gave birth to nineteenth-century asylumdom. To the contrary, I argue forcibly and explicitly for a very different set of conclusions.

> One must beware [as I've put it more than once], of the tendency to conclude that the mere existence of even a considerable degree of professional imperialism provides a sufficient explanation of the ever wider practical application of the term insanity....The initiative required to launch the process of casting out the undesirable from the community and into the asylum necessarily rested mostly in non-medical hands – whether this meant the lunatic's own family, or those in authority (employers, police, magistrates, and workhouse masters, as well as the occasional workhouse doctor). So that it is to this extra-professional world that one must look for the sources of a more expansive view of madness.[28]

And as for the claim that I portray nineteenth-century psychiatry as a powerful, imperialistic profession, I have, on the contrary, repeatedly stressed its weakness and heavily circumscribed powers, pointing out that even in the early twentieth century,

> alienism remained from many points of view a quite marginal specialty, uncertain of its own profile and prospects, and riven by sharp internal divisions and disputes....Mad-doctoring transformed remained a hobbled and stigmatised enterprise – handicapped not just by the limitations of its own knowledge and capacities, but also by its own internal divisions, and by the disdain and distrust that...have long marked society's attitudes to the mad and their keepers.[29]

What of the continuing opposition from Poor Law authorities, the community at large, and patients' families to placing lunatics in asylums? I have discussed at some length the often fierce resistance to and resentment of asylumdom one finds in many quarters, even as late as the 1870s and 1880s.[30] At the level of the family, moreover, I have pointed out that 'the relatives of the mad plainly possessed more ambivalent attitudes [than others] towards the asylum...both the comments of alienists in the admissions registers, and the fact that the stigma of confinement in county asylums was compounded by an association with the Poor Law, leave little doubt [of] that'.[31]

Finally, Andrews and I essentially agree about the differences between England and Scotland. *Museums of Madness*, it should be remembered, explicitly claimed to be (as its subtitle proclaimed) about the social organisation of insanity in nineteenth-century *England*. And subsequently (as I have partially indicated above), I have written directly on the peculiarities and particularities of Scottish responses to insanity, both in a lengthy introduction to the reprint edition of W.A.F. Browne's *What Asylums Were, Are, and Ought to Be*[32] and in substantial portions of *Masters of Bedlam*.[33] In practice, then, I think it is fair to say that the differences that exist between Andrews and myself on these issues are in reality more matters of nuance and emphasis than the fundamental conflicts over basic questions of interpretation he seems to think are present. On other fronts, meanwhile, his analysis of developments in Glasgow extends and deepens our knowledge in a variety of important ways. I was particularly struck by his analysis of the connections between the establishment of publicly funded parochial and district asylums from the 1860s onwards, and the expulsion of pauper patients from the older royal asylums, which now moved sharply up-market in terms of both facilities and clientele. (Here, I think one could potentially make useful and instructive comparisons with the very similar patterns one can observe in the United States among the so-called corporate asylums – places like the Mclean Asylum, the Pennsylvania Asylum, the Hartford Retreat, and the Bloomingdale Asylum.)[34] Salutary, too, are his emphases on the fallacies of speaking of pauper lunatics as though they constituted a single, homogeneous category; and his elaboration of a number of important aspects of 'the peculiarities of the Scots' when it came to handling the mad.

If lunacy reform was delayed and shaped in England by an aversion to the concentration of power at the national level that was extraordinarily widespread and well entrenched on both the structural and ideological levels, and if Scottish responses likewise reflected a rooted opposition to the spread of Sassenach approaches to poverty and dependency north of the border and the political capacity – displayed over decades – to block interference from Westminster, it must be emphasised that Ireland's status as a colony, ruled directly from Dublin Castle, had its own peculiar effects on the local fate of the insane. Mark Finnane's history of *Insanity and the Insane in Post-Famine Ireland*[35] emphasised some time ago that 'the especially powerful position of the state in early nineteenth century Ireland' allowed the English authorities 'to govern in a highly interventionist style [even] in the early nineteenth century'.[36] The result was an earlier and easier adoption of an asylum-based solution to the problems posed by the insane, and an expansion of the system at a more rapid rate than can be observed in either Scotland or England, so that 'by 1914 Ireland had a quite massive proportion of asylum beds'.[37]

Oonagh Walsh uses an intensive study of the case records of the Connaught District Asylum in a single year, 1893, to raise interesting questions about the confinement of the mad in one of the large pauper institutions the English created to confine crazy Irish men and women. Not least, she suggests that the patients at least occasionally were something more than simply passive victims, and that their relations, for their part, could be more active still in attempting to exploit the asylum system for their own advantage. Within limits, there is clearly something to both contentions. Still, I have to confess that I think there is a real risk that such arguments may be pushed too far. It is currently fashionable to insist on uncovering autonomy and agency where previously historians detected only subservience and control. And this may be salutary to a point, so long as we do not lose sight of massive asymmetries of power and privilege, and continue to recognise how partial, limited and constrained were the capacities and choices of those who made up the bulk of asylumdom's clientele – pauper patients and families alike.

Moving beyond the semi-colonial status of Ireland and the Irish, Shula Marks and Waltraud Ernst examine events in more far-flung imperial territories, the Cape Colony, South Africa, and India respectively. In South Africa, Marks shows, there was no systematic policy of repatriation, nor, till very late in the nineteenth century, any specialised colonial psychiatric institution. For much of the Victorian age, though 'the "moral management" of the insane had long been a touchstone of metropolitan progress', the colonists muddled along, pragmatically making use of prisons, gaols and beds in the infirmary for lepers and the chronically sick for their mad folk, and only haltingly beginning to adopt the asylum solution in the last twenty-five years of Victoria's long reign. Once launched down this pathway, however, here too the influence of the metropolis proved pervasive. In Marks's words, 'What is striking about Cape Town's Valkenberg Hospital built in the last decade of the nineteenth century is how similar its institutional history is to the story of the British county asylums – and how very different its context.' It is to that very different context that she turns at the last, seeking – as Jonathan Sadowsky has recently done for colonial Nigeria[38] – to spell out just what was distinctive about psychiatry transplanted to imperial climes.

Looking at 'the jewel in the crown', we see that policy here assumed very different forms, emphasising the point that imperialism had many guises and disguises. In India, within a larger and more elaborately structured colonial society, the symbolic values of the asylum as 'the most blessed manifestation of true civilisation the world can present',[39] led, as Waltraud Ernst shows, to early adoption of metropolitan customs in the management of madness – mostly for members of the Anglo-Indian community, but also, on a far smaller and uneven scale, for some of the 'natives' as well. Though at first these establishments were more important on a rhetorical than a practical level, Ernst argues that they were an essential prop for the preservation of the image and authority of colonial rule, not least by rendering the irrational (who might lower 'the European Character in the eyes of the Natives') invisible through incarceration – a strategy of isolation backed up by repatriation of those who failed to recover. Here was a more permanent method of placing such persons 'out of sight' as well as 'out of mind'.

Recording the past

The chapters in this volume thus offer a rich array of commentary upon and empirical findings about nineteenth-century responses to insanity. The flourishing state of current research in the field is, however, wholly dependent on the survival and accessibility of relevant materials – most especially, of course, the written record on which all historians are necessarily dependent; but also, for certain purposes, physical objects, most notably the built forms, the 'museums of madness' that for so long haunted the countryside and provided mute testimony to the emergence of segregative responses to the management of the mad. And on both of these issues, there are grounds for worry and concern.

I vividly recall, despite the passage of more than a quarter century, the variety of sites and settings in which I encountered the raw materials that formed the basis for *Museums of Madness*. Sometimes, as, for example, at St Crispins (the old Northampton County Lunatic Asylum), the records had been meticulously stored in a fire-proof vault, from which they were retrieved piecemeal over the course of my researches. At other times, as in the case of Roundway Hospital in Devizes (the old Wiltshire County Asylum), nineteenth-century records were stored higgledy-piggledy amid the debris of its late-twentieth-century operations, in a filthy basement amidst leaky pipes and scurrying representatives of the insect kingdom. Then there were places like St John's Hospital, Aylesbury (the Buckinghamshire County Lunatic Asylum), where prior to being granted access to an unusually rich array of records, as a callow graduate student I had to pass muster at an interview with the presiding medical officer (a scrutiny I suspect I might not survive today, given the hostility with which I have come to be regarded in certain psychiatric circles). And then, of course, there were the asylums whose records had already been transferred to county record offices and similar repositories, in part or in gross.

As these reflections indicate, much of my early work was conducted in the more or less comfortable/uncomfortable surroundings of a variety of asylums themselves, settings that allowed one a vicarious if sharply circumscribed and attenuated sense of what life in one of these warehouses of the unwanted must once have been like. Such encounters with the physicality of mass segregation and confinement, with the peculiar moral architecture which the Victorians constructed to exhibit and contain the dissolute and degenerate, are increasingly fugitive and fast-fading from the realm of possibility. One of the most striking parts of the conference at which these papers were presented was an afternoon visit to the three large nineteenth-century institutions that once served the county of Devon and the borough of Exeter. Their fates were various. One was still clinging to an ever-more tenuous existence as a treatment facility; another was in the process of conversion to luxury housing (its developers coyly disguising its stigmatising past); and the third, the old county asylum where John Charles Bucknill launched his career,[40] and one of the most striking and original pieces of moral architecture I have encountered, was derelict and deserted, contaminated by asbestos and hence left to moulder away, the prey of vandals intent on stripping the last vestiges of its integrity in the pursuit of items to resell at a profit. All three institutions were clearly destined in short order to find themselves consigned to the dustbin of history.

It is not just the buildings themselves, of course, that are in the throes of terminal decay or transformation. For these vast and straggling establishments once contained the records that are essential to the reconstruction of a world we have lost. Will these papers survive? Assuredly not in their entirety, for their preservation would require quantities of space and resources that will surely never be found. How then should we proceed? What criteria of selection should we offer the archivist, particularly as scholars increasingly try to link institutional records across sectors – the better to explore, for example, the interconnections between workhouse and pauper asylum, as Melling, Adair, and Forsythe have so cleverly begun to do? Here there are most assuredly no easy answers. Nor can one confidently anticipate that the historian's voice will weigh heavily in the balance when decisions are made about what to discard and what to preserve – or that our present generation can even adequately anticipate the issues and concerns that will animate future generations of scholars. Still, reasoned discussion and open debate are surely better than leaving the whole matter to the gnawing criticism of the mice, or the random depredations of weather and decay.

Let us all hope, then, that at a time when research in the history of psychiatry is flourishing as never before, and when the range and scope of the work being undertaken is expanding remarkably, all this effort will not be undercut by the demise of the institutions themselves, and with it, the destruction of the crucial records upon which we all in the last analysis are dependent. It would be particularly ironic were this destruction to happen at the moment when many historians seem to be returning to a rather more benign view of asylums than has prevailed for the last quarter century – part of a movement towards what Joseph Melling has termed 'late Whiggism'. It is an intellectual shift I confess I cannot entirely embrace or share, though I sympathise with those who recoil from the malign neglect our Orwellian political masters have dubbed 'community care', and agree that for some substantial fraction of the psychotic asylum care in its original sense is a virtual necessity. Yet I have too bleak a view of what the late Victorian bins became, and am too conscious of just how vulnerable asylumdom's captive population were when placed in the hands of a profession convinced of their biological degeneracy and inferiority, to feel at ease with what I fear is a romantic and rose-tinted nostalgia for that peculiar array of miniature worlds which we have now lost.

NOTES

1 See especially M. MacDonald, *Mystical Bedlam: Madness, Anxiety, and Healing in Seventeenth Century England*, Cambridge, Cambridge University Press, 1981; R. Porter, *Mind Forg'd Manacles: A History of Madness in England from the Restoration to the Regency*, London, Athlone, 1987.

2 That is not the same thing, of course, as saying that my work was or is 'Marxist', whatever that term meant then and now. (Cf. Gerald Grob, 'Marxian analysis and mental illness', *History of Psychiatry*, 1, 1990, pp. 223–32.) In important ways, I would suggest that my scholarship has always reflected themes that are far more readily seen as Weberian – as demonstrated, for instance, by my interest in the impact of rationalisation and political centralisation; in processes and consequences of occupational closure and professionalisation; in the importance of status as well as class, and in moral meanings and the activities of moral entrepreneurs.

3 My recent foray into what some see as the unlikely realm of sociological biography (A. Scull, C. MacKenzie, and N. Hervey, *Masters of Bedlam: The Transformation of the Mad-Doctoring Trade*, Princeton, Princeton University Press, 1997) is among other things an effort on my part to demonstrate that even a focus on the individual can be highly revealing about general social movements and processes.

4 See A. Scull, *Museums of Madness: The Social Organization of Insanity in Nineteenth Century England*, London, Allen Lane, 1979, *passim*, esp. pp. 34–42, 84–6, 99–101, 107.

5 See Leonard Smith, 'To cure those afflicted with the disease of insanity: Thomas Bakewell and Spring Vale Asylum', *History of Psychiatry*, 4, 1993, pp. 107–27.

6 See Scull, *Museums of Madness*, pp. 60–2, 110–11; A. Scull, *The Most Solitary of Afflictions: Madness and Society in Britain, 1700–1900*, London and New Haven, Yale University Press, 1993, pp. 88–91, 166–9.

7 See my own extended discussion of these issues in *The Most Solitary of Afflictions*, pp. 165–74.

8 Ibid.

9 See *The Most Solitary of Afflictions*, p. 303; Scull, MacKenzie and Hervey, *Masters of Bedlam*, pp. 176, 185, 200.

10 See Scull, *The Most Solitary of Afflictions*, pp. 267–9.

11 Ibid., pp. 313–14.

12 See N. Hervey, 'A slavish bowing down: the Lunacy Commission and the psychiatric profession 1845–60', in W.F. Bynum, R. Porter, and M. Shep-

herd, eds, *The Anatomy of Madness*, Vol. 2, London: Tavistock, 1985, pp. 98–131; Hervey, 'The Lunacy Commission 1845–60', unpublished Ph. D. dissertation, Bristol University, 1985. Forsythe *et al.* are surely wrong to see Hervey as one of those who see the Commissioners as weak and ineffectual. To the contrary, on my reading of his work, his findings are strongly supportive of the position they advance.

13 D.J. Mellett, 'Bureaucracy and mental illness: the Commissioners in Lunacy 1845–90', *Medical History*, 25, 1981, pp. 223-7 and *passim* and *The Prerogative of Asylumdom*, New York, Garland, 1982.

14 Some of the findings from Bartlett's pioneering research are presented in his chapter in the present volume.

15 See also the discussion in Scull, *The Most Solitary of Afflictions*, pp. 280–3.

16 Bynum, Porter, and Shepherd, eds, *The Anatomy of Madness*, Vol. 2, pp. 132–46.

17 Elaine Showalter, *The Female Malady: Women, Madness, and English Culture, 1830–1980*, New York, Pantheon, 1985.

18 Recent papers by the editors of this volume have raised some pertinent and penetrating criticisms of the arguments I advance there, and though I would want to quibble and debate them on some points of detail, Adair, Forsythe and Melling have indeed established that in important respects my interpretation 'seriously understates the complexity of the Poor Law as an institution which contributed to the mediation and construction of social relations in these decades.' R. Adair, B. Forsythe, and J. Melling, 'A danger to the public? Disposing of pauper lunatics in late-Victorian and Edwardian England', *Medical History*, 42, 1998, pp. 1–25 (quotation on p. 2); Forsythe, Melling, and Adair, 'The New Poor Law and the county pauper lunatic asylum: the Devon experience, 1834–1884', *Social History of Medicine*, 9, 1996, pp. 335–55.

19 See, in particular, their excellent papers 'The New Poor Law and the county pauper lunatic asylum – the Devon experience 1834–1884', *Social History of Medicine*, 9, 1996, pp. 335–55; 'A danger to the public? Disposing of pauper lunatics in late-Victorian and Edwardian England', *Medical History*, 42, 1998, 1–25; and 'Migration, family structure and pauper lunacy in Victorian England: admissions to the Devon County Pauper Lunatic Asylum, 1845–1900', *Continuity and Change*, 12, 3, 1997, pp. 373–401.

20 See the discussion in Scull, *The Most Solitary of Afflictions*, pp. 270–6.

21 Cf. Michel Foucault, *Histoire de la folie à l'âge classique*, Ch. 2. 'Le grand refermement', Paris, Gallimard, 1972.

22 M. Foucault, *Madness and Civilisation: A History of Insanity in the Age of Reason*, Vintage Books, 1973, pp. 261–2.

23 They may need to move smartly, lest in an age of decarceration, long-preserved records disappear along with the demise of the institutions themselves – a point to which I shall return below.

24 Scull, *The Most Solitary of Afflictions*, pp. 364–5.

25 Commissioners in Lunacy, *30th Annual Report*, 1876, pp. 74–6, 346–49.

26 See the discussion in Scull, MacKenzie and Hervey, *Masters of Bedlam*, pp. 93–5.

27 See ibid., pp. 183–5. For Dix's life and career, see the splendid modern biography by David Gollaher, *Voice for the Mad: The Life of Dorothea Dix*, New York, Free Press, 1995.

28 Scull, *The Most Solitary of Afflictions*, pp. 351–2 and *Museums of Madness*, pp. 239–40.

29 Scull, MacKenzie and Hervey, *Masters of Bedlam*, p. 274. See also Scull, *The Most Solitary of Afflictions*, p. 382, *Museums of Madness*, p. 258 and *Social Order/Mental Disorder: Anglo-American Psychiatry in Historical Perspective*, London, Routledge, 1989, pp. 22–3.
30 Scull, *The Most Solitary of Afflictions*, pp. 310–15.
31 Ibid., p. 309. I go on to point out, however, that 'once family tolerance had reached the breaking point, ties of blood may well have tended to accentuate rather than diminish the desire for seclusion, as families sought to hide what was unquestionably a source of profound shame and potential disgrace from public view and knowledge.' Ibid., pp. 309–10. In other words, attitudes towards the asylum were complex and often contradictory.
32 Andrew Scull, ed., *The Asylum As Utopia: W.A.F. Browne and the Mid-Nineteenth Century Consolidation of Psychiatry*, London, Routledge, 1990.
33 See chapters 4 and 6.
34 See the discussions in Nancy Tomes, *A Generous Confidence: Thomas Story Kirkbride and the Art of Asylum-Keeping, 1840–1883*, Cambridge, Cambridge University Press, 1983; and Scull, *Social Order/Mental Disorder*, Ch. 5.
35 Mark Finnane, *Insanity and the Insane in Post-Famine Ireland*, London, Croom Helm, 1981.
36 Ibid., p. 14.
37 Ibid., p. 222.
38 Jonathan Sadowsky, *Imperial Bedlam: Institutions of Madness and Colonialism in Southwest Nigeria*, Berkeley, University of California Press, forthcoming.
39 George E. Paget, *The Harveian Oration*, Cambridge, Deighton and Bell, 1866, pp. 34–5.
40 See Scull, MacKenzie and Hervey, *Masters of Bedlam*, Ch. 7.

SELECT BIBLIOGRAPHY OF THE HISTORY OF INSANITY

The following texts are selected from what is now a very large international literature on the history of insanity, of asylums and of psychiatry. They are largely confined to studies in social and cultural history rather than the wider social and medical sciences, which have their own voluminous collections of texts in these areas. Some of the best studies have been published in the form of articles and essays. The history of insanity and its treatment beyond western Europe and north America largely remains to be written, though significant research has recently been published. In addition to the collections listed below, the following journals include key contributions: *Medical History*, *Social History of Medicine*, *History of Psychiatry*, *Journal of Social History* and *History of Medicine*. These journals also provide a wider context for the analysis of insanity within the social and cultural history of medicine, as does the work of leading scholars such as Roy Porter.

Jonathan Andrews, Asa Briggs, Roy Porter, Penny Tucker and Keir Waddington, *The History of Bethlem*, London, Routledge, 1997.

Major reappraisal of the most infamous of all institutions for the insane, examining the history of the mythical Bethlem as well as its institutional life.

P. Bartlett and D. Wright, eds, *Outside the Walls of the Asylum: Historical Perspectives on 'Care in the Community' in Modern Britain and Ireland*, London, Athlone, 1999.

Recent scholarship emphasising the provisions for the insane beyond the boundaries of the asylum.

G.E. Berrios and H. Freeman, eds, *150 Years of British Psychiatry, 1841–1991*, London, Gaskell, 1991 and H. Freeman and G.E. Berrios, eds, *150 Years of British Psychiatry. Volume 2: The Aftermath*, London, Athlone, 1996.

Two major collections of essays written by a range of professionals and practitioners as well as historians of psychiatry.

W.F. Bynum, R. Porter and M. Shepherd, eds, *The Anatomy of Madness: essays in the history of psychiatry, Volume II*, London, Tavistock, 1985, and *Volume III*, London and New York, Routledge, 1988.

Last two volumes in substantial collections of important essays which remain key reference points for English and wider European and Asian research.

A. Digby, *Madness, Morality and Medicine: A Study of the York Retreat, 1796–1914*, Cambridge University Press, 1985.

An excellent early detailed analysis of the famous Quaker institution and moral treatment.

W. Ernst, *Mad Tales from the Raj. The European Insane in British India, 1800–1858*, London and New York, Routledge, 1991.

Rare account of colonial psychiatry. See also McCulloch, and Sadowsky.

M. Finnane, *Insanity and the Insane in Post-Famine Ireland*, London, Croom Helm, 1981.

An early critique of Scull (see also Grob) and the Foucauldian view of the asylum, which makes an important argument about the key role of the family in the institutionalisation of the insane.

Michel Foucault, *Madness and Civilisation: A History of Insanity in the Age of Reason*, Vintage Books, 1973.

One amongst the many texts by Foucault which have had a seminal influence on the study of insanity.

G.N. Grob, *Mental Institutions in America: Social Policy to 1875*, New York, Free Press, 1973.

The most important and thorough American scholarship on asylum development which provided an effective response to the radical and marxist-influenced studies of institutional change.

K. Jones, *Law, Lunacy and Conscience, 1744–1845*, London, Routledge and Kegan Paul, 1954 and *Asylums and After: A Revised History of the Mental Health Services From the Early 18th Century to the 1990s*, London, Athlone, 1993.

Two rather neglected but important narratives of progress in the care of the mentally ill. Criticised as Whiggish in tone by revisionist scholars but useful on reform and philanthropy.

J. McCulloch, *Colonial Psychiatry and 'the African Mind'*, Cambridge, 1995.

Important recent account following earlier work on Fanon.

M. MacDonald, *Mystical Bedlam: Madness, Anxiety, and Healing in Seventeenth Century England*, Cambridge, Cambridge University Press, 1981.

Path-breaking investigation of an English physician's practice in the early modern period, applying new computer techniques. A major work.

C. Mackenzie, *Psychiatry for the Rich: A History of the Private Ticehurst Asylum, 1792–1917*, London, Routledge, 1992.

One of the few studies of private asylums. See also Parry-Jones.

W.L. Parry-Jones, *The Trade in Lunacy: A Study of Private Madhouses in England in the Eighteenth and Nineteenth Centuries*, London, 1972.

A pioneering and widely cited study which remains one of the best treatments of private facilities.

R. Porter, *Mind Forg'd Manacles: A History of Madness in England from the Restoration to the Regency*, Athlone, London, 1987.

The best single text on the eighteenth century, demonstrating significant progress and diversity in what had often been considered a dark age for the treatment of the mad.

Jonathan Sadowsky, *Imperial Bedlam: Institutions of Madness and Colonialism in Southwest Nigeria*, Berkeley, University of California Press, forthcoming, 1999.

Major new discussion of institutions in west Africa.

A. Scull, *The Most Solitary of Afflictions: Madness and Society in Britain, 1780–1900*, Yale University Press, New Haven and London, 1993.
The most influential single account of the long nineteenth century. A reworking of the author's important *Museums of Madness*, originally published in 1979.
A. Scull, N. Hervey and C. Mackenzie, *Masters of Bedlam. The Transformation of the Mad-Doctoring Trade*, Princeton, Princeton University Press, 1966.
Gallery of vivid cameos of the leading psychiatrists of the nineteenth century.
A. Scull, ed., *Madhouses, Mad-Doctors and Madmen: The Social History of Psychiatry in the Victorian Era Philadelphia*, University of Philadelphia Press, 1981.
Includes important essays by Walton and other scholars.
E. Showalter, *The Female Malady: Women, Madness and English Culture, 1830–1980*, London, Virago, 1980.
An early exploration in the cultural history of madness. Remains the single most influential study of the relationship between gender and insanity in England.
N. Tomes, *A Generous Confidence: Thomas Story Kirkbride and the Art of Asylum-Keeping, 1840–1883*, New York, Cambridge University Press, 1983.
Model analysis of physician–patient relations.

INDEX

For Product Safety Concerns and Information please contact our EU
representative GPSR@taylorandfrancis.com
Taylor & Francis Verlag GmbH, Kaufingerstraße 24, 80331 München, Germany

www.ingramcontent.com/pod-product-compliance
Ingram Content Group UK Ltd.
Pitfield, Milton Keynes, MK11 3LW, UK
UKHW022111190926
475702UK00013B/1381
9781138868243